Lung Cancer

Cancer Treatment and Research

WILLIAM L. MCGUIRE, *series editor*

Osborne, C.K. (ed): Endocrine Therapies in Breast and Prostate Cancer. 1988. ISBN 0-89838-365-X
Lippman, M.E., Dickson, R. (eds): Breast Cancer: Cellular and Molecular Biology. 1988.
    ISBN 0-89838-368-4
Kamps, W.A., Humphrey, G.B., Poppema S. (eds): Hodgkin's Disease in Children: Controversies and
    Current Practice. 1988. ISBN 0-89838-372-2
Muggia, F.M. (ed): Cancer Chemotherapy: Concepts, Clinical Investigations and Therapeutic Advances.
    1988. ISBN 0-89838-381-1
Nathanson, L. (ed): Malignant Melanoma: Biology, Diagnosis, and Therapy. 1988. ISBN 0-89838-384-6
Pinedo, H.M., Verweij J. (eds): Treatment of Soft Tissue Sarcomas. 1989. ISBN 0-89838-391-9
Hansen, H.H. (ed): Basic and Clinical Concepts of Lung Cancer. 1989. ISBN 0-7923-0153-6
Lepor, H., Ratliff, T.L. (eds): Urologic Oncology. 1989. ISBN 0-7923-0161-7
Benz, C., Liu, E. (eds): Oncogenes. 1989. ISBN 0-7923-0237-0
Ozols, R.F. (ed): Drug Resistance in Cancer Therapy. 1989. ISBN 0-7923-0244-3
Surwit, E.A., Alberts, D.S. (eds): Endometrial Cancer. 1989. ISBN 0-7923-0286-9
Champlin, R. (ed): Bone Marrow Transplantation. 1990. ISBN 0-7923-0612-0
Goldenberg, D. (ed): Cancer Imaging with Radiolabeled Antibodies. 1990. ISBN 0-7923-0631-7
Jacobs, C. (ed): Carcinomas of the Head and Neck. 1990. ISBN 0-7923-0668-6
Lippman, M.E., Dickson, R. (eds): Regulatory Mechanisms in Breast Cancer: Advances in Cellular and
    Molecular Biology of Breast Cancer. 1990. ISBN 0-7923-0868-9
Nathanson, L. (ed): Malignant Melanoma: Genetics, Growth Factors, Metastases, and Antigens. 1991.
    ISBN 0-7923-0895-6
Sugarbaker, P.H. (ed): Management of Gastric Cancer. 1991. ISBN 0-7923-1102-7
Pinedo, H.M., Verweij, J., Suit, H.D., (eds): Soft Tissue Sarcomas: New Developments in the
    Multidisciplinary Approach to Treatment. 1991. ISBN 0-7923-1139-6
Ozols, R.F. (ed): Molecular and Clinical Advances in Anticancer Drug Resistance. 1991.
    ISBN 0-7923-1212-0
Muggia, F.M. (ed): New Drugs, Concepts and Results in Cancer Chemotherapy. 1991. ISBN 0-7923-1253-8
Dickson, R.B., Lippman, M.E. (eds): Genes, Oncogenes and Hormones: Advances in Cellular and
    Molecular Biology of Breast Cancer. 1992. ISBN 0-7923-1748-3
Humphrey, G., Bennett, Schraffordt Koops, H., Molenaar, W.M., Postma, A. (eds): Osteosarcoma in
    Adolescents and Young Adults: New Developments and Controversies. 1993. ISBN 0-7923-1905-2
Benz, C.C., Liu, E.T. (eds): Oncogenes and Tumor Suppressor Genes in Human Malignancies. 1993.
    ISBN 0-7923-1960-5
Freireich, E.J., Kantarjian, H. (eds): Leukemia: Advances in Research and Treatment. 1993. ISBN 0-7923-
    1967-2
Dana, B.W. (ed): Malignant Lymphomas, Including Hodgkin's Disease: Diagnosis, Management, and
    Special Problems. 1993. ISBN 0-7923-2171-5
Nathanson, L. (ed): Current Research and Clinical Management of Melanoma. 1993. ISBN 0-7923-2152-9
Verweij, J., Pinedo, H.M., Suit, H.D. (eds): Multidisciplinary Treatment of Soft Tissue Sarcomas. 1993.
    ISBN 0-7923-2183-9
Rosen, S.T., Kuzel, T.M. (eds): Immunoconjugate Therapy of Hematologic Malignancies. 1993.
    ISBN 0-7923-2270-3
Sugarbaker, P.H. (ed): Hepatobiliary Cancer. 1994. ISBN 0-7923-2501-X
Rothenberg, M.L. (ed): Gynecologic Oncology: Controversies and New Developments. 1994.
    ISBN 0-7923-2634-2
Dickson, R.B., Lippman, M.E. (eds): Mammary Tumorigenesis and Malignant Progression. 1994.
    ISBN 0-7923-2647-4

Lung Cancer

Advances in Basic and Clinical Research

Edited by

Heine H. Hansen
Department of Oncology 5074
Rigshospitalet
9 Blegdamsvej
DK-2100 Copenhagen
Denmark

KLUWER ACADEMIC PUBLISHERS
BOSTON / DORDRECHT / LONDON

0292370

Distributors

---

for North America: Kluwer Academic Publishers, 101 Philip Drive, Assinippi Park, Norwell, Massachusetts 02061 USA
for all other countries: Kluwer Academic Publishers Group, Distribution Centre, Post Office Box 322, 3300 AH Dordrecht, THE NETHERLANDS

Library of Congress Cataloging-in-Publication Data

Lung cancer: advances in basic and clinical research/edited by Heine H. Hansen.
    p. cm. — (Cancer treatment and research; v. 72)
    Includes bibliographical references and index.
    ISBN 0-7923-2835-3 (alk. paper)
    1. Lungs — Cancer. I. Hansen, Heine Hoi. II. Series.
    [DNLM: 1. Lung Neoplasms. W1 CA693 v. 72 1994/WF 658
    L96076 1994]
      RC280.L8L7673 1994
      616.99'424 — dc20
      DNLM/DLC
      for Library of Congress

                                94-10350
                                     CIP

Copyright

---

17 JUL 1997

Contents

Preface

Primary lung tumors are now a global health problem. Their incidence has risen dramatically during the last 5 to 6 decades, reflecting the popularity of cigarette smoking.

In this fifth volume dealing with lung cancer in the series on Cancer Treatment and Research, the main reason for this rising incidence is given in the first chapter by Hoffman and Hoffman (from the American Health Organization). Promising statistical evidence is presented, showing that in several developed countries, the consumption of cigarettes by adults has decreased markedly. However, worldwide cigarette consumption has not decreased but is on the rise, emphasizing that this public health problem deserves the greatest attention of the medical and scientific community.

Pastorino (Milan, Italy) presents experimental data showing that a number of substances, such as synthetic retinoids, antioxidants, etc., may function as modulators for cell growth by having anticarcinogenic abilities. Single trials on lung cancer chemoprevention in high-risk individuals are ongoing in both Europe and North America, including investigations in non-small cell lung cancer patients who have undergone complete resection.

The physiological and pharmacological elements of smoking habits are described by Tønnesen (Copenhagen, Denmark), who also presents data on the effect of nicotine substitutes on smoking cessation.

Recent developments on the biology of lung cancer are the focus of the next chapters. Srivastava and Kramer (Bethesda, MD, U.S.A.) shed light on the complex series of molecular, genetic, and histopathologic events leading to transformation of normal cells into malignant cells in lung cancer. The impact of the many extracellular factors and intracellular molecular events that are responsible for sustaining the growth of malignant lung tumors is also discussed by Sethi and Woll (Manchester, U.K.).

Among the major histologic types of lung cancer, adenocarcinoma has been rising significantly. The development of this type is the subject of a review by Noguchi and Shimosato (Tokyo, Japan). Senderovitz et al. (Copenhagen, Denmark) describe the special neuroendocrine characteristics of lung tumors and cover a series of neuroendocrine markers, such as NSE, chromogranin, synaptofysin, NCAM, etc., from both a histopathological and a clinical viewpoint.

With respect to management of lung cancer patients, there is a great need for better systemic therapy, including the development of in vivo and in vitro models for testing of antineoplastic agents. This topic is discussed by Kal (Rijswijk, The Netherlands) and Jensen and Sehested (Copenhagen, Denmark) who focus on non-small cell lung and small cell lung cancer, respectively. It is to be hoped that some of these model systems will facilitate a more rapid introduction of new cytostatic agents into the clinic.

One of the major obstacles in cytostatic treatment, responsible for the relatively dismal results obtained today, is multidrug resistance, as described by Broxterman and colleagues (Amsterdam, The Netherlands). The topic is intensively studied in the laboratory, but still with very few clinically relevant data.

With regard to diagnosis and staging of lung cancer, a number of new techniques have been developed, such as digital radiography, magnetic resonance imaging, and transesophageal ultrasonography applied in the diagnosis and staging of lung cancer (Kaplan and Goldstraw, London, U.K.).

Among the different therapeutic modalities, chest irradiation in small cell lung cancer is reviewed by Arriagada and colleagues (Paris, France), based on data from the authors' original studies and from a recent meta-analysis of literature data.

Another French colleague, Trillet-Lenoir (Lyon, France), brings us up to date on newer, large randomized trials using hematopoietic growth factors in small cell lung cancer, demonstrating a significant decrease in the morbidity of cytostatic treatment when concomittant hematopoietic growth factors are applied.

The effect on treatment results by one of the other recently developed biologic modifiers, interferon, is subjected to analysis by Mattson et al. (Helsinki, Finland), while Grant and Kris (New York, NY, U.S.A.) deal with the recent development of the new antineoplastic agents applied in lung cancer.

A rather rare type of lung cancer is the pulmonary blastoma, and Koss (Washington, DC, U.S.A.) gives us the latest information on this disease entity, including new insight into the histogenesis of the tumor.

Finally, Bernhard and Ganz (Bern, Switzerland/Los Angeles, CA, U.S.A.) describe the very many psychosocial issues faced by lung cancer patients at diagnosis and during treatment.

Altogether, these 17 chapters from 12 countries highlight some of the rapid developments taking place in basic and clinical research on lung cancer. Hopefully, these chapters not only give up-to-date information but also will stimulate further research into this manmade disease, which was almost unheard of a century ago.

Heine H. Hansen

List of Contributors

Rodrigo Arriagada, M.D., Department of Radiation Oncology, Institut Gustave-Roussy, Rue Camille Desmoulins, F-94805 Villejuif, France

Jürg Bernhard, Ph.D., Swiss Group for Clinical Cancer Research (SAKK), Konsumstrasse 13, CH-3007 Bern, Switzerland

Henk J. Broxterman, Ph.D., Department of Medical Oncology, Free University Hospital, De Boelelaan 1117, NL-1081 HV Amsterdam, The Netherlands

Patricia A. Ganz, M.D., UCLA Schools of Medicine and Public Health, Division of Cancer Control, Jonsson Comprehensive Cancer Center, 1100 Glendon Avenue, Suite 711, Los Angeles, CA 0024-3511, U.S.A.

Peter Goldstraw, F.R.C.S., Department of Thoracic Surgery, Royal Brompton National Heart & Lung Hospital, National Heart & Lung Institute, Sydney Street, London SW3 6HP, U.K.

Stefan C. Grant, M.B., B.Ch., Thoracic Oncology Service, Department of Medicine, Memorial Sloan-Kettering Cancer Center, 1275 York Avenue, New York, NY 10021, U.S.A.

Anne M. Hand, M.D., Ashfield, 47 Balcombe Road, Haywards Heath, West Sussex, RH 16 1PA, U.K.

Fred R. Hirsch, M.D., Medical Department P, Bispebjerg Hospital, DK-2400 Copenhagen, Denmark

Dietrich Hoffmann, Ph.D., Associate Director, American Health Foundation, 1 Dana Road, Valhalla, NY 10595, U.S.A.

Mrs. Ilse Hoffmann, American Health Foundation, 1 Dana Road, Valhalla, NY 10595, U.S.A.

Peter Buhl Jensen, M.D., Department of Oncology, The Finsen Institute/ Rigshospitalet, DK-2100 Copenhagen, Denmark

Henk B. Kal, M.D., TNO Radiological Service, Centre for Radiological Protection and Dosimetry, P.O. Box 5815, NL-2280 HV Rijswijk, The Netherlands

David Kaplan, F.R.C.S., C.T.H., Department of Thoracic Surgery, Royal Brompton National Heart & Lung Hospital, National Heart & Lung Institute, Sydney Street, London SW3 6HP, U.K.

Michael N. Koss, M.D., Department of Pulmonary and Mediastinal

Pathology, Armed Forces Institute of Pathology, Washington, DC 20306-6000, U.S.A.

Barnett S. Kramer, M.D., Executive Plaza North, Room 305, National Cancer Institute, National Institutes of Health Bethesda, MD 20892, U.S.A.

Mark G. Kris, M.D., Thoracic Oncology Service, Department of Medicine, Memorial Sloan-Kettering Cancer Center, 1275 York Avenue, New York, NY 10021, U.S.A.

Thierry Le Chevalier, M.D., Department of Medical Oncology, Institut Gustave-Roussy, Rue Camille Desmoulins, F-94805 Villejuif, France

Sabine C. Linn, M.D., Department of Medical Oncology, Free University Hospital, De Boelelaan 1117, NL-1081 HV Amsterdam, The Netherlands

Paula K. Maasilta, M.D., Department of Pulmonary Medicine, Helsinki University Central Hospital, Haartmaninkatu 4, SF-00290 Helsinki, Finland

Karin V. Mattson, M.D., Department of Pulmonary Medicine, Helsinki University Central Hospital, Haartmaninkatu 4, SF-00290 Helsinki, Finland

Masayuki Noguchi, M.D., 3rd Histopathology Section, Pathology Division, National Cancer Center Research Institute, Tsukiji 5-Chome, Chuoku, Tokyo, Japan

Ugo Pastorino, M.D., Department of Thoracic Surgery, Istituto Nazionale Tumori, Via g. Venezian, 1, I-20133 Milan, Italy

Jean-Pierre Pignon, M.D., Department of Medical Statistics, Institut Gustave-Roussy, Rue Camille Desmoulins, F-94805 Villejuif, France

Maxwell Sehested, M.D., Department of Pathology, Sundby Hospital, DK-2300 Copenhagen, Denmark

Thomas Senderovitz, M.D., Medical Department P, Bispebjerg Hospital, DK-2400 Copenhagen, Denmark

Tariq Sethi, M.D., Growth Regulation Laboratory, Imperial Cancer Research Fund, P O Box 123, Lincoln's Inn Fields, London WC2A 3PX, U.K.

Yukio Shimosato, M.D., Clinical Laboratory Division, National Cancer Center Hospital, Tsukiji 5-Chome, Chuoku, Tokyo 104, Japan

Birgit G. Skov, M.D., Department of Pathology, Glostrup Hospital, DK-2600 Copenhagen, Denmark

Sudhir Srivastava, M.D., Executive Plaza North, Room 305, National Cancer Institute, National Institutes of Health, Bethesda, MD 20892, U.S.A.

Philip Tønnesen, M.D., Dr. Med. Sci., Department of Pulmonary Medicine Y, Gentofte University County Hospital, DK-2900 Hellerup, Denmark

Véronique N. Trillet-Lenoir, M.D., Service de Pneumologie, Hospital Louis Predal, 28 Avenue Doyen Lepine, F-69394 Lyon Cedex 03, France

Carolien H.M. Versantvoort, M.D., Department of Medical Oncology, Free

University Hospital, De Boelelaan 1117, NL-1081 HV Amsterdam, The
Netherlands
Penella J. Woll, M.D., Department of Medical Oncology, Christie Hospital,
Wilmslow Road, Withington, Manchester M20 9BX, U.K.

1. Tobacco consumption and lung cancer

Dietrich Hoffmann and Ilse Hoffmann

Introduction

In 1912, Adler asked in the introduction to his book *Primary Malignant Growth of the Lungs and Bronchi*, 'Is it worthwhile to write a monograph on the subject of primary malignant lung tumors?' He concluded, 'There is nearly complete concensus of opinion that primary malignant neoplasms of the lungs are among the rarest forms of disease' [1]. In the following 70 years, however, there was a dramatic increase of primary lung cancer throughout the world. By 1985, lung cancer was the most frequently occurring cancer worldwide, with an estimated 896,000 new cases accounting for 11.8% of all cancer cases [2]. Figures 1 and 2 present the increase of lung cancer incidence in men in eight developed countries, namely, the U.S.A., the United Kingdom, West Germany, and France, and Canada, Italy, Sweden, and Japan, respectively [3–14].In the former U.S.S.R., lung cancer rose from about 31,400 reported cases in males and 8,800 in females in 1965 to 75,000 and 16,700, respectively, in 1984 [15]. In the U.S.A., lung cancer has been the leading cause of death from cancer in men since about 1960 and in women since about 1987 (figures 3 and 4).

Three factors have been incriminated in the significant increase in lung cancer: occupational exposure to carcinogens, urban air pollution, and tobacco smoking. There cannot be any question that certain occupational exposures increase the risk for lung cancer. The major occupationally occurring human lung carcinogens are asbestos, chromium and nickel vapors, arsenic, and iron oxide, as well as ionizing radiation (which includes exposure to radioactive ores), petroleum vapors, and bis(chloromethyl)ether. It has been estimated that the occupational contribution to total cancer incidence (not only lung cancer) in industrial countries amounts to between 1% and 5% [16,17].

A number of epidemiological studies have indicated that urban pollution may contribute to the higher lung cancer incidence rates in developed countries. Doll and Peto [17] have estimated that around 1980, about 2% (range 1% to less than 5%) of all cancer deaths in the U.S.A. were attributable to air pollution. Hammond and Horn [18,19] in their large-scale

Heine H. Hansen, (ed), Hansen: Lung Cancer.
© *1994 Kluwer Academic Publishers. ISBN 0-7923-2835-3. All rights reserved.*

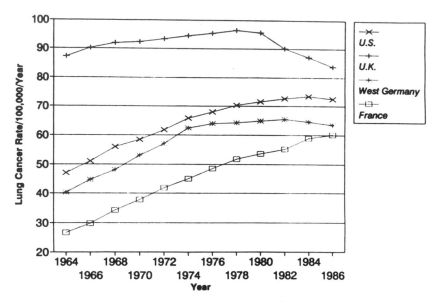

Figure 1. Lung cancer incidence rates in males, 1964–1986, for the U.S.A., U.K., West Germany, and France [3–14].

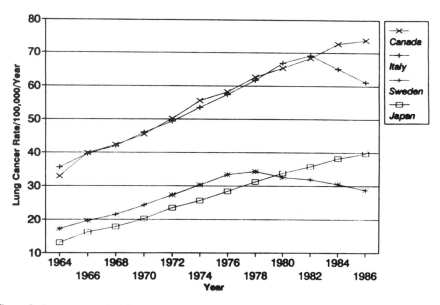

Figure 2. Lung cancer incidence rates in males, 1964–1986, for Canada, Italy, Sweden, and Japan [3–14].

2

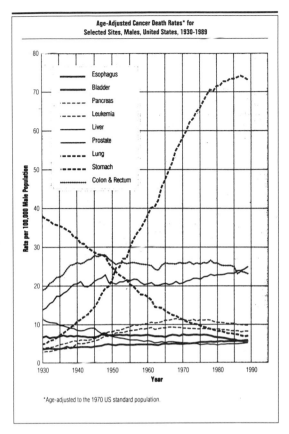

Figure 3. Age-adjusted cancer death rates for nine selected sites, U.S.A., 1930–1988, Males [32].

prospective study with the American Cancer Society, observed an urban factor that indicated that city residents have a somewhat higher risk for bronchiogenic carcinoma than people living in rural areas (figure 5). However, the urban factor for lung cancer may not be due to urban air pollutants entirely, but could result from other variables, including the better reporting of lung cancer cases in cities, lung cancer patients moving into urban residence prior to death, differences in smoking habits and patterns between residents in urban and rural areas, and/or occupational differences in the two areas. In 1989, Pershagen [20] reviewed the major cohort and case–control studies on lung cancer in urban areas of developed countries. These data were standardized for smoking. He concluded, 'Urban air pollution and exposure near some types of industries may be related to an increased risk of lung cancer' [20].

Tobacco smoking has been clearly recognized as the major cause of lung cancer in developed countries since the first reports by the Royal College of

3

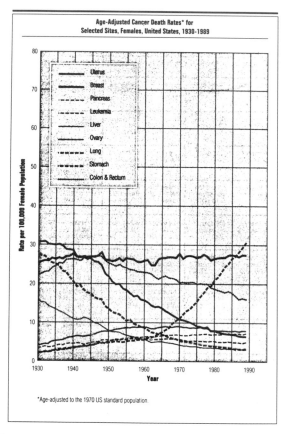

Figure 4. Age-adjusted cancer death rates for nine selected sites, U.S.A., 1930–1988, Females [32].

Physicians of London in 1962 and by the U.S. Surgeon General of the Public Health Service in 1964 [21,22]. During the past two decades, lung cancer has also strongly increased in several developing countries, clearly due to cigarette smoking [2,23]. In most developed countries, tobacco smoking is held responsible for at least 70% to 80% of all lung cancers [16,23]. Shopland et al. [24] from the U.S. National Cancer Institute estimated that in the U.S.A., 90.3% of the 92,000 deaths from lung cancer in men and 78.5% of the 51,000 lung cancer deaths in women in 1991 were caused by cigarette smoking. Cigar and pipe smoking are also causally related to cancer of the lung, although not to the same extent as cigarette smoking [25].

4

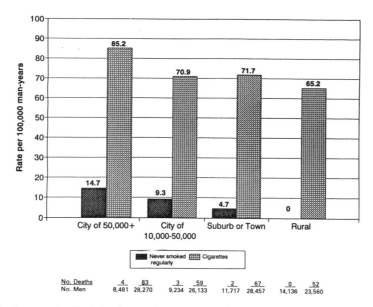

| No. Deaths | | 4 | 83 | 3 | 59 | 2 | 67 | 0 | 52 |
| No. Men | | 8,481 | 28,270 | 9,234 | 26,133 | 11,717 | 28,457 | 14,136 | 23,560 |

Figure 5. Age-standardized death rates for well-established bronchiogenic carcinoma, exclusive of adenocarcinoma, by rural–urban classification. Rates of cigarette smokers are compared with those for men who never smoked regularly [18,19].

Tobacco consumption

Since tobacco smoking, and especially the smoking of cigarettes, has been causally associated with lung cancer, and since the lung cancer incidence rates have dramatically increased, it is important to record the changes in cigarette consumption during the last 70 years to fully understand this phenomenon. Figure 6 reflects the increase of cigarette consumption per adult since 1921 for the U.S.A. and the United Kingdom, since 1935 for France, and since 1950 for West Germany [26,27]. In all four countries, a steep increase in cigarette consumption occurred beginning between 1930 and 1950. In the U.S.A. and the U.K., this increase continued until 1960–1970 and then gradually leveled off; beginning about 1975–1980, per capita cigarette consumption decreased. France and West Germany did not record further increases of cigarette use after 1990. In Sweden, the increase in cigarette consumption halted between 1975 and 1980, reaching a maximum of 2,000 cigarettes per year per adult. Italy reached the highest per capita annual consumption in 1985 with about 2,430 cigarettes (figure 7). These data compare with a maximal annual per capita use of about 3,900 cigarettes in the U.S.A. between 1975 and 1980 (figure 6), about 3,350 cigarettes in Canada in 1975, and about 3,500 cigarettes in Japan in 1980 [26,27].

Cigar consumption has been declining since 1964, when it reached a maximum of 75 cigars per adult in the U.S.A. In Germany, cigar con-

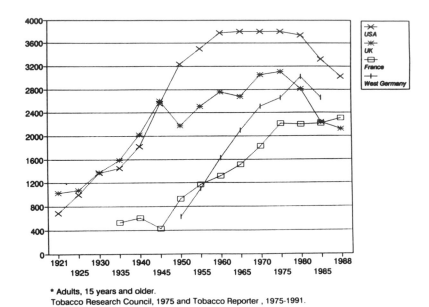

* Adults, 15 years and older.
Tobacco Research Council, 1975 and Tobacco Reporter , 1975-1991.

Figure 6. Adult consumption of cigarettes in the U.S.A., U.K., France, and West Germany [26,27]. Adult = 15 years or older.

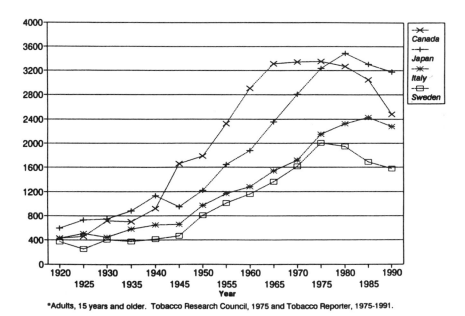

*Adults, 15 years and older. Tobacco Research Council, 1975 and Tobacco Reporter, 1975-1991.

Figure 7. Adult consumption of cigarettes in Canada, Japan, Italy, and Sweden [26,27]. Adult = 15 years or older.

sumption declined beginning in 1957 to about 25 cigars per adult in 1988. In Canada, the maximum of 41 cigars per adult in 1971 fell to 11 cigars per adult in 1988 [26,27]. However, there are some countries where cigars and cigarillos are especially popular. This fact may be of consequence in respect to the lung cancer incidence rates. In Denmark, for example, where the smoking of cigarillos is widespread, the annual adult consumption of cigars and cigarillos in 1965 amounted to 320; however, it has decreased since then to about 90 per adult [26,27].

Consumption of coarse-cut, loose tobacco such as that used for pipe smoking has also significantly diminished in developed countries. As a case in point, Germany recorded in 1934 the use of 390 g pipe tobacco per adult, and in 1980 only about 40 g. However, use of fine-cut tobacco for hand-rolled cigarettes has significantly increased in those developed countries where loose tobacco is not taxed to the same extent as are manufactured cigarettes. In 1987, fine-cut, loose cigarette tobacco consumption increased per adult in the U.K. to about 100 g, in 1986 in Sweden to about 200 g, in Canada to about 500 g, and in the Netherlands to 1,450 g [26,27]. Since at present a manufactured cigarette contains only about 0.75 g tobacco, these data would raise number of cigarettes consumed per adult per year (figures 6 and 7) in the U.K. by about 135 cigarettes, in Sweden by 270 cigarettes, in Canada by 670 cigarettes, and in the Netherlands by 1,900 cigarettes. However, in general, hand-rolled cigarettes deliver significantly more tar, nicotine, carbon monoxide, and other toxic smoke components than do most manufactured cigarettes.

The epidemiology of smoking and lung cancer

In 1961, Wynder and Day [28] proposed three postulates for the causation of non-communicable diseases, including cancer:
1. The greater and the more prolonged the exposure to the factor, the greater the risk of the population involved.
2. The epidemiological pattern should be consistent with the distribution of the factor.
3. Removal or reduction of the risk factors for a given population group should be followed by a reduction in the incidence of disease.

More than 100 epidemiological studies from developed and developing countries have demonstrated a dose–response relationship between number of cigarettes smoked and the risk for cancer of the lung [25,29,30]. Figures 8 and 9 depict the mortality ratios derived from two U.S. prospective studies for males and females, respectively, in relation to daily cigarette consumption [31,32]. Clearly, the epidemiological data satisfy the first postulate for a causative association between cigarette smoking and lung cancer [28]. Laboratory studies support the epidemiological findings by documenting a dose–response relationship between exposure to cigarette smoke and pul-

7

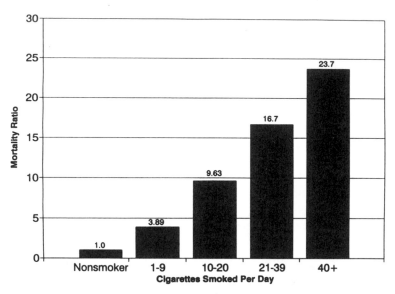

Figure 8. Lung cancer mortality ratio for males by cigarettes smoked per day [29].

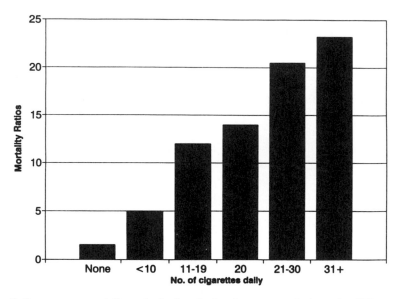

Figure 9. Lung cancer mortality ratio for females by cigarettes smoked per day [29].

monary adenoma in mice [33] and tumors of the upper respiratory tract in hamsters [34], and also between applications of total particulate matter (TPM) of cigarette smoke to the skin of mice and rabbits and the tumor yield at the site of application [35].

8

One observation that does not appear to fully support postulate 1 above is that after adjusting for number of cigarettes smoked per day and for age at which smoking has begun, Japanese cigarette smokers have a lower risk for lung cancer than cigarette smokers in the U.S., Canada, the United Kingdom, and Sweden 29] [see (figures 2 and 7). Three explanations have been suggested: the depth of inhalation may come into play; so may the preference of the Japanese for cigarettes with charcoal-containing filter tips (more than 70% of all cigarettes sold in Japan have charcoal filter tips, compared to only a few percent of cigarettes on the markets of the other countries); and differences in diet between the Japanese and the residents of other countries may also be an underlying factor. A combination of these three factors has also been considered. This discrepancy concerning Japanese cigarette smokers deserves further detailed study.

Postulate 2 is supported by the observation that the depth of inhalation (figure 10 [36]) as well as the age at onset of cigarette smoking (figure 11 [31]) determine the risk for lung cancer. Cigar and pipe smokers face a significantly higher risk for lung cancer than do nonsmokers, yet they have a lower risk for lung cancer than do cigarette smokers [25]. At first, these results appear to be in disagreement with laboratory data, which have shown that the TPM of cigar smoke contains higher levels of carcinogenic agents than does cigarette smoke [35,36]. However, this discrepancy can be explained, at least partially, by the fact that primary cigar and pipe smokers have the tendency to avoid deep inhalation of the smoke. The latter concept is supported by the fact that cigar and pipe smokers have at least the same risk for cancer of the oral cavity as cigarette smokers [25,29,30].

Postulate 3 is clearly satisfied for tobacco smoking and lung cancer. Doll and Peto [17] as well as other epidemiologists [25,29,30] have shown that cessation of smoking leads to a gradual reduction of risk for lung cancer. After 15 to 20 years of cessation, the ex-smoker reaches a plateau for lung cancer risk that is very low, yet remains 10% to 100% higher than that for a person who never smoked. Furthermore, as will be discussed later in the section titled "Reduction in Exposure," a long-term smoker of filter cigarettes faces a 30%–50% lower risk of developing lung cancer than does the smoker of cigarettes without filter tips [25,37,38]. Both observations, the risk reduction for lung cancer in ex-smokers and the decrease for lung cancer in long-term smokers of filter cigarettes, sustain postulate 3 above.

Changes in the distribution of histologic types of lung cancer

In the first large-scale case–control study on smoking and lung cancer in the U.S. in 1950, only 35 out of 599 male cigarette smokers died from lung adenocarcinoma; the remaining 564 cases were diagnosed as having squamous cell carcinoma. Thus, the ratio of these two types of lung cancer was 1:16 [39]. In 1974, the same investigators reported for male smokers

9

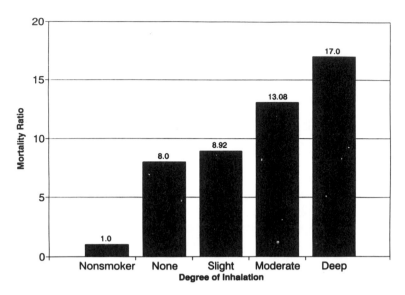

Figure 10. Lung cancer mortality ratio for males by degree of inhalation [29].

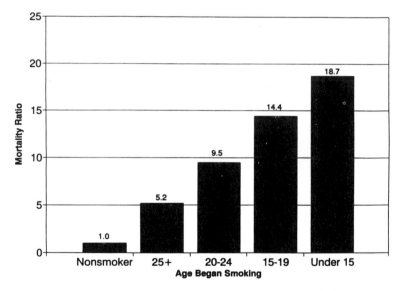

Figure 11. Lung cancer mortality ratio for males by age begun smoking [29].

with lung cancer a ratio of 1:2.5; in 1985 this ratio was 1:1.4 [38]. A detailed study on the histology of the lung cancer of patients at Baptist Memorial Hospital in Memphis, Tennessee, covering 22 years (1964–1985), revealed gradual changes of the nature of tumors during this time span

10

among all male lung cancer cases. In 1964, 56% had squamous cell carcinoma and 4% adenocarcinoma (1:17); in 1985, there were 37% with squamous cell carcinoma and 27% with adenocarcinoma (1:1.4). During this time, small cell carcinoma in the male lung cancer patients changed from 4% to 17% and large cell carcinoma from 36% to 29%. During these 22 years, in female lung cancer patients, the incidence of squamous cell carcinoma changed from 6% to 23%, adenocarcinoma from 41% to 40% (1:0.14 to 1:0.58), small cell carcinoma from 6% to 30%, and large cell carcinoma from 47% to 7% [40]. Similar observations of changes of histological types of lung cancer were reported in three additional studies from the U.S. [41–43]. The National Cancer Institute examined the lung cancer cases in five geographic areas of the United States, encompassing 7% of the U.S. population, comparing cancer incidences as well as ratios of squamous cell carcinoma to adenocarcinoma for the periods 1967–1971 and 1984–986 [44]. On the basis of 1970 standards for categories, the lung cancer incidence rates in white males within this population rose from 67.3 to 84.1 (+25%), in black males from 86.1 to 126.9 (+47%), in white females from 14.2 to 35.7 (+121%), and in black females from 15.3 to 40.2 (+163%). Squamous cell carcinoma and adenocarcinoma in this population increased in white males by 25% and 111% (1:2.3 to 1:1.4), in black males by 50% and 151% (1:2.8 to 1:7) in white females by 156% and 220% (1:0.76 to 1:0.65), and in black females by 209% and 221% (1:0.89 to 1:0.86) (see table 1).

Table 1. Trends in the incidence of adenocarcinoma (A) and squamous cell carcinoma (S) of the lung in five geographic areas of the U.S.A., 1969–1971 to 1984–1986[a,b]

	1969–1971		1984–1986		
	No. of cases	Ratio A:S	No. of cases	Ratio A:S	% Change
White males					
Adenocarcinoma	1,638	1:2.3	3,685	1:1.4	111
Squamous cell carcinoma	3,767		5,100		25
Black males					
Adenocarcinoma	193	1:2.8	633	1:1.7	151
Squamous cell carcinoma	543		1,070		50
White females					
Adenocarcinoma	747	1:0.76	2,572	1:0.65	120
Squamous cell carcinoma	566		1,658		156
Black females					
Adenocarcinoma	75	1:0.89	340	1:0.86	221
Squamous cell carcinoma	67		291		209

[a] On the basis of data by Devesa et al. [44].
[b] Geographical areas: Atlanta, Connecticut, Detroit, Iowa, and San Francisco–Oakland.

Several questions arise. First, why did pulmonary adenocarcinoma increase to a much greater extent than squamous cell carcinoma of the lung, especially in males? Second, why did pulmonary adenocarcinoma occur more frequently than squamous cell carcinoma in women — quite opposite to the observation in men? Third, why were the lung cancer incidence rates among U.S. blacks, and especially among black men, significantly higher than among U.S. whites?

Regarding the first question, a working hypothesis has emerged that will be discussed later. It relates to the modification of the makeup of cigarettes during the past four decades, which has caused changes in smoking intensity for the consumer. The answer to the second question, why pulmonary adenocarcinoma occur more frequently in women than squamous cell carcinoma, remains unclear; however, it has been speculated that the female endocrine system plays a decisive role in the induction of adenocarcinoma [45]. In regard to the third question, studies have shown that even after adjusting for the number of cigarettes smoked daily and for the starting age at the onset of the smoking habit, black Americans still have a higher lung cancer incidence than white Americans [46]. Several points have been considered as reasons for this, including differences in the type of cigarettes smoked, degree of smoking intensity, and diet; none of these points has so far been substantiated.

The physicochemical nature of tobacco smoke

The carcinogenic potency of an inhaled aerosol is greatly influenced by its physicochemical nature. The burning of tobacco generates mainstream smoke (MS) during puff drawing, and sidestream smoke (SS) during smouldering between puffs. The physicochemical nature of the types of smoke is dependent on various factors. These include the type of tobacco and its cut, the temperatures prevailing during puff drawing (860–900°C) or smouldering (500–600°C), and the availability of oxygen — i.e., the reducing characteristics of the burning zone — and also the physical design of the tobacco product (e.g., length, diameter, paper, wrapper or pipe bowl, variety of cigarette paper, filter tip, and porosity).

The composition of the processed tobacco in cigarettes influences the chemistry, toxicity, and carcinogenicity of the smoke. Cigarettes sold in the U.S., Japan, and most Western European countries utilize blends of bright, burley, and Oriental tobaccos, while cigarettes made in the United Kingdom and Finland contain predominantly bright tobaccos. Both types of cigarettes deliver weakly acidic MS (pH 5.5–6.2) in which nicotine is present in protonated form in the particulate matter. In France and in some parts of Italy, North Africa, and Middle and South America, a high proportion of the cigarette brands contain only burley or black tobacco. In the smoke

12

of these cigarettes, which is neutral to weakly alkaline (pH 6.8–7.5), a significant portion of the nicotine is present in the vapor phase in an unprotonated form. The smoke of cigars is neutral to alkaline (pH 6.5–8.0), and like the MS of burley cigarettes, it contains unprotonated nicotine in the vapor phase [47]. Unprotonated nicotine is more quickly absorbed through the buccal mucosa than protonated nicotine [48]. The pH of MS of cigarettes and cigars is decisively influenced by the concentration of ammonia in the smoke [49], which is primarily governed by the nitrate content of the tobacco. Thus, burley tobaccos that are rich in nitrate [50] deliver weakly alkaline smoke.

The MS emerges from the mouthpiece of a cigarette as an aerosol and weighs between 400 and 500 mg. It contains about 1×10^{10} particles per ml (the highest reported concentration of particles in polluted urban air is 5×10^5 per ml), which range in diameter from 0.1 to 1.0 µm (mean diameter 0.2 µm) and which are dispersed in a vapor phase (particles up to 2.5 µm are considered to be lung damaging [51]). About 95% of the MS of a nonfilter cigarette is comprised of 400 to 500 individual gaseous components, with nitrogen, oxygen, and carbon dioxide as major constituents (table 2). Today we know that the particulate matter contains at least 3500 individual components (table 3) [52,53].

All combustion products contain free radicals; in the case of tobacco smoke, these are highly reactive oxygen- and carbon-centered types in the vapor phase, and relatively stable radicals in the particulate phase. The principal latter type appears to be a quinone/hydroquinone complex that has the potential to reduce molecular oxygen to superoxide and eventually to hydrogen peroxide and hydroxy radicals [54,55]. Some studies have implicated the free radicals in cigarette smoke to be partially responsible for the reduced levels of certain antioxidants (such as vitamin E and ascorbic acid) when compared to the levels in nonsmokers. The radicals are also considered to be responsible for oxidative damage in the lung of cigarette smokers [56,57].

For the chemical analysis, the smoke is arbitrarily separated into a vapor phase and a particulate phase. If more than 50% of a given smoke component appears in the vapor phase of fresh smoke it is considered a volatile smoke component; all others are particulate phase components. Tables 2 and 3 list the major types of components identified and their estimated components in the smoke of one cigarette [25,30,35,38–60]. The quantitative analytical data for cigarette smoke constituents are derived from machine smoking, with one 35-ml puff per minute for a puff duration of two seconds. However, these smoking parameters do not fully reflect the human cigarette-smoking habits of today. For example, a smoker of a low-nicotine cigarette may take up to five puffs per minute with puff volumes of up to 50 ml [61–64].

The data presented in tables 2 and 3 are important in regard to the biological activity of smoke constituents. However, the lists are by no means

Table 2. Major constituents of the vapor phase of the mainstream smoke of nonfilter cigarettes

Compound	Concentration/cigarette (% of total effluent)
Nitrogen	280–320 mg (56–64%)
Oxygen	50–70 mg (11–14%)
Carbon dioxide	45–65 mg (9–13%)
Carbon monoxide	14–23 mg (2.8–4.6%)
Water	7–12 mg (1.4–2.4%)
Argon	5 mg (1.0%)
Hydrogen	0.5–1.0 mg
Ammonia	10–130 µg
Nitrogen oxides (NO_x)	100–600 µg
Hydrogen cyanide	400–500 µg
Hydrogen sulfide	20–90 µg
Methane	1.0–2.0 mg
Other volatile alkanes [20][a]	1.0–1.6 mg[b]
Volatile alkenes [16]	0.4–0.5 mg
Isoprene	0.2–0.4 mg
Butadiene	25–40 µg
Acetylene	20–35 µg
Benzene	6–70 µg
Toluene	5–90 µg
Styrene	10 µg
Other volatile aromatic hydrocarbons [29]	15–30 µg
Formic acid	200–600 µg
Acetic acid	300–1,700 µg
Propionic acid	100–300 µg
Methyl formate	20–30 µg
Other volatile acids [6]	5–10 µg[b]
Formaldehyde	20–100 µg
Acetaldehyde	400–1,400 µg
Acrolein	60–140 µg
Other volatile aldehydes [6]	80–140 µg
Acetone	100–650 µg
Other volatile ketones [3]	50–100 µg
Methanol	80–180 µg
Other volatile alcohols [7]	10–30 µg[b]
Acetonitrile	100–150 µg
Other volatile nitriles [10]	50–80 µg[b]
Furan	20–40 µg
Other volatile furans [4]	45–125 µg[b]
Pyridine	20–200 µg
Picolines [3]	15–80 µg
3-Vinylpyridine	7–30 µg
Other volatile pyridines [25]	20–50 µg[b]
Pyrrole	0.1–10 µg
Pyrrolidine	10–18 µg
N-Methylpyrrolidine	2.0–3.0 µg
Volatile pyrazines [18]	3.0–8.0 µg
Methylamine	4–10 µg
Other aliphatic amines [32]	3–10 µg

[a] Parentheses show the number of individual compounds identified in a given group.
[b] Estimate.

Table 3. Major constituents of the particulate matter of the mainstream smoke of nonfilter cigarettes

Compound	µg/Cigarette
Nicotine	100–3,000
Nornicotine	5–150
Anatabine	5–15
Anabasine	5–12
Other tobacco alkaloids [17][a]	n.a.
Bipyridyls [4]	10–30
n-Hentriacotane [n-$C_{31}H_{64}$]	100
Total nonvolatile hydrocarbons [45][b]	300–400[b]
Naphthalene	2–4
Naphthalenes [23]	3–6[b]
Phenanthrenes [7]	0.2–0.4[b]
Anthracenes [5]	0.05–0.1[b]
Fluorenes [7]	0.6–1.0[b]
Pyrenes [6]	0.3–0.5[b]
Fluoranthenes [5]	0.3–0.45[b]
Carcinogenic polynuclear aromatic hydrocarbons [11][c]	0.1–0.25
Phenol	80–160
Other phenols [45][b]	60–180[b]
Catechol	200–400
Other catechols [4]	100–200[b]
Other dihydroxybenzenes [10]	200–400[b]
Scopoletin	15–30
Other polyphenols [8][b]	n.a.
Cyclotenes [10][b]	40–70[b]
Quinones [7]	0.5
Solanesol	600–1,000
Neophytadienes [4]	200–350
Limonene	30–60
Other terpenes [200–250][b]	n.a.
Palmitic acid	100–150
Stearic acid	50–75
Oleic acid	40–110
Linoleic acid	150–250
Linolenic acid	150–250
Lactic acid	60–80
Indole	10–15
Skatole	12–16
Other indoles [13]	n.a.
Quinolines [7]	2–4
Other aza-arenes [55]	n.a.
Benzofurans [4]	200–300
Other O-heterocyclic compounds [42]	n.a.
Stigmasterol	40–70
Sitosterol	30–40
Campesterol	20–30
Cholesterol	10–20
Aniline	0.36
Toluidines	0.23
Other aromatic amines [12]	0.25
Tobacco-specific N-nitrosamines [6][c]	0.34–2.7
Glycerol	120

[a] Parentheses show the number of individual compounds identified.
[b] Estimate.
[c] For details, see figure 6.
n.a.: not available.

15

a complete annotation of all smoke constituents detected to date. Tobacco contains at least 30 metals [35,60,65]. Per cigarette, one finds 38 mg potassium, 22 mg of calcium, and 5.5 mg of magnesium as the major metals. Since less than 1% of these metals are transferred from the tobacco into the smoke [66], toxicologically important ones, such as nickel and cadmium, are present only in minute amounts and are therefore not listed in table 3. Deleted from the tables are also agricultural chemicals and pesticides, even though residues of such agents are known to occur on the tobacco leaf and are partially transferred into the smoke. Because of the differences in the nature and amounts of these agents used in individual tobacco-growing countries, and since applications to the tobacco plant change from year to year [67,68], tables 2 and 3 do not list these chemicals in the smoke. Nevertheless, it is fairly certain that commercial tobaccos contain up to a few parts per million of DDT, DDD, and maleic hydrazide; less than 20% of these are transferred into MS.

The increasing market share of cigarettes with low smoke yields shows that these products are 'consumer acceptable.' This acceptability has been achieved by enhancing the smoke flavor through selection of aromatic tobacco varieties for the cigarette tobacco blend, adding extracts from tobacco or other plants, and/or adding synthetic flavor components [69]. Except for menthol ($\leqslant$500 µg/cigarette [70]), flavor additives are trade secrets; thus, there is little information as to the chemical nature and concentrations of such flavor additives and their possible toxicity and carcinogenicity. Coumarin, a known animal carcinogen [71], has in the past been used as a flavor additive; however, the use of certain additives in tobacco products has been discontinued in many countries.

Tobacco carcinogenesis

The objective of studies in tobacco carcinogenesis is to identify tumor initiators, tumor promoters, cocarcinogens, and organ-specific carcinogens in tobacco products; to explore their formation during tobacco growing, processing, and smoking; to investigate their mode of metabolic activation; and to develop biomarkers for the uptake and metabolism of the major toxic and carcinogenic agents by tobacco chewers and smokers. Since millions of men and women throughout the world continue to smoke cigarettes despite intensive public health information and education about the health hazards of tobacco use, research must also be concerned with the reduction of the toxicity and carcinogenicity of tobacco smoke and with the possibility of inhibiting the initiation and progression of tumors in persons who have a long history of smoking.

Bioassays

The long-term exposure of mice to cigarette smoke diluted with air leads to adenocarcinoma in the lung [33], in Syrian golden hamsters to a dose-related induction of benign and malignant tumors in the upper respiratory tract, especially in the larynx [34], and in rats to benign and malignant tumors of the lung [72]. Separating cigarette smoke by a filter into particulate matter and gas phase, and exposing mice to the air-diluted gas phase alone, induces lung adenocarcinoma similar to those seen with whole smoke [33]. However, in hamsters, the gas phase alone does not induce tumors in the respiratory tract. These data indicate that in inhalation studies with mice, hamsters, and rats, whole cigarette smoke is carcinogenic in the respiratory tract; although the vapor phase alone does not contain sufficient amounts of carcinogens to induce squamous cell carcinoma, it does contain agents that elicit pulmonary adenocarcinoma.

Tumor initiators, tumor promoters, and cocarcinogens

The total particulate matter (TPM) of cigarette smoke, also called tar, is carcinogenic on mouse skin, on the skin of rabbits, and in the connective tissue of rats [35]. Fractionation studies have shown that only the neutral fraction of TPM, especially its fraction B (2% of whole TPM) and subfraction BI (0.6% of whole TPM), is carcinogenic. However, neither the neutral fraction alone nor fractions B or BI account for more than part of the carcinogenic activity of the whole tar [73,74]. When the BI subfraction is assayed on mouse skin together with the weakly acidic fraction (9%–10% of the whole tar), which by itself is inactive, one observes 75% to 80% of the activity of the whole tar [73,74]. Thus, fraction BI contains a concentrate of tumor initiators, and the weakly acidic fraction harbors tumor promoters and/or cocarcinogens. Chemical-analytical studies have revealed that BI contains the polynuclear aromatic hydrocarbons (PAHs), a number of which are known carcinogens, and when applied in minute amounts, these are active as tumor initiators. In the weakly acidic fraction, phenolic compounds are enriched; several of these are known tumor promoters or known cocarcinogens, as is the case for catechol and methylcatechols [75–77]. Table 4 lists the concentrations of the identified carcinogenic PAHs, aza-arenes, the known tumor promoters, and cocarcinogens in the smoke of one cigarette. We consider the PAHs to act as contact carcinogens in tobacco carcinogenesis. This concept is supported by studies that have shown that intratracheal instillation of carcinogenic PAH leads to squamous cell carcinoma of the bronchi but not to pulmonary adenocarcinoma [78,79].

Table 5 lists additional animal carcinogens that have been identified in tobacco smoke in minute amounts. Formaldehyde and acetaldehyde are exceptions, since they are present in cigarette smoke in considerable amounts and may be active as tumor-enhancing agents in lung carcinogenesis.

Table 4. Tumor initiators, tumor promoters and cocarcinogens in tobacco smoke

Compounds	Mainstream smoke (per cigarette)	IARC-evaluation of evidence of carcinogenicity[a]	
		In laboratory animals	In humans
Tumor initiators			
PAHs			
Benz(a)anthracene	20–70 ng	Sufficient	
Benzo(b)fluoranthene	4–22 ng	Sufficient	
Benzo(j)fluoranthene	6–21 ng	Sufficient	
Benzo(h)fluoranthene	6–12 ng	Sufficient	
Benzo(a)pyrene	20–40 ng	Sufficient	Probable
Chrysene	40–60 ng	Sufficient	
Dibenz(a,h)anthracene	4 ng	Sufficient	
Dibenzo(a,i)pyrene	1.7–3.2 ng	Sufficient	
Dibenzo(a,l)pyrene	Present	Sufficient	
Indeno(1,2,3-cd)pyrene	4–20 ng	Sufficient	
5-Methylchrysene	0.6 ng	Sufficient	
Aza-arenes			
Dibenz(a,h)acridine	0.1 ng	Sufficient	
Dibenz(a,j)acridine	3–10 ng	Sufficient	
7H-Dibenzo(c,g)carbazole	0.7 ng	Sufficient	
Tumor promoters			
Phenol	80–120 μg		
o-Cresol	20–30 μg		
m-Cresol	10–20 mg		
p-Cresol	30–60 μg		
Cocarcinogens			
Catechol	50–330 μg		
3-Methylcatechol	10–20 μg		
4-Methylcatechol	15–25 μg		

[a] No designation indicates that an evaluation by the International Agency for Research on Cancer (IARC) has not been carried out.

Organ-specific carcinogens

Studies in occupational cancer have shown that some chemicals induce tumors at specific sites. Certain aromatic amines are bladder carcinogens; vinyl chloride induces angiosarcoma of the liver; and some inhalants cause cancer of the lung. Experimental studies have demonstrated that independent of site and route of application, certain types of N-nitrosamines induce esophageal cancer, others pancreas cancer, or others pulmonary adenocarcinoma in laboratory animals.

Table 6 lists organ-specific carcinogens and their concentrations in cigarette smoke. Polonium-210 is a known lung carcinogen; however, its significance in tobacco smoke as an inducer of lung tumors has been questioned.

Table 5. Minor carcinogens in cigarette smoke

Compounds	Mainstream smoke (per cigarette)	IARC-evaluation of evidence of carcinogenicity[a]	
		In laboratory animals	In humans
Formaldehyde	70–100 μg	Sufficient	
Acetaldehyde	18–1,400 μg	Sufficient	
Crotonaldehyde	10–20 μg		
Benzene	12–60 μg	Sufficient	Sufficient
Acrylonitrile	3.2–15 μg	Sufficient	Limited
2-Nitropropane	0.73–1.21 μg	Sufficient	
Ethylcarbamate	20–38 ng	Sufficient	
Hydrazine	24–43 ng	Sufficient	Inadequate
Arsenic	40–120 ng	Inadequate	Sufficient
Nickel	0–600 ng	Sufficient	Limited
Chromium	4–70 ng	Sufficient	Sufficient
Cadmium	41–62 ng	Sufficient	Limited
Lead	35–85 ng	Sufficient	Inadequate

[a] No designation indicates that an evaluation by the International Agency for Research on Cancer (IARC) has not been carried out.

Uranium miners who are exposed to significantly higher levels of polonium-210 were found to be at risk for lung cancer [80]. In 1987, the U.S. National Council on Radiation Protection and Measurement ascribed about 1% of the risk for lung cancer after 50 years of cigarette smoking to the role of polonium-210 inhaled with the smoke [81]. Although the levels of aromatic amines in cigarette smoke, such as 2-naphthylamine and 4-aminobiphenyl, are low, epidemiological and biochemical studies consider the aromatic amines important contributors to the increased risk of cigarette smokers for cancer of the urinary bladder [82–84].

Of special interest in tobacco carcinogenesis are the N-nitrosamines, which are formed by nitrosation of nicotine and of minor Nicotiana alkaloids during tobacco processing and during smoking [36]. To date, seven tobacco-specific N-nitrosamines (TSNAs) have been identified in tobacco products (figure 12). Of these, N'-nitrosonornicotine (NNN), 4-(methylnitrosamino)-1-(3-pyridyl)-1-butanone (NNK), and 4-(methylnitrosamino)-1-(3-pyridyl)-1-butanol (NNAL) are powerful animal carcinogens, N'-nitrosoanabasine (NAB) is moderately active as a carcinogen, and N'-nitrosoanatabine (NAT), 4-(methylnitrosamino)-4-(3-pyridyl)-1-butanol (iso-NNAL), and 4-(methylnitrosamino)-4-(3-pyridyl)butyric acid (iso-NNAC) appear to be inactive [85]. The concentrations of TSNAs in tobacco products are alarmingly high. The U.S. National Academy of Science has estimated that in 1986 to 1987, a U.S. nonsmoker was on a daily basis exposed to about 1 μg of carcinogenic N-nitrosamines, while a one-pack-a-day smoker was

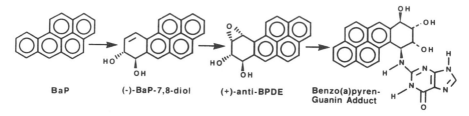

Figure 13. Benzo(a)pyrene (BaP): metabolic activation and binding to DNA [92].

BaP (-)-BaP-7,8-diol (+)-anti-BPDE Benzo(a)pyren-Guanin Adduct

Although tobacco smoke contains a considerable number of carcinogens (tables 4–6), this overview will only discuss those that have been associated with an increased risk for lung cancer, namely, the carcinogenic polynuclear aromatic hydrocarbons (PAHs) and the tobacco-specific N-nitrosamines (TSNAs).

PAHs. The carcinogenic PAHs in tobacco smoke are considered to be major contributors to the increased risk of smokers for bronchiogenic carcinoma. In humans, these procarcinogens are metabolically activated to reactive species by the P450 1A1 enzyme [91]. A major carcinogenic PAH in combustion products is benzo(a)pyrene (BaP). It is metabolically activated via 7,8-dihydroxy-7,8-dihydro BaP to its ultimate carcinogenic form, (+)7α,8β-dihydroxy-9β,10β-epoxy-7,8,9,10-tetrahydroBaP. The latter is known to react with DNA (figure 13) [92]. However, the major metabolic change of PAHs is the detoxification to phenolic compounds, in the case of BaP to 3-hydroxy BaP by P450 2C and 3A enzymes [93]. The ultimate reactive forms of PAHs covalently bind with DNA; this activates proto-oncogenes and inhibits tumor suppressor genes. In laboratory animals, the carcinogenic potency of several types of genotoxic carcinogens, including PAHs, is usually correlated with their potential to form adducts with DNA [94,95].

Studies using the ^{32}P-post-labeling method have shown that the DNA from lung tissue of smokers and nonsmokers contains multiple adducts, with levels and patterns varying greatly between individuals. However, DNA adducts measured with the ^{32}P-labeling method in tissues of the lung and larynx have generally demonstrated an association with cigarette smoking [96,97]. DNA–PAH. adducts in peripheral blood leukocytes have been utilized as biomarkers of exposure to carcinogenic PAHs. In the case of lung cancer patients, current smokers show significantly higher levels PAH–DNA adducts than current smoker controls [98]. 1-Hydroxypyrene appears to be a useful biomarker to measure the uptake of PAHs [99].

TSNAs. Of the tobacco-specific N-nitrosamines, NNK and its metabolic reduction product, NNAL (figure 12), induce primarily pulmonary adenoma

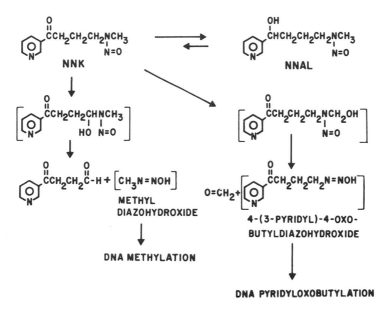

Figure 14. Metabolism of 4-(Methylnitrosamino)-1-(3-pyridyl)-1-butanone (NNK) [85].

and adenocarcinoma in mice, rats, and hamsters. In vitro studies with several different animal tissues and tissues from human lung, liver, and other organs, and microsomal preparations from human lung and liver as well as in vivo studies with mice and rats have delineated three major pathways for the metabolism of NNK (figure 14). In mice, rats, and monkeys, a major metabolite is NNAL and its glucuronide conjugate [98,99]. The pathway of primary importance of NNK carcinogenicity is α-hydroxylation. NNK is α-hydroxylated either at the methyl or methylene group; these hydroxy NNK-derivatives decompose under formation of methane diazohydroxide and pyridyloxobutane diazohydroxide as well as the corresponding aldehydes, 4-oxo-4-(3-pyridyl)butanal and formaldehyde. Methane diazohydroxide reacts with DNA to form methylated bases, including the promutagenic O^6methylguanine (O^6mG) and 7-methylguanine, while pyridyloxobutane diazohydroxide forms pyridyloxobutylated DNA. After NNK administration and upon acid treatment of DNA adducts, 4-hydroxy-1-(3-pyridyl)-1-butanone (HPB) is released; this can be quantified to determine the level of DNA adduct formation [85]. O^6-mG produces guanine-cytosine (GC) to adeninethymine (AT) transitions, i.e., changes in the DNA from one purine to another purine or from one pyrimidine to another pyrimidine.

The HPB-releasing DNA adducts have been quantified in lung tissues from smokers and nonsmokers, and methylated DNA has been assessed in lungs. The levels of methylated DNA were greater in smokers than in nonsmokers [100]. This may in part be due to the exposure to and activation

23

of NNK, although other methylating compounds such as N-nitrosodimethylamine are also present in tobacco smoke.

Smokers' urine contains NNAL and NNAL-glucuronide [101]. The levels of these two NNK metabolites correlate well with the exposure of smokers to NNK as well as with the levels in urine of cotinine, a major metabolite of nicotine. The determination of the levels of NNAL and NNAL-glucuronide in the urine and HPB-releasing adducts in the blood of a given smoker enables an estimation of the rate of metabolic activation of the tobacco-specific carcinogen NNK relative to the dose of NNK absorbed by an individual smoker, and may be indicative of relative cancer risk.

Relevance to humans

The relevance of a rodent carcinogen to the induction of cancer in humans can be evaluated by considering the following six aspects:
1. The type of tumor induced in rodents vs. the human tumor
2. The dose required to induce tumors in rodents vs. the estimated dose in humans
3. Comparisons of the metabolic activation and detoxification of carcinogens in rodents and humans
4. Comparisons of DNA or protein adduct formation in rodents and humans
5. Comparisons of mutations in rodent vs. human tumors
6. Epidemiologic evidence

PAHs. The most frequently occurring type of lung cancer in smokers is squamous cell carcinoma [38–44]. As discussed earlier, the major contact carcinogens in tobacco smoke are the PAHs. In rodents, application to the lung of PAHs or of a PAH concentrate from cigarette tar leads exclusively to squamous cell carcinoma [78,79,102].

Tumors of the trachea and bronchi of hamsters are induced upon intratracheal instillation of a single dose of 5 mg BaP on Fe_2O_3, which corresponds to approximately 50 mg/kg body weight (0.2 mmol/kg), or upon chronic administration of a total dose of 7.5 mg BaP on Fe_2O_3 (75 mg/kg, 0.3 mmol/kg) [103]. A smoker who consumes 40 cigarettes per day for 40 years would be chronically exposed to approximately 12 mg of BaP or about 0.17 mg/kg (0.8 µmol/kg). On the basis of mg/kg total body weight, these calculations are perhaps too conservative for a locally acting carcinogen such as BaP. Furthermore, BaP is only one of 11 known carcinogenic PAHs identified in cigarette smoke (table 4). These exposure estimates and the determinations of the tumorigenic potential of PAH in bioassays strongly suggest that PAHs play a significant role in the induction of squamous cell carcinoma in the lungs of smokers.

As discussed earlier, the P450 1A1 [91] required for the metabolic activation and detoxification of carcinogenic PAHs is comparable in rodents and

24

humans, and the ultimate carcinogenic forms of BaP and of other carcinogenic PAHs are identical. The isolation of 7,8,9,10-tetrahydroxy-7,8,9,10-tetrahydroBaP from human urine, after hydrolysis of tetrols covalently bound to macromolecular species and/or conjugated, proves that BaP and other carcinogenic PAHs are metabolically activated to dihydroxyepoxides in humans as in rodents [104]. With respect to the binding of carcinogenic PAHs to the DNA of lung tissues, it is noteworthy that 11 out of 13 DNA samples from smokers and 2 out of 3 DNA samples from exsmokers contained benzo(a)pyrenediol-epoxide adducts in the lung tissue adjacent to the cancer [105].

We have only limited knowledge about mutations in the lungs of smokers that may be induced by carcinogenic PAHs. In two reports on adduct formations in smokers' lungs, only four cases of squamous cell carcinoma of the lung were listed as containing activated *ras*-proto-oncogenes [106,107]. A number of publications have reported on mutations of the tumor suppressor gene p53 in squamous cell carcinoma of smokers [108–110]. In one case, p53 mutations were observed in 6 out of 8 cancers. However, the reported mutations were detected on various codons and caused both transitions and transversions. There are no reports on comparisons of p53 gene mutations in squamous cell carcinoma of smokers' lung and p53 mutations in lung tumors of rodents induced by BaP or other carcinogenic PAHs.

Coke oven workers who are exposed to aerosols with high PAH content are known to be at increased risk for squamous cell carcinoma of the lung [111]. Of the six established criteria for the relevance of experimental data to human cancer induction by a carcinogen or group of carcinogens, the carcinogenic PAHs fulfill at least five, thus supporting the concept that these hydrocarbons contribute to the increased risk of smokers for squamous cell carcinoma of the lung.

TSNAs. As cited earlier, it is well established that adenocarcinoma of the lung is the major tumor induced by NNK in mice, rats, and Syrian golden hamsters, independent of route of administration [85,87–90]. In men who smoke cigarettes, pulmonary adenocarcinoma is the second most frequently occurring type of lung cancer; in women who smoke, it is the most common type of lung cancer [38–44]. Extensive dose–response studies with NNK have been carried out in rats using multiple subcutaneous injections [85,87, 89,90]. The lowest dose required to induce pulmonary tumors in rats was 0.4 mg/rat or 1.8 mg/kg [89]. Individuals who smoke 40 cigarettes per day for 40 years receive a total dose of about 100 mg or 1.4 mg/kg of NNK [36]. This estimate has been supported by quantifying the NNK metabolites NNAL and NNAL-glucuronide in smokers' urine [101]. The mean level of these metabolites in the 24-hour urine voids was 11.4 mmol at an average daily cigarette consumption of 23 cigarettes. At exposure to 40 cigarettes per day for 40 years, the collective urinary excretion of the NNK metabolites amounts to approximately 1 mg/kg. Thus, the lowest dose of NNK required to induce pulmonary tumors in rats (1.8 mg/kg) lies near the range of human exposure (1.0–1.4 mg/kg).

α-Hydroxylation of the carcinogenic TSNAs, including NNK, is a major pathway for the metabolic activation not only in rodents but also in cultured human lung and human lung microsomes. However, relative to the enzymatic reduction of NNK to NNAL, there is substantially less α-hydroxylation in human lung tissue than in rodents (figure 14) [85,112,113]. It appears that the most active isozyme in human lung tissue and microsomes for the oxidative matabolism of NNK is P450 1A2, similar to the case in rodents, although the P450 1A1 and 2B1 are also active in rodents [114–116]. Other P450 isozymes are likely playing a role in the oxidative metabolism of NNK in human lung tissue [113].

As outlined in figure 14, the enzymatic α-hydroxylation of the methylene group in NNK leads to methyl diazohydroxide. The latter reacts with DNA to form methylated bases, including O^6-methylguanine (O^6mG) and 7-methylguanine [89,117,118]. The α-hydroxylation of the methyl group leads to pyridyloxobutane diazohydroxide (figure 14), which forms pyridyloxobutylated DNA. In rodents after treatment with NNK, O^6mG is an important adduct in NNK carcinogenesis [119,120]. In the lungs and tracheas of smokers, the levels of the methylated bases, and especially of 7-methylguanine, are higher than in nonsmokers [121]. However, NNK may not be the only methylating agent; other smoke constituents also have methylating potential. In the lung of rodents, pyridyloxobutylated DNA and hemoglobin adducts have been identified upon treatment with NNK [118]. In tissues from the peripheral lung and tracheobronchial tissues, the levels of pyridyloxobutylated DNA were much higher in cigarette smokers than in nonsmokers [100]. The pyridyloxobutylated hemoglobin adduct, which is formed upon treatment of rodents with NNK, as well as with NNN, was detected in a subset of smokers [122]. These findings are consistent with the concept that NNK is metabolically activated in some smokers, leading to DNA and hemoglobin adducts in a manner similar to that seen in the lungs and blood of rodents.

In mice and Syrian golden hamsters, NNK-induced adenocarcinoma of the lung contain activated K-*ras* genes, with mostly guanine–adenine (G–A) transitions on codon 12 [123,124]. Comparative studies of activated K-*ras* genes in lung tumors induced by methylating and pyridyloxobutylating agents in mice have shown that the methylating agent causes exclusively G–A transitions, while the pyridyloxobutylating agent causes mainly guanine–thymine (G–T) transversions [125], i.e., changes from a purine to a pyrimidine or vice versa. From a total of 141 lung adenocarcinoma specimens from smokers or exsmokers, 41 tested positive for a point mutation in codon 12 (30%), compared to only 2 out of 40 tumors in patients who never smoked (5%). The mutations in smokers were approximately 80% G–T transversions and 20% G–A transitions [126]. The G–T transversions detected in K-*ras* genes in human lung adenocarcinoma could be a result of the NNK-pyridyloxobutylation pathway. However, it is also possible that other DNA-damaging agents in tobacco smokes such as carcinogenic PAHs, aldehydes, secondary nitroalkanes, and carcinogenic aromatic amines could have induced G–T transversions [125,127].

Although the epidemiologic evidence is strong that cigarette smoking is causally associated with pulmonary adenocarcinoma, it appears to be a rather insurmountable task to pinpoint a single group of agents from the complex inhalant, which contains at least 4,000 compounds, as the most significant contributor to a specific type of malignant tumor. However, only tobacco chewers and smokers are exposed to the TSNAs. Unlike the PAHs and aromatic amines, TSNAs do not occur in occupational environments. While the carcinogenic PAHs have been incriminated as the causative agent for lung cancer in coke oven workers and aromatic amines are held responsible for bladder cancer in dye workers, we have no such leads for TSNAs as human carcinogens. Despite these obstacles, there are considerations that could support the concept that NNK contributes to the increased risk of cigarette smokers for adenocarcinoma of the lung. One approach would be molecular epidemiology studies in which the relationship of specific DNA or Hb adduct levels with adenocarcinoma could be determined. The second aspect relates to the more rapid increase of pulmonary adenocarcinoma than of squamous cell carcinoma during the past four decades in the lung cancer patterns in developed countries (see 'Changes in Distribution of Histologic Types of Cancer,' above). Concurrently with this development, the percentage of filter cigarettes increased from less than 1% of all manufactured cigarettes to 90%–95%, and the tar and nicotine yields of cigarettes decreased from more than 35 mg and 2.5 mg to less than 14 mg and 1.2 mg, respectively, as measured under standard laboratory conditions [128,129]. The lower smoke yields of cigarettes were achieved not only by utilizing efficient filter tips but also by effecting a more complete combustion of the tobacco column. The changes toward more complete combustion were the result of the use of more porous paper, expanded as well as reconstituted tobaccos, and tobacco blends with increased nitrate content [29,129]. These changes have led to a smoke aerosol with decreased levels of PAHs and increased levels of TSNAs (figure 15). Most importantly, the smoker of cigarettes with low nicotine yields tends to increase smoking intensity by taking more frequent puffs and by drawing larger puff volumes [61–64]. The result is a significantly higher smoke yield of NNK [130,131], the smoke component suspected to be a major contributor to the increased risk for pulmonary adenocarcinoma in smokers.

The data presented here are consistent with the hypothesis that NNK is one cause of adenocarcinoma in smokers. Specifically with respect to adenocarcinoma in smokers, a stronger argument can be made for NNK as a cause than for any other carcinogen in tobacco smoke.

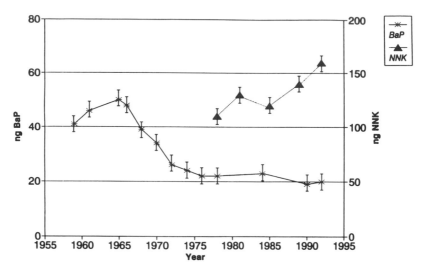

Figure 15. BaP and NNK in mainstream smoke of a leading U.S. nonfilter cigarette, 1959–1992.

Reduction of exposure

Epidemiological studies have clearly demonstrated a dose–reponse relationship between cigarette consumption and squamous cell carcinoma of the lung and pulmonary adenocarcinoma (figures 8, 9, and 11) [29–31,37–44]. Inhalation studies with mice have shown that increased smoke exposure is followed by an increased rate of pulmonary adenoma [33]. In hamsters, the dose response is seen in an increase of benign and malignant squamous epithelial tumors in the upper respiratory tract [34]. Cessation of smoking is the only safe way to eliminate the risk for lung cancer. Quitting the smoking habit at any age reduces lung cancer mortality [132]. However, cigarette modifications that reduce smoke yields are seen as practical steps towards reducing the lung cancer risk of those cigarette smokers who will not or cannot give up smoking. As discussed earlier, the changes in the makeup of commercial cigarettes in developed countries during the last 40 years have led to a major reduction of tar and nicotine yields in cigarette smoke [128,129]. This reduction has been achieved not only by the use of filter tips but also by modifying the tobacco blend and by increasing the porosity of the cigarette paper [129]. Figure 16 documents the gradual reduction of the U.S. sales-weighted average tar and nicotine yields between 1955 and 1980, with arrows indicating the first introduction of specific changes in the makeup of the U.S. blended cigarette [133]. The increasing use of perforated filter tips, which during puff drawing reduce the velocity of the air that streams through the burning cone, has also led to a selective reduction of some toxic, volatile smoke components such as carbon monoxide, hydrogen

28

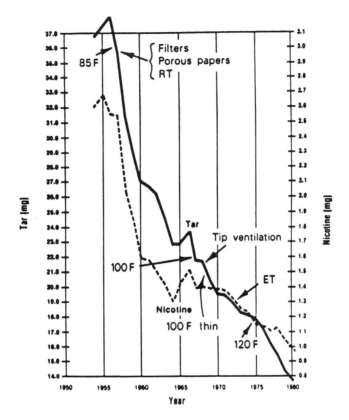

Figure 16. U.S. sales-weighted average tar and nicotine yields [129]. RT, reconstituted tobacco; ET, expanded tobacco; F, cigarettes with filter tips; numbers, lengths of filter cigarettes in millimeters. Arrows denote years in which specific changes were first introduced.

cyanide, and nitrogen oxide [134] as measured in smoke generated by machine smoking under standard conditions (one puff/minute, a puff duration of two seconds, a puff volume of 35 ml). These standardized smoking conditions represented the average smoking pattern of a smoker of high-yield cigarettes manufactured before 1955. When smoking present-day low-yield filter cigarettes, the smoker tends to increase smoking intensity by drawing puffs up to 4 or 5 times per minute with puff volumes up to 50 ml [61–64] to satisfy his or her nicotine needs. Consequently, many smokers of low-yield cigarettes are exposed to higher amounts of tar, nicotine, and toxic and tumorigenic agents than are determined by machine smoking of cigarettes. Nevertheless, epidemiological studies from various developed countries have shown that the long-term smoker of filter cigarettes (>10 years) has a 30%–50% lower risk for lung cancer than the long-term smoker of nonfilter cigarettes [30,37,38].

During the past few decades, we have witnessed in male smokers a shift

29

in the ratio of squamous cell carcinoma to pulmonary adenocarcinoma of the lung from about 1:16 to 1:1.4 [38–44]. A working hypothesis tries to explain this phenomenon by suggesting that the more intense smoking by consumers of filter cigarettes compared to consumers of nonfilter cigarettes and the deeper inhalation of the aerosol by the smoker of a low-yield cigarette is a major reason for the disproportionate increase in lung adenocarcinoma over squamous cell carcinoma. Furthermore, analyses of smoke obtained under standardized conditions has shown that the NNK yield in the smoke of a U.S. blended cigarette has increased over the years (figure 15). The more intense smoking of filter cigarettes will further increase the actual exposure to NNK [130,131]. Since NNK is suspected to be an important contributor to the increased risk of cigarette smokers for lung adenocarcinoma, and since the smoke yields of NNK rise with increasing nitrate content of the tobaccos [135], the tobaccos used for the cigarettes should ideally have low nitrate contents, although this change may be counterproductive with respect to smoke yields of carcinogenic PAHs.

As mentioned previously, the only way to avoid smoking-related diseases, including lung cancer, is to refrain from smoking. Because millions of people continue to smoke, development of less harmful cigarettes should not be rejected per-se. A leading U.S. newspaper wrote in an editorial in 1989, 'Obviously, no smoking is better than smoking, but the best should not be the enemy of the good. There is a strong social case for encouraging manufacturers to develop cigarettes that will sell' [136]. One may agree with this point of view as long as society still condones the smoking of cigarettes, cigars, and pipes.

Chemoprevention

Since millions of people throughout the world continue to smoke cigarettes, and due to the limited success of smoking-cessation efforts, the concept of chemoprevention of tobacco-related cancers is an attractive goal. The chemoprevention of lung cancer is still very young; nevertheless, it is unique because of the clearly defined major causative factor.

In 1992 the U.S. National Cancer Institute sponsored a total of 12 phase I (toxicity screening) and 22 phase II and III (small and large scale) clinical trials with chemopreventive agents, including β-carotene, 13-cis-retinoic acid, retinol, and calcium compounds. Several of these 34 clinical trials were concerned with chemoprevention of cancer of the upper aerodigestive tract and with cancer of the lung in smokers, especially prevention of second primary tumors [137]. Basically, there are two types of chemopreventive agents, namely, the blocking agents that prevent carcinogens from reaching or reacting with target sites and the tumor suppressors that inhibit the development of the neoplastic process in cells [138,139]. Blocking agents are generally considered to be those that block the effect of genotoxic agents;

however, among these are also some agents that inhibit tumor promotion. The latter group interferes primarily with the arachidonic acid cascade [138,139].

One goal of the research on chemopreventive agents in tobacco carcinogenesis has been to inhibit the formation in rodents of lung tumors induced by tobacco-specific carcinogens, specifically NNK, and to delineate their mechanisms of action in model assays. The majority of the agents tested for their chemopreventive effect in NNK-treated animals are micronutrients (table 7). So far, none of them have reached phase I of clinical trials; however, their low toxicity, coupled with data from assays in mice and rats on the inhibition of NNK-induced lung tumors, appears promising and should lead to clinical trials [140–147]. With one exception, these agents are effective because they inhibit the metabolic activation of the tobacco-specific carcinogen NNK and/or its DNA-alkylation in the lungs of rats and mice. The exception relates to the major polyphenol in green tea, (−)epigallocatechin gallate (EGCG), which suppresses oxidative DNA damage by NNK.

Postscript

The increasing incidence of lung cancers in cigarette smokers throughout the world will remain a major health problem for years to come. This public health problem deserves the greatest attention of the medical and scientific community. However, some promising statistical evidence shows that in several developed countries the consumption of cigarettes by adults has remarkably decreased. These data should allow a forecast of a reduction in the lung cancer rates, at least in younger cohorts. A number of factors have had a major impact on the declining cigarette consumption. These include public health information campaigns and education on the ill effects of smoking, the availability of smoking cessation clinics, the restriction of smoking in public places, and the increasing taxation of tobacco products. It is hoped that these efforts will be continued in developed countries and that the developing countries will learn from these experiences. Further development of low-yield cigarettes with less toxicity and carcinogenicity of the smoke should also be pursued. Worldwide, the cigarette consumption has not decreased but instead is on the rise. In developed countries, there are many smokers who will not or cannot give up their tobacco habit. A recent development, the chemoprevention of tobacco-related cancers, deserves full support, if only to learn the long-term effects of chemopreventive agents upon a well-defined large population group, namely, cigarette smokers. These studies will not only delineate the underlying mechanisms of chemoprevention but will also lead to the development of new agents that have efficacy in chemoprevention of various types of cancer.

Beyond these ongoing programs in the prevention of smoking-related

Table 7. Effect of chemopreventive agents inhibiting NNK carcinogenesis in laboratory animals

NNK total dose (µmol)	Chemopreventive agent			Species, sex	Tumor incidence (%)	Tumor multiplicity	Reference
	Route of admin.	Name	Level (µmol)				
500	s.c.	Control		F-344 rats, male	80[a] 38[b] 28[c]	—	[140]
		Phenylethyl-ITC	3 g/diet (21 wks)		43[a] 35[b] 18[c]		
10	i.p.	Phenylethyl-ITC	4 × 5	A/J mice, female	93[a]	4.1[a]	[141]
			4 × 1		100[a]	6.5[a]	
		Phenylpropyl-ITC	4 × 5		11[a]	0.2[a]	
			4 × 1		75[a]	1.2[a]	
		PhenylbutylITC	4 × 5		11[a]	0.2[a]	
			4 × 1		42[a]	0.8[a]	
			4 × 0.2		100[a]	4.2[a]	
		Phenylpentyl-ITC	4 × 5		25[a]	0.3[a]	
			4 × 1		53[a]	0.9[a]	
			4 × 0.2		100[a]	3.0[a]	
		Phenylhexyl-ITC	4 × 5		5[a]	0.1[a]	
			4 × 1		0	0	
			4 × 0.2		70[a]	1.2[a]	
		Control	—		100[a]	7.9[a]	

Dose	Route	Treatment	Dose	Species				Ref
500	s.c.	Sinigrin	3 g/diet (21 wks)	F-344 rats	79[a]		—	[142]
		Control			80[a]			
10	i.p.	Indole-3-carbinol	100	A/J mice, female	95[a]		61[a]	[143]
		Control	500		100[a]			
47	p.o.	Ellagic acid	4 g/diet	A/J mice, female	100[a]		6.5[a]	[144]
		BHA	5 g/diet		96[a]		10.7[a]	
		Control			68[a]		7.5[a]	
39	p.o.	D-limonene	25 mg	A/J mice, female	100[a]		1.9[a]	[145]
		Lemon oil	25 mg		—	0	15.7[a]	
		Orange oil	25 mg		—	0	13.3[a]	
		Control			—	0	7.4[a]	
					—	0	8.2[a]	
					100[a]		44.8–50.8[a]	
							0.25–2.8[d]	
9.7	p.o.	D-limonene	25 mg	A/J mice, female	—		2.5[a]	[146]
		Control			100[a]		11.2[a]	
9.7	p.o.	Diallyl sulfide	3 × 200 mg		38[a]		0.6[a]	
10		Control		A/J mice, female	100		7.2[a]	[147]
(136)		Control			100[a]		7.6[a]	
	p.o.	XSC	5 ppm/diet		100[a]		4.1[a]	
		XSC	10 ppm/diet		90[a]		3.3[a]	
		XSC	15 ppm/diet		85[a]		1.8[a]	

[a] Lung tumors.

[b] Liver tumors.

[c] Nasal cavity tumors.

[d] Tumors of the forestomach.

ITC, isothiocyanate; EGCG, (−)epigallocatechin gallate; XSC, 1,4-phenylene-bis(methyleneselenocyanate); drinkg, drinking.

cancer, there remain a number of intriguing questions that deserve answers. As discussed earlier in this overview, we need to search for an explanation for the fact that in female cigarette smokers, lung adenocarcinoma occurs more frequently than squamous cell carcinoma, and why the situation is just the reverse in male smokers. The disproportionate increase of adenocarcinoma over squamous cell carcinoma in male cigarette smokers during recent decades may in part be due to the introduction of low-yield cigarettes beginning about 1965 to 1970. The resulting modifications in smoke chemistry, together with more intense smoking of the low-tar, low-nicotine cigarettes, have altered the qualitative and quantitative aspects of exposure to smoke toxins and smoke carcinogens. Other unanswered questions concern the high lung cancer incidence rates in certain groups (African-Americans vs. Caucasians) and the relatively low lung cancer incidence rates in some countries (Japan vs. the U.S.A. and Western Europe). Issues relating to smoking and lung cancer that were not discussed in this chapter include the role of micronutrients as modifiers of tobacco carcinogenesis. Although epidemiological studies imply that micronutrients, including several vitamins, may reduce the risk of tobacco-related cancer, scientific knowledge about the effects and mechanisms of these suspected chemopreventive agents is only beginning to emerge. A recent model study has shown that rats on a low-fat diet (5% corn oil) that were treated with NNK developed lung cancer later and had a lower incidence rate of pancreas cancer than rats treated with the same dose of NNK but maintained on a high-fat diet (23.5% corn oil) [148]. These bioassay data support the concept that a high-fat diet may further increase the smoker's risk for cancer of the lung [149–152]. It needs to be studied whether this modifying effect of the fat in the diet on tobacco carcinogenesis is a result of specific unsaturated fatty acids or of the fat diet per se.

Perhaps the greatest challenges in the smoking–lung-cancer domain lie in the development and application of biomarkers for identifying those tobacco smokers who are at especially high risk for lung cancer and for cancer at other sites. A beginning has been made by identifying and quantifying adducts of PAHs and TSNAs with DNA and hemoglobin and by determining 1-hydroxypyrene, and NNAL and NNAL-glucuronides in the urine of smokers. It is hoped that this aspect of biochemical epidemiology will be further developed in both prospective and retrospective studies with cigarette smokers as a new approach to risk assessment.

Acknowledgments

The authors appreciate the editorial assistance of Jennifer Johnting. Our studies are supported by grants CA-29580 and CA-17613 from the U.S. National Cancer Institute.

References

1. Adler I. 1912. Primary Malignant Growths of the Lungs and Bronchi. Longmans, Green & Co.: New York.
2. Parkin DM, Pisani P, Ferlay J. 1993. Estimates of the worldwide incidence of eighteen major cancers in 1985. Int J Cancer 54:594–606.
3. Silverberg E, Holleb AI. 1974. Cancer around the world, 1964–65/ CA Cancer J Clin 21:26–27.
4. Silverberg E, Holleb AI. 1971. Cancer around the world, 1966–67. CA Cancer J Clin 24:16–17.
5. Silverberg E. Holleb AI. 1975. Cancer around the world, 1968-69. CA Cancer J Clin 25:16–17.
6. Silverberg E, Holleb AI. 1976. Cancer around the world, 1970–71. CA Cancer J Clin 26:26–27.
7. Silverberg E, Holleb AI. 1978. Cancer around the world, 1972–73. CA Cancer J Clin 28:28–29.
8. Silverberg E, Holleb AI. 1980. Cancer around the world, 1974–75. CA Cancer J Clin 30:34–35.
9. Silverberg E, Holleb AI. 1982. Cancer around the world, 1976–77. CA Cancer J Clin 32:26–27.
10. Silverberg E, Holleb AI. 1984. Cancer around the world, 1978–79. CA Cancer J Clin 34:18–19.
11. Silverberg E, Holleb AI. 1986. Cancer around the world, 1980–81. CA Cancer J Clin 36:20–121.
12. Silverberg E, Holleb AI. 1988. Cancer around the world, 1982–83. CA Cancer J Clin 38:18–19.
13. Silverberg E, Holleb AI. 1989. Cancer around the world, 1984–86. CA Cancer J Clin 39:16–17.
14. Boring CC, Squires TS, Tong T. 1991. Cancer around the world, 1986–88. CA Cancer J Clin 43:22–23.
15. Zaridze DG, Gurevicius R. 1986. Lung cancer in the USSR: Patterns and trends. In Tobacco, A Major International Health Hazard, DG Zaridze and R Peto (eds.). IARC Sci Publ 74:87–101.
16. Wynder EL, Gori GB. 1977. Contribution of the environment to cancer incidence: An epidemiologic exercise. J Natl Cancer Inst 58:825–832.
17. Doll R, Peto R. 1981. The causes of cancer: Quantitative estimates of avoidable risks of cancer in the United States today. J Natl Cancer Inst 66:1193–1308.
18. Hammond EC, Horn D. 1958. Smoking and death rates — report on 44 months of follow-up of 187,783 men. I. Total mortality. JAMA 166:1159–1172.
19. Hammond EC, Horn D. 1958. Smoking and death rates — report on 44 months of follow-up of 187,783 men. II. Death rates by cause. JAMA 166:1294–1308.
20. Pershagen, G. 1990. Air pollution and cancer. In Complex Mixtures and Cancer Risk, H Vainio, M Sorsa, and AJ Michael (eds.). IARC Monogr 104:240–251.
21. Royal College of Physicians, London. 1962. Smoking and Health. Pitman: London.
22. U.S. Surgeon General. 1964. Smoking and Health. U.S. Public Health Service Publ. No. 1103, Washington, DC.
23. Zaridze DG, Peto R. 1986. Tobacco: A major international health hazard. IARC Sci Publ 74.
24. Shopland DR, Eyre H-J, Pechacek TF. 1991. Smoking-attributable cancer mortality in 1991: Is lung cancer now the leading cause of death among smokers in the United States? J Natl Cancer Inst 83:1142–1148.
25. U.S. Surgeon General. 1989. Reducing the health consequences of smoking. Twenty five years of progress. U.S. Department of Health Human Services Publ No (CDC) 89-8411.

26. Lee PN. 1975. Tobacco consumption in various countries. Research Paper 6, 4th ed. Tobacco Research Council, London.
27. Cigarette consumption in various countries 1972–1992 (editorial). Tobacco J Int.
28. Wynder EL, Day E. 1961. Some thoughts on the causaition of chronic disease. JAMA 175:997–999.
29. U.S. Surgeon General. 1982. The health consequences of smoking. Cancer. U.S. Depatrent of Health Human Services Publ No (PHS) 82–50179.
30. International Agency for Research on Cancer. 1986. IARC Monographs on the Evaluation of the Carcinogenic Risk of Chemicals to Humans. Vol. 38, Tobacco Smoking. IARC: Lyon, France.
31. Kahn HA. 1966. The Dorn study of smoking and mortality among U.S. veterans: Report on eight and one-half years of observation. Natl Cancer Inst Monogr 19:1–125.
32. American Cancer Society. 1988. Cancer Facts and Figures. American Cancer Society: New York.
33. Leuchtenberger C, Leuchtenberger R. 1970. Effects of chronic inhalation of whole fresh smoke and its gas phase on pulmonary tumorigenesis in Snell's mice. U.S. Atomic Energy Comm Symp Ser 21:329–346.
34. Dontenwill W, Chevalier H-J, Harke H-P, Lafrenz U, Rekzeh G, Schneider B. 1973. Investigations of the effects of chronic cigarette smoke inhalation in Syrian golden hamsters. J Natl Cancer Inst 51:1781–1832.
35. Wynder EL, Hoffmann D. 1967. Tobacco and Tobacco Smoke: Studies in Experimental Carcinogenesis. Academic Press: New York.
36. Brunnemann KD, Hoffmann D. 1991. Analytical studies on N-nitrosamines in tobacco and tobacco smoke. Recent Adv Tobacco Sci 17:71–112.
37. Stellman SD, Garfinkel L. 1989. Lung cancer risk is proportional to cigarette tar yield. Evidence from a prospective study. Prev Med 18:518–525.
38. Zang E, Wynder EL. 1992. Cumulative tar exposure. A new index for estimating lung cancer risk among cigarette smokers. Cancer 70:69–76.
39. Wynder EL, Graham EA. 1950. Tobacco smoking as a possible factor in bronchiogenic carcinoma. A study of six hundred and eighty four proved cases. JAMA 143:329–336.
40. El-Torky M, El-Zeky F, Hall CJ. 1990. Significant changes in the distribution of histologic types of lung cancer. A review of 4928 cases. Cancer 65:2361–2367.
41. Dodds L, Davis S, Polissar L. 1986. A population-based study of lung cancer incidence trends by histologic type, 1974–81. J Natl Cancer Inst 76:21–29.
42. Wu AH, Henderson BE, Thomas DC, Mack TM. 1986. Secular trends in histologic types of lung cancer. J Natl Cancer Inst 77:53–56.
43. Beard CM, Jedd MB, Woolner LB. 1988. Fifty-year trend in incidence rates of bronchiogenic carcinoma by cell type in Olmsted County, Minnesota. J Natl Cancer Inst 80:1404–1407.
44. Devesa SS, Shaw GL, Blot WJ. 1991. Changing patterns of lung cancer incidence by histologic type. Cancer Epidemiol Biomarkers Prev 1:29–34.
45. Chaudhuri PK, Thomas PA, Walker MJ, Briele HA, Das Gupta TKD, Beattie CW. 1982. Steroid receptors in human lung cancer cytosols. Cancer Lett 16:327–332.
46. Hebert JR, Miller DR, Toporoff ED, Teas J, Barone J. 1991. Black–white differences in United States Cancer Rates: A discussion of possible dietary factors to explain large and growing divergencies. Cancer Prev 1:141–156.
47. Brunnemann KD, Hoffmann D. 1974. The pH of tobacco smoke. Food Cosmet Toxicol 12:115–124.
48. Armitage AK, Turner DM. 1970. Absorption of nicotine in cigarette and cigar smoke through the oral mucosa. Nature 226:1231–1232.
49. Brunnemann KD, Hoffmann D. 1975. Chemical studies on tobacco smoke XXXIV. Gas chromatographic determination of ammonia in cigarette and cigar smoke. J Chromatogr Sci 13:159–163.

50. Neurath G, Ehmke H. 1964. Untersuchungen über den Nitratgehalt des Tabaks. Beitr Tabakforsch 2:333–344.

51. Kotin P, Falk HL. 1963. Atmospheric factors in the pathogenesis of lung cancer. Adv Cancer Res 7:475–514.

52. Dube MF, Green CR. 1982. Methods of collection of smoke for analytical purposes. Recent Adv Tobacco Sci 8:42–102.

53. Roberts DL. 1988. Natural tobacco flavor. Recent Adv Tobacco Sci 14:49–81.

54. Nakayama T, Kodama M, Nagata C. 1984. Generation of hydrogen peroxide and superoxide anion radical from cigarette smoke. Gann 75:95–98.

55. Pryor W, Stone K. 1993. Oxidants in cigarette smoke. Radicals, hydrogen peroxide, peroxynitrate and peroxynitrite. Ann NY Acad Sci 686:12–28.

56. Knekt P. 1993. Vitamin E and smoking and the risk of lung cancer. Ann NY Acad Sci 686:280–288.

57. Chow CK. 1993. Cigarette smoking and oxidative damage in the lung. Ann NY Acad Sci 686:289–298.

58. Green CR. 1977. Some relationship between tobacco leaf and smoke composition. Proc Am Chem Soc Symp Recent Advances in the Chemical Composition of Tobacco and Tobacco Smoke, New Orleans, LA, pp. 426–470.

59. Wahlberg I, Enzell CR. 1987. Tobacco isoprenoids. Natural Product Rep 4:237–276.

60. Tso TC. 1990. Production, Physiology and Biochemistry of the Tobacco Plant. Ideals Inc., Beltsville, MD.

61. Russell MAH. 1980. The case for medium-nicotine, low-tar, low-carbon monoxide cigarettes. In A Safe Cigarette? GB Gori and FG Bock (eds.). Banbury Rep 3:297–310.

62. Herning RI, Jones RT, Bachman J, Mines AH. 1981. Puff volume increases when low-nicotine cigarettes are smoked. Br Med J 283:187–189.

63. Kozlowski LT, Rickert WS, Pope MA, Robinson JC, Frecker RC. 1982. Estimating the yield to smokers of tar, nicotine, and carbon monoxide from the 'lowest yield' ventilated filter-cigarettes. Br J Addict 77:159–165.

64. Haley NJ, Sepkovic DW, Hoffmann D, Wynder EL. 1985. Cigarette smoking as a risk factor for cardiovascular disease VI. Compensation with nicotine availability as a single variable. Clin Pharmacol Ther 38:164–170.

65. Norman V. 1977. An overview of the vapor phase semi-volatile and nonvolatile components of cigarette smoke. Recent Adv Tobacco Sci 3:28–58.

66. Jenkins RW Jr, Goldey C, Williamson TG. 1985. Neutron activation analysis in tobacco and tobacco smoke studies: 2R1 cigarette composition, smoke transference and butt filtration. Beitr Tabakforsch 13:59–65.

67. Wittekindt W. 1986. Recommended plant protecting agents — current strategies in 22 important tobacco exporting countries. Beitr Tabakforsch 13:271–280.

68. Sheets TJ. 1991. Pesticides on tobacco: Perceptions and realities. Recent Adv Tobacco Sci 17:33–68.

69. Leffingwell JC, Leffingwell D. 1988. Chemical and sensory aspects of tobacco flavor — An overview. Recent Adv Tobacco Sci 14:169–218.

70. Perfetti TA, Gordon HH. 1985. Just noticeable difference studies of mentholated cigarette products. Tobacco Sci 29:57–66.

71. International Agency for Research on Cancer. 1976. Coumarin. IARC Monogr 10:113–119.

72. Dalbey WE, Nettesheim D, Griesemer R, Caton JE, Guerin MR. 1980. Chronic inhalation of cigarette smoke by 344 rats. J Natl Cancer Inst 64:383–390.

73. Hoffmann, D, Wynder EL. 1971. A study of tobacco carcinogenesis XI. Tumor initiators, tumor accelerators and tumor promoting activity of condensate fractions. Cancer 27:848–864.

74. Dontenwill W, Chevalier HJ, Harke HPV, Klimisch HJ. 1976. Experimentelle Untersuchungen über die krebserzeugende Wirkung von Zigarettenrauch-Kondensaten an der

Mâusehaut. VI. Mitteilung: Untersuchungen zur Fraktionierung von Zigarettenrauch-Kondensat. Z Krebsforsch 85:1655–1161.

75. Hecht SS, Thorne RL, Maronpot RR, Hoffmann D. 1975. A Study of Tobacco Carcinogenesis XIII. Tumor promoting subfractions of the weakly acidic fraction. J Natl Cancer Inst 55:1329–1336.

76. Van Duuren BL, Goldschmidt BM. 1976. Cocarcinogenic and tumor promoting agents in tobacco carcinogenesis. J Natl Cancer Inst 56:1237–1242.

77. Hecht SS, Carmella S, Mori H, Hoffmann D. 1981. Role of catechol as a major cocarcinogen in the weakly acidic fraction of smoke condensate. J Natl Cancer Inst 66:163–169.

78. Blacklock JW. 1957. The production of lung tumors in rats by 3,4-benzopyrene, methylcholanthrene and condensate from cigarette smoke. Br J Cancer 11:181–191.

79. Deutsch-Wenzel R, Brune H, Grimmer G, Dettbarn G, Misfeld J. 1983. Experimental studies in rat lungs on the carcinogenicity and dose-response relationships of eight frequently occurring environmental polycyclic aromatic hydrocarbons. J Natl Cancer Inst 71:539–544.

80. Harley NH, Cohen BS, Tso TC. 1980. Polonium-210. A questionable risk factor in smoking-related carcinogenesis. Banbury Rep 3:93–104.

81. National Council on Radiation Protection and Measurement. 1987. Ionizing radiation exposure of the population of the United States. NCRP Rep 93, Bethesda, MD.

82. Doll R. 1971. Cancers related to smoking. Proc. 2nd World Conf. Smoking and Health. Pitman: London, pp. 10–23.

83. Bryant MS, Vineis P, Skipper PL, Tannenbaum SR. 1988. Hemoglobin adducts of aromatic amines: associations with smoking status and type of tobacco. Proc Natl Acad Sci USA 85:9788–9791.

84. Bartsch H, Malaveille C, Friesen M, Kadlubar FF, Vineis F. 1993. Black (air-cured) and blond (flue-cured) tobacco cancer risk IV. Molecular dosimetry studies implicate aromatic amines as bladder carcinogens. Eur J Cancer, 1199–1207.

85. Hecht SS, Hoffmann D. 1989. The relevance of tobacco-specific nitrosamines to human cancer. Cancer Surv 8:273–294.

86. National Research Council. 1981. The Health Effects of Nitrate, Nitrite, and N-Nitroso Compounds. NRC: Washington, DC, chapter 7.

87. Rivenson A, Hoffmann D, Prokopczyk B, Amin S, Hecht SS. 1988. A study of tobacco carcinogenesis XLII. Induction of lung and pancreas tumors in F344 rats by tobacco-specific and Areca-derived N-nitrosamines. Cancer Res 48:6912–6917.

88. LaVoie EJ, Prokopczyk G, Rigotty J, Czech A, Rivenson A, Adams JD. 1987. Tumorigenic activity of the tobacco-specific nitrosamines 4-(methylnitrosamino)-1-(3-pyridyl)-1-butanone (NNK) 4-(methylnitrosamino)-4-(3-pyridyl)-1-butanol (NNAL) and N′-nitrosonornicotine (NNN) on topical application to Sencar mice. Cancer Lett 37:277–283.

89. Belinsky SA, Foley JF, White CM, Anderson MW, Maronpot R. 1990. Dose–response relationship between O^6-methylguanine formation in Clara cells and induction of pulmonary neoplasia in the rat by 4-(methylnitrosamino)-1-(3-pyridyl)-1-butanone. Cancer Res 50:3772–3780.

90. Hoffmann D, Djordjevic MV, Rivenson A, Zang E, Desai D, Amin S. 1993. A study of tobacco carcinogenesis LI. Relative potencies of tobacco-specific N-nitrosamines as inducers of lung tumors in A/J mice. Cancer Lett 71:25–30.

91. Guengerich FP, Shimada T. 1991. Oxidation of toxic and carcinogenic chemicals by human cytochrome P-450 enzymes. Chem Res Toxicol 4:391–407.

92. Dipple A, Moschel RC, Bigger CAH. 1984. Polynuclear aromatic carcinogens. In Chemical Carcinogens, CE Searle (ed.). Am Chem Soc Monogr 182:41–163.

93. Yun C-H, Shimada T, Guengerich FP. 1992. Roles of human liver cytochrome P450 2C and 3A enzymes in the 3-hydroxylation of benzo(a)pyrene. Cancer Res 52:1868–1874.

94. Pellkonen O, Vahakangas KN, Nebert DW. 1980. Binding of polycyclic aromatic hydrocarbons to DNA. Comparison with mutagenesis and tumorigenesis. J Toxicol Environ Health 6:1009–1020.

95. Hall M, Grover PL. 1990. Polycyclic hydrocarbons: metabolism, activation and tumor initiation. In Chemical Carcinogenesis and Mutagenesis, Vol. 1, CS Cooper and PL Grover (eds.). Berlin: Springer-Verlag, pp. 327–372.

96. Perera P, Mayer J, Jaretzki A, Hearne S, Brenner D, Young TL, Fischman HK, Grimes M, Grantham S, Tang MX. 1989. Comparison of DNA adducts and sister chromatid exchange in lung cancer cases and controls. Cancer Res 49:4446–4451.

97. Hansen AM, Poulsen OM, Christensen JM. 1993. Determination of 1-hydroxypyrene in human urine by high-performance liquid chromatography. J Anal Toxicol 17:38–44.

98. Morse MA, Eklind K, Toussant M, Amin SG, Chung F-L. 1990. Characterization of a glucuronide metabolite of 4-(methylnitrosamino)-1-(3-pyridyl)-1-butanone (NNK) and its dose-dependent excretion in the urine of mice and rats. Carcinogenesis 11:1819–1823.

99. Hecht SS, Trushin N, Reid-Quinn CA, Burak ES, Jones AB, Southers JL, Gombar CT, Carmella SG, Anderson LM, Rice JM. 1993. Metabolism of the tobacco-specific nitrosamine 4-(methylnitrosamino)-1-(3-pyridyl)-1-butanone in the patas monkey: pharmacokinetics and characterization of glucuronide metabolites. Carcinogenesis 14:229–236.

100. Foiles PG, Akerkar SA, Carmella SG, Kagan M, Stoner GD, Resau JH, Hecht SS. 1991. Mass spectrometric analysis of tobacco-specific nitrosamine-DNA adducts in smokers and nonsmokers. Chem Res Toxicol 4:364–368.

101. Carmella SG, Akerkar S, Hecht SS. 1993. Metabolites of the tobacco-specific nitrosamine 4-(methylnitrosamino)-1-(3-pyridyl)-1-butanone in smokers' urine. Cancer Res 53:721–724.

102. Davis BR, Whitehead JK, Gill ME, Lee PN, Butterworth AD, Rose JJ. 1975. Response of rat lung to tobacco smoke condensate or fractions derived from it administered repeatedly by intratracheal instillation. Br J Cancer 31:453–461.

103. Saffiotti U, Montesano R, Sellakumar AR, Cefis F, Kaufman DG. 1972. Respiratory tract carcinogenesis induced in hamsters by different dose levels of benzo(a)pyrene and ferric oxide. J Natl Cancer Inst 49:1199–1204.

104. Weston A, Bowman ED, Carr P, Rothman N. Strickland PT. 1993. Detection of metabolites of polycyclic aromatic hydrocarbons in human urine. Carcinogenesis 14:1053–1055.

105. Alexandrov K, Rojas M, Geneste O, Castegnaro M, Camus A-M, Petruzzelli S, Giuntini C, Bartsch H. 1992. An improved fluorometric assay for dosimetry of benzo(a)pyrene diol-epoxide-DNA adducts in smokers' lung: Comparisons with total bulky adducts and aryl hydrocarbon hydroxylase activity. Cancer Res 52:6248–6253.

106. Reynolds SH, Anna CK, Brown KC, Wiest JS, Beattie EJ, Pero RW, Iglehart JD, Anderson MW. 1991. Activated protooncogenes in human lung tumors from smokers. Proc Natl Acad Sci USA 88:1085–1089.

107. Husgafvel-Pursiainen K, Hackman P, Ridanpää M, Anttila S, Karjalainen A, Partanen T, Taikina-Aho O, Heikkila L, Vainio H. 1993. K-ras mutations in human adenocarcinoma of the lung: association with smoking and occupational exposure to asbestos. Int J Cancer 53:250–256.

108. Chiba I, Takahashi T, Nau MM, D-Amico A, Curiel DT, Mitsudomi T, Buckhagen DJ, Carbone D, Piantadosi S, Koga H, Reissman PT, Slamon DJ, Holmes EC, Minna JD. 1990. Mutations in the p53 gene are frequent in primary, resected non-small cell lung cancer. Oncogene 5:1603–1610.

109. Suzuki H, Takahashi T, Kuroishi T, Suyama M, Ariyoshi Y, Takahashi T, Ueda R. 1992. p53 mutations in non-small lung cancer in Japan. Association between mutations and smoking. Cancer Res 52:734–736.

110. Miller CW, Simon K, Aslo A, Kok K, Yokota, Buys HCM, Terada M, Koeffler HP. 1992. p53 Mutations in human lung tumors. Cancer Res 52:1695–1698.

111. International Agency for Research on Cancer. 1984. Coke production. IARC Monogr 34:101–131.

112. Castonguay A, Stoner GD, Schut HAJ, Hecht SS. 1983. Metabolism of tobacco-specific N-nitrosamines by cultured human tissues. Proc Natl Acad Sci USA 80:6694–6697.

113. Smith TJ, Guo Z, Gonzalez FJ, Guengerich FP, Stoner GD, Yang CS. 1992. Metabolism

of 4-(methylnitrosamino)-1-(3-pyridyl)-1-butanone in human lung and liver microsomes and cytochromes P-450 expressed in hepatoma cells. Cancer Res 52:1757–1763.

114. Smith TJ, Guo Z, Thomas PE, Chung F-L, Morse MA, Eklind K, Yang CS. 1990. Metabolism of 4-(methylnitrosmino)-1-(3-pyridyl)-1-butanone in mouse lung microsomes and its inhibition by isothiocyanates. Cancer Res 50:6817–6822.

115. Devereux TR, Anderson MW, Belinsky SA. 1988. Factors regulating activation and DNA alkylation of 4-(N-methyl-N-nitrosamino)-1-(3-pyridyl)-1-butanone and nitrosodimethylamine in rat lung and isolated lung cells, and the relationship to carcinogenicity. Cancer Res 48:4215–4221.

116. Guo Z, Smith TJ, Ishizaki H, Yang CS. 1991. Metabolism of 4-(methylnitrosamino)-1-(3-pyridyl)-1-butanone (NNK) by cytochrome P450IIB1 in a reconstituted system. Carcinogenesis 12:2277–2282.

117. Hecht SS, Trushin N, Castonguay A, Rivenson A. 1986. Comparative tumorigenicity and DNA methylation in F344 rats by 4-(methylnitrosamino)-1-(3-pyridyl)-1-butanone and N-nitrosodimethylamine. Cancer Res 46:498–502.

118. Murphy SE, Palomino A, Hecht SS, Hoffmann D. 1990. Dose–response study of DNA and hemoglobin adduct formation by 4-(methylnitrosamino)-1-(3-pyridyl)-1-butanone in F344 rats. Cancer Res 50:5446–5452.

119. Hecht SS, Spratt TE, Trushin N. 1988. Evidence for 4-(3-pyridyl)-4-oxobutylation of DNA in F344 rats treated with the tobacco-specific nitrosamines 4-(methylnitrosamino)-1-(3-pyridyl)-1-butanone and N'-nitrosonornicotine. Carcinogenesis 9:161–165.

120. Peterson LA, Hecht SS. 1991. O^6-Methylguanine is a critical determinant of 4-(methylnitrosamino)-1-(3-pyridyl)-1-butanone tumorigenesis in A/J mouse lung. Cancer Res 51:5557–5564.

121. Mustonen R, Schoket B, Hemminki K. 1993. Smoking-related DNA adducts: ^{32}P-postlabeling analysis of 7-methylguanine in human bronchial and lymphocyte DNA. Carcinogenesis 14:151–154.

122. Carmella SG, Kagan SS, Kagan M, Foiles PG, Palladino G, Quart AM, Quart E, Hecht SS. 1990. Mass spectrometric analysis of tobacco-specific nitrosamine hemoglobin adducts in snuff dippers, smokers, and nonsmokers. Cancer Res 50:5438–5445.

123. Belinsky SA, Devereux TR, White CM, Foley JF, Maronpot RR, Anderson MW. 1991. Role of Clara cells and type II cells in the development of pulmonary tumors in rats and mice following exposure to a tobacco-specific nitrosamine. Exp Lung Res 17:263–278.

124. Oreffo VIC, Lin H-W, Padmanabhan R, Witschi HP. 1993. K-ras and p53 point mutations in 4-(methylnitrosamino-1-(3-pyridyl)-1-butanone-induced hamster lung tumors. Carcinogenesis 14:451–455.

125. Ronai Z, Gradia S, Peterson LA, Nagao M, Makino H, Hecht SS. 1993. Analysis of K-ras and p53 mutations in lung tumors induced by 4-(methylnitrosamino)-1-(3-pyridyl)-1-butanone (NNK), 4-(acetoxymethylnitrosamino)-1-(3-pyridyl)-1-butanone (NNKOAc) or acetoxy-methylmethylnitrosamine (AMMN). Proc Am Assoc Cancer Res 34:170.

126. Rodenhuis S, Slebos RJC. 1992. Clinical significance of ras oncogene activation in human lung cancer. Cancer Res Suppl. 52:2665s–2669s.

127. Singer B, Essigmann JM. 1991. Site-specific mutagenesis: retrospective and prospective. Carcinogenesis 12:949–955.

128. Kiryluk S, Wald N. 1989. Trends in cigarette smoking habits in the United Kingdom. In Nicotine, Smoking and the Low Tar Programme, N Wald and P Froggatt (eds.). Oxford University Press: Oxford, UK, pp. 53–69.

129. Hoffmann D, Hoffmann I, Wynder EL. 1991. Lung cancer and the changing cigarette. IARC Sci Publ 105:449–459.

130. Fischer S, Spiegelhalder B, Preussmann R. 1989. Influence of smoking parameters on the delivery of tobacco-specific nitrosamines in cigarette smoke. A contribution to relative risk evaluation. Carcinogenesis 10:1059–1066.

131. Djordjevic MV, Sigountos CW, Brunemann KD, Hoffmann D. 1990. Tobacco-specific

nitrosamine delivery in the mainstream smoke of high- and low-yield cigarettes smoked with varying puff volumes. Proc CORESTA Symp, pp. 54–62.

132. Halpern MT, Gillespie BW, Warner KE. 1993. Patterns of absolute risk of lung cancer mortality in former smokers. J Natl Cancer Inst 85:457–464.

133. Norman V. 1982. Changes in the smoke chemistry of modern day cigarettes. Recent Adv Tobacco Sci 8:141–177.

134. Norman V. 1974. The effect of perforated tipping paper on the yields of various smoke components. Beitr Tabakforsch 7:282–287.

135. Brunnemann KD, Masaryk J, Hoffmann D. 1983. The role of tobacco stems in the formation of N-nitrosamines in tobacco and mainstream and sidestream smoke. J Agric Food Chem 31:1221–1224.

136. Safer cigarettes. 1989. New York Times, March 3, p. A38.

137. Kelloff GJ, Boone CW, Malone WF, Steele VE. 1992. Chemoprevention clinical trials. Mutat Res 267:291–295.

138. Wattenberg LW. 1992. Inhibition of carcinogenesis by minor dietary constituents. Cancer Res 52:2085s–2091s.

139. Wattenberg LW. 1993. Inhibition of carcinogenesis by nonnutrient constituents in the diet. In Food and Cancer Prevention: Chemical and Biological Aspects, KW Waldron, IT Johnson, and GR Fenwich (eds.). The Royal Society of Chemistry: Cambridge, UK, pp. 12–23.

140. Morse MA, Wang C-X, Stoner GD, Mandal S, Conran PB, Amin SG, Hecht SS, Chung F-L. 1989. Inhibition of 4-(methylnitrosamino)-1-(3-pyridyl)-1-butanone-induced DNA adduct formation and tumorigenicity in the lung of F344 rats by dietary phenethyl isothiocyanates. Cancer Res 49:549–553.

141. Morse MA, Eklind KI, Amin SG, Hecht SS, Chung F-L. 1989. Effects of alkyl chain length on the inhibition of NNK-induced lung neoplasia in A/J mice by arylalkyl isothiocyanates. Carcinogenesis 10:1757–1759.

142. Morse MA, Wang C-X, Amin SG, Hecht SS, Chung F-L. 1988. Effect of dietary sinigrin or indole-3-carbinol on O^6-methylguanine-DNA-transmethylase activity and 4-(methylnitrosamino)-1-(3-pyridyl)-1-butanone-induced DNA methylation and tumorigenicity in F344 rats. Carcinogenesis 9:1891–1895.

143. Morse MA, LaGreca SD, Amin SG, Chung F-L. 1990. Effects of indole-3-carbinol on lung tumorigenesis and DNA methylation induced by 4-(methylnitrosamino)-1-(3-pyridyl)-1-butanone (NNK) on the metabolism and disposition of NNK in A/J mice. Cancer Res 2613–2617.

144. Pepin P, Rossignol G, Castonguay A. 1990. Inhibition of NNK-induced lung tumorigenesis in A/J mice by ellagic acid and butylated hydroxyanisole. Cancer J 3:266–273.

145. Wattenberg LW, Coccia JB. 1991. Inhibition of 4-(methylnitrosamino)-1-(3-pyridyl)-1-butanone carcinogenesis in mice by D-limonene and citrus fruit oils. Carcinogenesis 12:115–117.

146. Hong J-Y, Wang ZY, Smith TJ, Zhou S, Shi S, Pan J, Yang CS. 1992. Inhibitory effects of diallyl sulfide on the metabolism and tumorigenicity of the tobacco-specific carcinogen 4-(methylnitrosamino)-1-(3-pyridyl)-1-butanone (NNK) in A/J mouse lung. Carcinogenesis 13:901–904.

147. El-Bayoumy K, Upadhyaya P, Desai DH, Amin S, Hecht SS. 1993. Inhibition of 4-(methylnitrosamino)-1-(3-pyridyl)-1-butanone tumorigenicity in mouse lung by the synthetic organoselenium compound, 1,4-phenylenebis(methylene)seleno-cyanate. Carcinogenesis 14:1111–1113.

148. Hoffmann D, Rivenson A, Abbi R, Wynder EL. 1993. A study of tobacco carcinogenesis L. Effect of the fat content of the diet on the carcinogenic activity of 4-(methylnitrosamino)-1-(3-pyridyl)-butanone in F344 rats. Cancer Res 53:2758–2761.

149. Wynder EL, Hebert JR, Kabat GC. 1987. Association of dietary fat and lung cancer. J Natl Cancer Inst 79:631–637.

150. Hebert JR, Kabat GC. 1991. Distribution of smoking and its association with lung cancer: implications for studies on the association of fat with cancer. J Natl Cancer Inst 83:872–874.
151. Xie JX, Lesaffre E, Kasteloot H. 1991. The relationship between animal fat intake, cigarette smoking and lung cancer. Cancer Cause Control 2:79–83.
152. Goodman MF, Hankin JH, Wilkens LR, Kolonel LN. 1992. High-fat foods and the risk of lung cancer. Epidemiology 3:288–299.

2. Lung cancer chemoprevention

Ugo Pastorino

Introduction

Cancer chemoprevention is in a phase of extensive development, and the results achieved so far are particularly promising in the field of lung and upper aerodigestive tract carcinogenesis.

Of the clinical trials in this area, only a few have been concluded; the majority are ongoing on healthy subjects as well as on cancer patients. These trials are expected to provide substantial information about crucial aspects of chemoprevention: optimal selection of target populations, choice of preventive agent(s), dose and duration of treatment, and definition of specific endpoints. At the experimental level, it is essential to assess the nature and extent of biological effects on human carcinogenesis, in terms of reduction and/or delay of new primary tumors in the target field. At the clinical level, it is important to define the overall benefit of prevention measures — namely, an improvement of survival — having adjusted for competing factors such as tobacco smoking in the intervention phase, non-cancer morbidity and mortality, or recurrence of prior disease.

Biologic characterization of lung carcinogenesis has significantly improved as a consequence of chemoprevention research. A number of cytogenetic and molecular biology studies have been performed on the normal bronchial epithelium and the tumor specimens of patients undergoing pulmonary resection for single or multiple lung cancer, showing that specific and consistent genetic changes may be indentified in the various steps of aerodigestive tract carcinogenesis. Based on this finding, we have now the chance to design a new generation of small-scale clinical trials using genetic biomarkers to identify optimal candidates for specific chemoprevention programs, and also to monitor the results of intervention in the short and intermediate term.

Heine H. Hansen, (ed), Hansen: Lung Cancer.
© *1994 Kluwer Academic Publishers. ISBN 0-7923-2835-3. All rights reserved.*

Epidemiologic aspects

Primary versus pharmacological prevention

Widespread control of tobacco consumption and reduction of environmental exposure to known carcinogens remain the major goals for lung cancer prevention. Lung cancer incidence rates have been constantly declining in the United States and England since the mid-1970s, as a consequence of effective tobacco control achieved during the two prior decades. It has been estimated by the National Cancer Institue that approximately 800,000 tobacco-related deaths were either postponed or prevented by primary prevention measures between 1964 and 1985 [1]. Specific smoking cessation trials now involve a few million heavy smokers in the United States through the NCl Smoking, Tobacco, and Cancer Program (STCP), with a special emphasis on high-risk social or ethnic groups [2].

Nonetheless, even if further reductions in tobacco consumption take place in most Western countries, the overall lung cancer mortality will remain very high for many years to come.

A recent study on worldwide incidence rates has estimated a total of nearly 900,000 new cases of lung cancer in 1985 [3], with an overall increase of 36% from 1980 to 1985. Areas where incidence is declining (North America and northern Europe) account for only 25% of the total burden, while lung cancer incidence and tobacco epidemic are growing in the majority of developing countries. As an example, if the major Eastern countries were ever to reach the actual incidence rates of North America, China alone would provide over 500,000 new cases of lung cancer per year.

For these reasons, chemoprevention should never be considered a substitute for primary prevention, but only a potential complement. In fact, in subjects who have already quit smoking, reversal or antagonism of promotion and/or progression stages might help in reducing lung cancer mortality. In addition, biologic and clinical research related to chemoprevention may contribute to clarify some of the complex aspects of epithelial carcinogenesis and individual susceptibility to tobacco exposure, with ultimate benefits in the collateral fields of early diagnosis and adjuvant treatments.

Dietary factors in lung cancer

Based on the evidence of geographic and historical trends in cancer incidence, human epidemiologic studies have tried to correlate the risk of lung cancer with environmental factors other than tobacco consumption. Among these, dietary deficiency of vitamins, micronutrients, or specific foods has emerged as a potential modifier of lung cancer risk. Unlike other sites of disease, in lung cancer the epidemiologic data are quite consistent in favor of a protective effect of specific groups of substances. Table 1 summarizes the results of case–control or cohort studies on dietary intake of vitamin A-

44

Table 1. Case-control studies on dietary intake of vitamin A-related foods and subsequent-risk of lung cancer

Author	Cases	Dietary component	Relative Risk low vs high[a]	Ref.
Bjelke	36	Vitamin A	2.6	[4]
Mettlin	292	Vitamin A	1.5-1.7	[5]
Mc Lennan	233	Green vegetables	2.2	[6]
Gregor	104	Vitamin A	1.5-1.3	[7]
Hirayama	807	Green/yellow veg.	1.4	[8]
Shekelle	33	Beta-carotene	3.0-5.5-7.0	[9]
Kvale	153	Vitamin A	1.6	[10]
Hinds	261	Vitamin A	1.6-1.4-2.0	[11]
Ziegler	763	Beta-carotene	1.3	[12]
Samet	447	Vitamin A	1.1-1.4	[13]
Middleton	514	Vitamin A	1.5	[14]
Pisani	417	Carrots	1.8-2.0	[15]
Le Marchand	332	Beta-carotene	1.9	[16]

[a] For all given classes.

related foods and lung cancer risk. A relative deficiency in vitamin A or beta-carotene intake is associated with an average 1.5- to 2-fold increase in the risk of lung cancer [4-16]. The available studies on serum or plasma levels of the same substances are more controversial. The majority of papers reported a higher risk of lung cancer related to low beta-carotene levels in the blood, while most studies on blood retinol levels did not show a significantly lower value in lung cancer patients as compared to controls [17-29].

A protective effect against lung cancer has been hypothesized also for substances belonging to the group of antioxidants, such as selenium or vitamin E (alpha-tocopherol), both in terms of dietary consumption [23,25] and serum levels [18]. A recent epidemiologic study has shown that the risk of cancer of the oral cavity is reduced by approximately 50% in subjects taking supplemental vitamin E compared to those not taking the supplement, thus demonstrating for the first time a protective effect of dietary vitamin E supplementation [30].

Although the challenge of defining individual habits is somewhat frustrated by the low accuracy of dietary questionnaires, the epidemiological studies support the hypothesis that a different intake of common dietary components could modulate the risk of lung cancer [31].

Experimental chemoprevention

Experimental data provide a solid body of evidence on the feasibility of lung cancer chemoprevention [32,33]. They include nearly all the available systems for testing anticarcinogenic activity, in vitro and in vivo. Among the various substances with potential chemopreventive properties, the most deeply investigated agents are still retinol (vitamin A) and its synthetic derivatives, also called retinoids.

The experimental activity of retinoids has been summarized in a few extensive reviews, showing the wide spectrum of mechanisms of action that is peculiar to these substances [34,35].

Retinoids exert a strong regulatory effect upon the physiologic mechanisms of cell proliferation and differentiation [36–42]. Experimentally, they are able to inhibit malignant transformation [44–48] and suppress tumor promotion [49–52], particularly in the presence of indirect carcinogens, such as benzopyrene or methylcholantrene [53–56]. The antipromotion effect of retinoids is of great interest in human lung cancer chemoprevention due to their potential for interfering with the late stages of tumor progression. Under specific conditions, retinoids have shown a direct antineoplastic effect [57,58] as well as inhibition of sarcoma and epidermal growth factors [59,60]. Another potential mechanism of action is represented by the enhancement of immune response to cancer, both cell mediated [35,61] and antibody mediated [62,63].

The discovery of specific nuclear retinoic acid receptors (RARs) has dramatically increased our knowledge of the mechanisms of action of retinoids [64–67]. RARs belong to the superfamily of ligand-activated nuclear receptors for steroid and thyroid hormones. They are DNA-binding, transcription-modulating proteins, whose expression may be induced by retinoic acid administration [68–70]. Three subtypes of RARs have been identified: RARs-α, RAR-β, and RAR-γ. The RAR-α gene is located on chromosome 17q21, the RAR-β gene on chromosome 3p24, and the RAR-γ gene on chromosome 12q13 [71]. The concept of upregulation or downregulation of RARs may explain how retinoids can interfere with epithelial cell growth or inhibit progression of premalignant cells to cancer, and offers a rational basis for selection of receptor-specific retinoids in chemoprevention [72,73].

The other group of agents with a potentially strong protective effect is represented by antioxidants, including selenium, beta-carotene, alpha-tocopherol (vitamin E), and N-acetyl-cysteine. Antioxidants may inhibit the process of carcinogenesis at various steps: from metabolic inactivation or detoxification of chemical carcinogens to prevention of DNA damage by free-radical scavenging [74–77].

Dietary selenium has proven effective in preventing carcinogenesis in various animal models, including mammary gland, colon, skin, and lung [78,79].

Beta-carotene, a natural precursor of vitamin A, has also proven effective in experimental chemoprevention studies [80–83], although its activity may be explained by conversion into retinol. In fact, the specific antioxidant activity of beta-carotene and other carotenoids such as cathaxanthine has been unequivocally demonstrated only for UV-induced skin tumors in mice [81].

In recent years, a novel interest has arisen concerning N-acetyl-cysteine (NAC), an aminothiol and synthetic precursor of intracellular cysteine and glutathione (GSH), widely used in the past as a mucolytic drug and antidote against acetaminophen-induced hypatotoxicity [82]. Due to its nucleophilic and antioxidant properties, NAC has proven effective in decreasing the direct mutagenicity of several chemical compounds in the *Salmonella* test, inhibiting the mutagenicity of nitrosation products, and enhancing thiol concentration in intestinal bacteria [83,84]. At the nuclear level, NAC was able to inhibit the in vivo formation of carcinogen–DNA adducts, reduce carcinogen-induced DNA damage, and protect nuclear enzymes, such as poly(ADP-ribose) polymerase [85]. Of interest, benzo[a]pyrene diolepoxide (BPDE)–DNA adducts in rats exposed either to intratracheal benzo[a]pyrene or cigarette smoke were prevented by NAC not only in the lung but also in the heart and aorta, thus suggesting a protective effect against cardiovascular disease [86]. As for cancer chemoprevention, it has been demonstrated that NAC inhibits urethane-induced lung tumors in mice [87] and colon carcinogenesis with 1,2 dimethylhydrazine in rats [88].

Another distinct field of research concerns combination schedules for cancer chemoprevention [89]. Using the model of adenosquamous lung carcinoma induced in Syrian golden hamsters with N-nitrosodiethylamine (DEN), a carcinogen requiring metabolic activation, Moon has demonstrated that the combination of N-(4-hydroxyphenyl)retinamide (4-HPR) plus selenium (Se) plus α-tocopherol (vitamin E) was five times more effective in preventing lung cancer than any of these agent alone [90]. In the same system, retinol and beta-carotene were ineffective when administered alone, while their concurrent administration reduced the incidence of adenosquamous lung cancers as well as dysplasias. These data, although still preliminary, are promising for their practical implications for clinical chemoprevention.

Development of preventive agents

Natural Retinol

Natural retinol, or vitamin A, was made available for experimental testing and clinical practice over 50 years ago. The widespread interest in retinol as a modulator of cell growth was generated by its physiologic properties, which are evident from the very early phases of fetal development. In fact, in higher animals, vitamin A is essential for vision, reproduction, and maintenance of differentiated epithelia and mucus secretion [36,42]. In the field of lung carcinogenesis, one of the early observations demonstrated that bronchial metaplasia could be induced in the tracheal hamster epithelium by vitamin A deprivation or benzopyrene instillation, both being preventable by retinol administration [53].

Retinol, as well as other retinoids, has shown a definite clinical anticancer activity in different epithelial tumors, particularly in skin cancer. A number of published studies have demonstrated that these substances, whether administered topically or orally, can achieve a complete remission in a high proportion of patients with basal cell and advanced squamous cell carcinoma [33,49,91].

Unfortunately, most of the old studies were hardly interpretable because of methodological problems and insufficient quality of data. One particularly confusing aspect is that of side effects and toxicity of vitamin A. The longlasting concern about retinol toxicity, so common among the medical community, does not appear to be substantiated by clinical data. In nearly 50 years of clinical application in ophthalmology and dermatology, there were only a few cases of serious intoxication and no deaths attributable to the so-called hypervitaminosis A syndrome [92,93].

With natural retinol, a daily dose of 25,000 IU has been considered adequate for large-scale intervention trials on healthy individuals, where side effects must be absent or negligible. For adjuvant trials in cancer patients, a much higher dose (300,000 IU/day) can be selected, based on efficacy data derived from other diseases [94–97]. Among the different types of vitamin A, the emulsified retinol palmitate has shown optimal absorption properties and bioavailability, compared with the equivalent oily solution [98]. Data from two randomized clinical trials confirm the essential safety of emulsified retinol palmitate, given at high dose for a relatively long period of time (1–2 years) [99]. With this schedule, one should expect typical side effects, such as mucocutaneous dryness, desquamation, or cheilitis. Transient liver enlargement and rise of serum triglycerides are also frequently observed.

Synthetic retinoids

Starting from the late 1960s, industrial laboratories have made an enormous effort to produce synthetic analogues with higher, or more selective, activity and lower toxicity than natural vitamin A. In this research process, over 1500 new retinoids have been produced and biologically tested [100]. Two biological assays were used to test the different retinoids: the in vitro reversal of tracheal keratinization on hamsters raised on vitamin A-deficient diet, and in vivo ability to reverse skin papillomas in mice [52,101]. The results were analyzed by Bollag in terms of therapeutic index, that is, the ratio between dose causing hypervitaminosis A and dose causing anti-papilloma effects in mice.

Of the few compounds with high therapeutic index, only 13-*cis*-retinoic acid and etretinate ultimately entered medical practice to undergo thorough clinical investigation. Unfortunately, the toxicological profile in humans was less favorable than was anticipated from the animal data [102–104].

The results of randomized placebo-controlled trials conducted at the M.D. Anderson Cancer Center on patients with oral leukoplakia have proven beyond any doubt that 13-*cis*-retinoic acid is an effective drug. However, the degree of toxicity observed in these patients was substantial, and prevented long-term administration at full dosage [105]. As a matter of fact, natural retinol, with or without beta-carotene, is currently being used in most chemoprevention studies on healthy populations [106,107]. Another synthetic retinoid of potential interest for lung cancer prevention is N-(4-hydroxyphenyl) retinamide (4-HPR). The research on 4-HPR has been initially focused on breast cancer chemoprevention due the elective concentration of this compound in the mammary gland of treated animals [108], and its ability to inhibit chemically induced mammary carcinoma in rats [109]. Moreover, 4-HPR appeared to be safer than other retinoids with respect to genotoxicity [110].

On the basis of this experimental evidence, a large randomized clinical trial has been activated at the National Cancer Institute of Milan in 1987 on patients with resected breast cancer, with the aim of preventing a new primary cancer in the contralateral breast. This trial has confirmed the excellent tolerability of 4-HPR, given orally at the daily dose of 200 mg. The only concern, in terms of side effects, was related to lowered serum retinol levels [111] and impaired dark adaptation in a significant proportion of treated patients [112,113]. Although clinical data on the direct efficacy of 4-HPR against cancer or premalignant diseases are still lacking, a concurrent study conducted in the same institute on patients surgically treated for oral leukoplakia has shown a significant reduction in the incidence of new leukoplakia lesions [114].

Antioxidants

The experimental data accumulated in the last decade have boosted the interest in antioxidants as potential inhibitors of the early phases of lung carcinogenesis. Natural antioxidants, such as beta-carotene and alpha-tocopherol (vitamin E), are attractive for their tolerability and lack of clinical side effects (except for moderate yellowing of the skin). They are currently under testing in several large clinical trials being conducted in healthy populations; the results of these trials are expected in the coming years. Clinical data on the efficacy of beta-carotene are presently limited to the model of oral leukoplakia, where beta-carotene has shown better tolerability but lower activity than retinol or 13-*cis*-retinoic acid [115–117].

N-acetyl-cysteine (NAC) has been used for nearly 30 years as a mucolitic agent in the treatment of chronic obstructive pulmonary disease (COPD), and large randomized studies have demonstrated a significant reduction in the frequency of acute bronchitis, superimposed viral infections, and progression of pulmonary damage [118,119]. However, the distinct cytoprotective effect of NAC against several toxic agents goes far beyond the mucolitic activity. In fact, NAC given at high doses is the elective antidote for hepatorenal toxicity in acute acetaminophen (paracetamol) poisoning [120,121]. Such clinical experience, combined with the data on experimental cancer prevention, strongly supports a thorough investigation of NAC in phase III chemoprevention trials.

New preventive agents

In the United States, the National Cancer Institute (NCI) established in 1982 a comprehensive chemoprevention program aimed at identifying and testing the ability of specific dietary components and drugs to reduce human cancer incidence [107]. This program includes preclinical screening of new agents, assessment of efficacy and safety, and conduct of clinical trials in humans. Of the nearly 1000 substances with putative preventive activity, over 100 agents are now under investigation in vitro and in vivo, and a few of them are ready to be tested in phase II and III studies. Among this new generation of chemopreventive agents, a few appear promising for lung cancer chemoprevention purposes [122,123].

Oltipraz and other dithiolethiones are synthetic compounds initially reported as constituents of cruciferous vegetables and were widely used in the 1980s as antischistosomal drugs [124]. Collateral studies on their mechanisms of action demonstrated a strong antioxidant, radio and chemoprotective properties, and a significant inhibition of carcinogenesis at various sites, such as the lung, GI, liver kidney, and bladder [125–127]. Oltipraz appears to be protective against early induction phases of carcinogenesis, with definite exposure to known genotoxic procarcinogens such as cigarette smoking for upper aerodigestive tract tumors or aflatoxin B1 for hepatocellur carcinoma [128]. Initial experience with chronic administration of low doses of the drug has shown that major toxicity is represented by phototoxicity and heat intolerance occurring in a high proportion of cases [129]; however, further studies are in progress to assess the optimal dose and duration.

Difluoromethylornithine (DFMO), a specific inhibitor of ornithine decarboxylase (OCD), has been widely investigated for its chemopreventive potential related to polyamine depletion [130]. In fact, DFMO is a potent anticarcinogen in various animal models and sites such as skin, oral cavity, stomach, colon, bladder, and prostate [131–133]. Unfortunately, long-term use of DFMO causes significant ototoxicity both in animals and in humans, with a frequency of otogenic seizures exceeding 50% in animals treated with DFMO [134]. Dose de-escalating regimens (from 3 to 0.29/m2/day), as well as specific antidotes, are now under clinical testing [135].

Ellagic acid (EA) and phenethyl-isothiocyanates (PEITC) are truly natural dietary components present in various fruits, nuts, and cruciferous vegetables. Both EA and PEITC are 'blocking agents,' meaning that they induce enzyme detoxification and inhibit carcinogen activation [136]. EA also shows antioxidant and DNA scavenger properties. In vivo studies showed a strong inhibition of tumorigenesis in mouse lung and skin, as well as in rat esophagus [137–140].

An obvious question for future clinical trials is how to profit from the best of these new agents. In theoretical terms, the administration of various subtances with different mechanisms of action may represent a more effective approach to anticarcinogenesis. This concept of polychemoprevention is clearly supported by the experience of cancer chemotherapy. Simultaneous or sequential regimens are equally valid options to be tested. The final aim is to improve the efficacy and reduce the toxicity of chemoprevention programs.

Randomized clinical trials

Primary chemoprevention in healthy individuals

Primary lung cancer chemoprevention trials in healthy individuals are mainly based on epidemiologic and experimental data. These studies aim at interfering with the early phases of lung carcinogenesis by counteracting a hypothetical deficiency of putative protective agents, such as beta-carotene, retinol (vitamin A), or alpha-tocopherol (vitamin E). The target population is represented by otherwise healthy individuals at high risk of developing lung cancer because of previous heavy exposure to smoking, asbestos, or other carcinogens. The doses selected for preventive agents are relatively low in order to avoid significant side effects, to obtain high recruitment and compliance rates, and to allow a double-blind setting. A major concern is to reduce to the minimum the risk of harmful effects for the population under treatment and to guarantee a long-term tolerability of the intervention plan.

Table 2 summarizes the ongoing trials on lung cancer chemoprevention in high-risk individuals, funded by the National Cancer Institute [107]. The largest study is being conducted in cooperation with the National Public Health Institute of Finland to test the effects of oral administration of beta-carotene (20 mg/day) and alpha-tocopherol (vitamin E, 50 mg/day) in a population of heavy smokers with low expected intake of crucial micronutrients [141]. The study involves 29,000 men, aged 50 to 69, randomized with a 2×2 factorial design into four separate treatment groups, to receive either beta-carotene or vitamin E or both. The factorial design was selected to evaluate two intervention plans in a single large trial with a minimal increase in cost. The analysis of this trial is under way, and the results will be available by the end of 1993. The other large study is being conducted in the United States on 22,000 male physicians, ages 40 to 84, who are taking beta-carotene (50 mg/alternate days) or aspirin (325 mg/alternate days) to investigate a potential preventive effect against cancer incidence at any site

Table 2. Primary lung cancer chemoprevention trials supported by NCI

Investigator	Target	Agent	Dose	Size (pts)
Albanes (Finland)	Smokers 50–69 yr	Beta-carotene Vitamin E	20 mg/day 50 mg/day	29,000
Hennekens (Harvard)	Male physicians 40–84 yr	Beta-carotene Aspirin	50 mg/alt. days 325 mg/alt. days	22,000
Goodman (Seattle)	Smokers 50–69 yr	Beta-carotene Retinol	30 mg/day 25,000 IU/day	13,000
Omenn (Seattle)	Asbestos workers smokers, 45–69 yr	Beta-carotene Retinol	30 mg/day 25,000 IU/day	4,000
McLarty (Tyler)	Asbestos workers	Beta-carotene Retinol	50 mg/day 25,000 IU/alt. day	600

against or myocardial infarction [142]. In its aspirin branch, this trial has already demonstrated a significant reduction of myocardial infarction, but no difference in mortality. A new, similar trial, named the Women's Health Study, is expected to randomize 40,000 female nurses, aged 50 and older, to beta-carotene, vitamin E, and aspirin.

Treatment of precancerous lesions

A high level of interest and expectation for chemoprevention of pre-malignant lesions in the upper aerodigestive tract has been generated by the studies in oral leukoplakia. In the last decade, oral leukoplakia has represented the most reliable clinical model to test the direct efficacy of chemopreventive agents in the short term. In this field, the trials conducted at the M.D. Anderson Cancer Center are of fundamental importance because of the strict methodological criteria applied: randomized, double-blind setting, pathological assessment of pre-random status, and response to treatment. The first study demonstrated that 13-*cis*-retinoic acid (1–2 mg/kg daily/3 mos) could achieve major regression of leukoplakia in 67% of patients (vs. 10% for placebo), but relapse occurred in most cases soon after the end of treatment [105]. A further study of isotretinoin was then designed to overcome the problems of significant toxicity and high relapse rate. In this trial, patients received an induction treatment with high-dose isotretinoin (1.5 mg/kg per day) for a three-month induction period and were then randomized to a nine-month maintenance therapy with either low-dose isotretinoin (0.5 mg/kg/d) or beta-carotene (30 mg/d). This study showed that low-dose isotretinoin was more effective than beta-carotene in maintaining clinical/histological remission (relapse rate of 6% vs. 58%), thus demonstrating that low-dose isotretinoin was an effective and well-tolerated maintenance therapy for oral premalignancy [117]. A recent study has demonstrated that vitamin E is also effective against oral leukoplakia or dysplasia [143]. Of 43 evaluable patients treated with alpha-tocopherol (400 IU twice daily for 24 weeks), 20 (46%) had clinical responses and nine (21%) had histologic responses.

Based on the favorable results achieved in oral premalignancy, a new study was conducted at the M.D. Anderson Cancer Center on heavy-smoker volunteers with bronchial metaplasia. Eighty-seven chronic smokers with bronchial dysplasia and/or metaplasia greater than 15%, as assessed by multiple bronchoscopic biopsies (six sites), were randomized to either 13-*cis*-retinoic acid (1 mg/kg/day) or placebo. Bronchoscopic reevaluation at six months, available for 67 subjects, showed a similar decrease in the frequency of squamous metaplasia in both arms of the study (55 vs. 59%), being more pronounced in those who had stopped smoking [144]. This study, although negative in terms of efficacy of the applied treatment, has already provided substantial information on the natural history of bronchial metaplasia, which underlines the importance of properly controlled trials. On the other hand, the biologic and clinical significance of squamous metaplasia still needs to be clarified.

Prevention of second primary tumors

As a consequence of improved survival and accurate clinical evaluation and follow-up, achieved in modern clinical trials, second primary tumors have emerged as an important clinical entity in many diseases [145,146]. Multiple primary tumors may occur in the upper aerodigestive tract due to wide-spread exposure of this epithelium to common etiologic factors such as tobacco smoking and other environmental carcinogens. Dietary habits may also play a role as modifiers of the individual risk of cancer. This clinical evidence finds its biologic rationale in the concept of 'field cancerization,' which suggests that repeated exposure of the entire epithelial surface to carcinogenic insults may result in the occurrence of multiple, independent premalignant or malignant foci [147].

In patients cured for a cancer of the oral cavity, larynx, lung, esophagus, and bladder, the incidence of second primary tumors in all sites is 10% to 35%, depending on the site, histologic type, and stage of the index tumor, and corresponds to an incidence of 2% to 6% per year [148–150]. Second primary lung cancers account for a large proportion of these events, in the range of 8% to 20% overall [151–155]. In patients with a good initial prognosis, the occurrence of synchronous or metachronous tumors represents a significant cause of treatment failure. In fact, most of these second primary tumors occur in the lung and are often unresectable at the time of diagnosis.

Compared to healthy subjects, patients cured for a prior cancer show a higher motivation to accept the extra burden of a chemoprevention plan as an extension of long-term follow-up planned for their index tumor. Moreover, side effects are better tolerated, and higher doses can be given in order to achieve a potential adjuvant effect against primary cancer relapse.

For all the above reasons, patients curatively treated for a prior cancer of the upper aerodigestive tract are an ideal population to test the efficacy of chemopreventive agents (retinoids, vitamins, and antioxidants), either alone or in combination with other adjuvant treatments [32,33].

The pioneer study on chemoprevention of second primary tumors was conducted by Hong [156] on patients with squamous cell carcinoma of the head and neck. All patients had been previously treated with, therapy, or both, and were disease-free at study entry. After stratification by tumor site (oral cavity, oropharynx, hypopharynx, or larynx) and prior treatment (surgery, radiation, combined), patients were randomized to receive either isotretinoin (50 to 100 mg/m2/day) or placebo for 12 months. The study was closed in 1990, having enrolled a total of 103 cases. The endpoints of this study were recurrence of primary disease and development of second primary tumors. After a median follow-up of 32 months, the first analysis showed that retinoid treatment significantly reduced the incidence of second primary tumors [156]. Only two patients (4%) on the retinoid arm developed second primary tumors versus 12 patients (24%) on the placebo arm ($p = 0.005$). Most second primaries (13/14, 93%) occurred in the head and neck, esophagus, or lung. Treatment-related toxicity was significant, and 33% (16/49) of the isotretinoin patients could not complete the 12-month schedule. A recent updated analysis, with a 54-month median follow-up, confirmed the reduction in second primary tumors — 7 patients (14%) on the retinoid arm versus 16 patients (31%) on the placebo arm — but the difference was less striking ($p = 0.04$) [157].

This placebo-controlled and randomized trial remains a major breakthrough in human cancer chemoprevention research and a basis for future studies on head and neck and lung cancer patients. A concurrent study was conducted from 1985 to 1991 by a French cooperative group (GETEC): 323 patients with a cured (T1-2 N0-1) squamous cancer of the oral cavity and oropharynx were randomized to receive a synthetic retinoid (Etretinate, oral 25 mg daily, 24 months) or placebo. The endpoint of this study was total survival. The analysis of this trial has been performed recently, and formal publication is under way. Preliminary reports are negative in terms of efficacy: both survival and occurrence of second primary tumors are similar in the two arms [158].

The first randomized clinical trial on lung cancer patients began in 1985 at the National Cancer Institute of Milan. Patients with pathological stage 1 (T1–T2, N0, M0) non-small cell lung carcinoma after complete surgical resection were selected for this study. Patients were randomly assigned to either vitamin A treatment (oral 300,000 IU daily, 12 to 24 months) or control without treatment, stratified according to the center, cell type (squamous versus nonsquamous), and previous cancer at another site (absent versus cured). Endpoints of this study were relapse of prior cancer, occur-

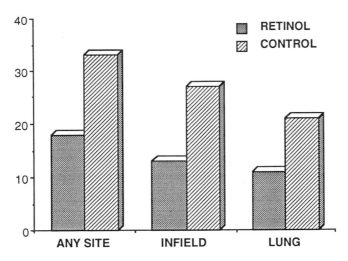

Figure 1. Results of the randomized trial on lung cancer chemoprevention, conducted at the National Cancer Institute of Milan. Distribution of second primary tumors by site: overall, in the chemoprevention field, and in the lung only.

rence of new primary cancers, and survival. The accrual was closed in 1989 with 307 evaluable patients, and the results of multivariate analysis, based on a 46-month median follow-up, have been recently published [159]. In summary, 56 pailients (37%) patients in the treated arm and 75 (48%) in the control arm developed either recurrence or new primary tumors. Eighteen patients (12%) developed a second primary tumor in the treated group, and 29 patients developed 33 (21%) second primary tumors in the control group. Figure 1 shows the distribution of second primary tumors by site. The time to relapse and/or new primary (disease-free interval) is illustrated in figure 2. The estimated disease-free proportion at five years was 64% vs. 51% in favor of the treatment arm; the difference was close to statistical significance ($p = 0.054$, Logrank test) and just significant when adjusted for primary tumor classification ($p = 0.038$, Cox regression model). A statistically significant difference in favor of treatment was observed with reference to time to new primaries in the field of prevention, i.e., tobacco-related tumors ($p = 0.045$, Logrank test). The estimated proportion free of new primary tumors in the field was 89% vs. 80%, respectively ($p = 0.045$, figure 3). In our trial, the absence of improvement in overall survival may be partially due to noncancer mortality (identical in the two arms), as well as to salvage treatment. In fact, salvage surgery for new primary tumors was applied to 44% of cases (8 of 18) in the retinol arm and 69% in the control arm (20 of 29). As for second primary lung cancer, the excess of cases observed in the control arm was somewhat balanced by the high frequency of salvage resection (figure 4), while the number of unresectable cases was similar in the two arms.

55

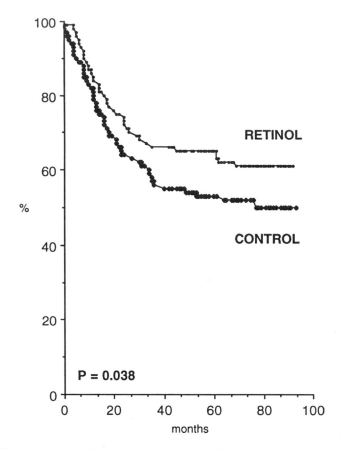

Figure 2. Time to relapse and/or new primary cancer (disease-free interval) in the Milan trial. Results of multivariate analysis with Cox regression model ($p = 0.038$).

In terms of toxicity and side effects, high-dose vitamin A has proved to be a relatively safe treatment, well tolerated for a period of one to two years, with an overall compliance rate of nearly 80%.

In conclusion, this study has demonstrated that high-dose vitamin A is effective in reducing the number of new primary malignancies related to tobacco consumption and may improve the disease-free interval in patients curatively resected for stage I lung cancer. The impact of such a treatment on survival needs to be further explored.

Based on the experience accumulated in the first lung cancer trial, a new European cooperative study was set up in 1988 as a joint venture of the EORTC Lung Cancer and Head and Neck Cancer Cooperative Groups [160] in order to test the combination of two agents with different preventive properties: retinol palmitate and n-acetyl-cysteine (NAC). EUROSCAN was aimed at preventing second primary tumors in patients treated for upper

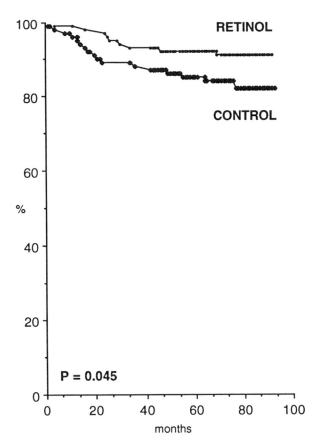

Figure 3. Time to new primaries in the field of prevention, i.e., tobacco-related tumors, in the Milan trial ($p = 0.045$).

aerodigestive cancer. Eligible patients were those previously treated for squamous cancer of the larynx (Tis, T1-2-3, N0-1), squamous cancer of the oral cavity (T1-2, N0-1), or non-small cell lung cancer (pT1-2, N0-1 and T3 NO). Four treatment arms were planned in a 2 × 2 factorial design, to increase efficiency and power: 1) retinol palmitate and NAC, 2) retinol palmitate, 3) NAC, and 4) no treatment. Randomization has taken place after surgery and/or completion of radiotherapy, without any fixed limit of time. Stratification has been by sex, prior or concurrent chemotherapy, squamous versus nonsquamous histology (lung cancer), supraglottic or glottic location of laryngeal cancer, and smokers versus never smokers. Retinol palmitate was administered at the daily oral dose of 300,000 IU for the first 12 months, followed by 150,000 IU for 12 additional months. NAC was administered at the daily dose of 600 mg for two years. Minimal follow-up included physical examination every three months and chest x-ray every six

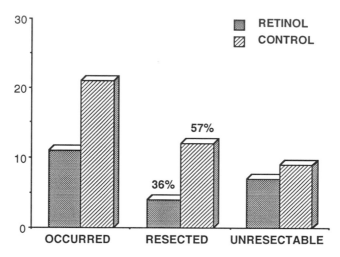

Figure 4. Second primary lung cancers in the Milan trial. Total number of cases, cases which underwent salvage resection, and unresectable cases in the two arms.

months. Endpoints of this study are relapse of prior cancer, occurrence of new primary cancers, and survival. By April 1993, all 2000 planned patients had entered the trial, but it was decided to prolong the accrual up to 2500 patients. The different mechanisms of action of the two agents, the large population, and the various types of disease selected increase the chances of success of this clinical trial, which is expected to go on for at least ten years.

The interest generated by the above trials has convinced the main American cooperative groups to engage in the field of second primary tumor prevention, and two large studies started in 1992 [161]. The first is promoted by the Radiation Therapy Oncology Group (RTOG) in conjunction with the Community Clinical Oncology Program (CCOP) and the M.D. Anderson Cancer Center on patients with stage I and II head and neck cancer. The second is promoted by the U.S. Intergroup on resected stage I non-small cell lung carcinoma. Each trial should enter over 600 patients, to be treated with oral 13-*cis*-retinoic acid at the dose of 30 mg/day.

Biologic selection of high-risk individuals

In the choice of target populations for prevention trials, the epidemiologic selection of high-risk individuals (i.e., heavy smokers) has the obvious counterpart of huge sample sizes and extremely long periods of follow-up. Clinical selection of patients cured of a prior cancer has slightly improved the performance of chemoprevention trials, but the power of detecting significant differences is reduced by overwhelming factors such as primary cancer relapse, comorbidity, and misclassification of ultimate endpoints.

Biologic definition of high-risk subjects is currently one of the crucial aspects in the development of chemoprevention research. In fact, to increase the cost–benefit ratio of intervention plans, specific subpopulations of very high-risk individuals should be identified for each type of cancer on the basis of constitutive or acquired abnormalities detectable in the target tissues. New cytogenetic and molecular biology techniques are very effective tools to detect early changes, associated with a specific risk of cancer, in target tissues such as tracheobronchial epithelium.

Multiple cytogenetic abnormalities have been described in lung cancer, particularly deletions in the short arm of chromosomes 1, 3, 7, 8, 9, 11, and 17 [162–167]. The frequency of rearrangements in each chromosome is somewhat different according to the type and source of biological samples (cell lines vs. short-term cultures, primary tumor vs. distant metastases), but some changes (3p, 17p) are quite consistent in the various studies. Oncogene amplification and/or overexpression is detectable in a high proportion of cases, particularly involving erbB1 (EGFR) in squamous carcinoma [165, 168–171]. K-ras and erbB2 (neu) in adenocarcinoma [172–179] and myc in small cell carcinoma [180–183]. Deletion, mutation, or altered expression of tumor suppressor genes represent the other important markers of genetic damage, mainly involving rb1 in small cell carcinoma [184,185], RARβ in non-small cell carcinoma [186–189], and tp53 in all types [190–197]. Such genetic changes have shown a correlation with tumor stage and patient survival, thus making biological markers a potential, independent prognostic factor in lung cancer [171,198,199].

What is of peculiar interest for chemoprevention purposes is the fact that significant genetic changes may be detectable, with various degrees of severity, in bronchial dysplasia as well as in pathologically normal mucosa [200,201]. A recent report of our experience, conducted on 65 cases of lung cancer resected in an early stage, has shown that the normal bronchial epithelium, collected at distant sites from the primary tumor, bears multiple genetic abnormalities [202]. As illustrated in table 3, a rearranged karyotype was detected in 20% of the evaluable cases, overexpression of EGFR in 39%, and her2/neu in 14%, while the overall frequency of genetic changes of any type in the normal epithelium was 46% (30/65).

The occurrence of genetic changes in the normal bronchial mucosa was associated with various clinical and pathologic features of the patients (table 4). For instance, overexpression of her2/neu was significantly higher in patients with adenocarcinoma ($p=0.0048$), suggesting that her2/neu overexpression is an early and specific marker in these patients. Moreover, patients with multiple tumors of the upper aerodigestive tract, either synchronous or metachronous, showed a much higher frequency of genetic changes as compared to those with single or multiple tumors in other sites (60% vs. 32%, $p=0.019$). These data indicate that specific genetic abnormalities may be detectable in the various stages of lung tumorigenesis, in a sequence of events that goes from normal epithelium to bronchial metaplasia

Table 3. Genetic changes in normal bronchial samples of lung cancer patients

Abnormality	N. evaluable	N. positive	%
Cytogenetic (any)	63	13	20
chr 3p		6	
chr 7p		6	
chr 17		3	
EGFR	51	20	39
HER2/NEU	51	7	14
Any changes	65	30	46

Modified from [202].

Table 4. Frequency of genetic changes in normal bronchial mucosa according to selected clinical features (% of positive)

Abnormality	Histologic type		Multiple tumors		Follow-up	
	Squamous	Adeno	Yes	No	Ned	Rec
Cytogenetic (any)	26	17	28	15	13	40[a]
3p	9	13	18	3	10	10
EGFR	43	40	56	33	37	67
HER2/NEU	0	30[a]	28	5[a]	20	0
Any changes	34	56	60	32[a]	38	67

[a] $p < 0.05$.
Ned = no evidence of disease; Rec = lung cancer recurrence.

and dysplasia, carcinoma in situ, and early-stage invasive cancer, as well as locally advanced and metastatic lung cancer (table 5).

In practical terms, it is conceivable that a panel of specific markers, including chromosome deletions (3p, 7p, 17), p53 staining, and EGFR and *neu* amplification, will be used to select future candidates for chemoprevention programs. In fact, with the actual development of immonostaining techniques for fresh and paraffin-embedded tissues, fluorescence in situ hybridization (FISH), and PCR for selective chromosome testing, even small samples collected through bronchoscopic biopsies, brushing, or sputum cytology will become suitable for the screening of high-risk individuals.

Endpoints in lung cancer chemoprevention

There is little doubt that the ultimate goal of prevention trials is the improvement of long-term survival. Nonetheless, due to the enormous re-

Table 5. Sequence of genetic events in lung carcinogenesis

Pathologic status	Chromosomal changes (%)	p53 immunostaining	p53 molecular
Normal mucosa	Simple rearrangements (20%) (3p, 7, 11, 17)	Negative	Negative
Bronchial metaplasia		Spots only	Undetectable
Bronchial dysplasia	Same + 17p mutations	Positive	Mutations
In situ carcinoma		Positive	Mutations
Early invasive cancer	Complex karyotypes (60%) (3p, 7, 8, 9, 11, 17, HSR/DMs)	Extensively positive	Mutations
Metastatic cancer	More complex karyotypes (100%)	Extensively positive	Mutations

sources and time needed to demonstrate a survival benefit, overall survival is not the ideal endpoint to answer practical questions such as optimal agent selection, dose and duration of treatment, latency, and maintenance of the biological effect.

As already pointed out, even in the favorable case of significant reductions in the occurrence of new primary tumors, survival may not be improved, as a consequence of comorbidity, noncancer mortality, and effective salvage surgery applied to incident cancers, particularly in the context of well-conducted clinical trials.

New primary tumors are the main endpoint for chemoprevention trials, but stricter criteria should be defined with respect to target sites and differential diagnosis. From our point of view, only tumors occurring in the target field of chemoprevention should be considered as relevant endpoints. For upper aerodigestive tract tumors, this concept applies to tobacco-related cancers (oral cavity, pharynx, larynx, lung, esophagus, and bladder), or in other words those neoplastic events occurring as a consequence of the field cancerization process. For instance, there is no reason to consider leukemias, sarcomas, or cancer of the stomach, colon, or even skin as failures of this chemoprevention program.

In patients cured of a prior cancer in the same area, the differential diagnosis between recurrence and second primary tumor has been based in the past on site (distance from prior cancer), histologic type (same vs. different), and temporal sequence (time elapsed from prior cancer). All the above criteria were affected by individual cultural biases and poor specificity of standard histopathology and have proven unreliable whenever confronted with modern diagnostic tools.

A recent study testing p53 gene mutations in 31 primary head and neck cancers and the corresponding second primary cancers of the upper aerodigestive tract, has demonstrated one or more mutations in 21 of 31 cases [203]. All the p53 mutations observed in the initial tumor were different

Table 6. Intermediate biomarkers in lung cancer chemoprevention

Genetic markers	Micronuclei
	Ploidy and DNA content
	Chromosome deletions/translocations
	Oncogene activation
Differentiation markers	Squamous markers (keratins, involucrin)
	Blood group antigens
Proliferation markers	Proliferating Cell Nuclear Antigen (PCNA)
	Thymidine Labeling Index
	Retinoic Acid Receptors (RARs)
	Epidermal Growth Factor Receptor (EGFR)
	Transforming Growth Factor-β (TGF-β)

from those of the second or third primary cancer, in terms of presence or specific codon location. This study not only supported the concept that second cancers arise as independent events but also provided evidence that p53 mutation is an effective test for differential diagnosis of multiple primary tumors. Our recent experience has confirmed this observation in lung cancer patients. In a series of cases of multiple synchronous lung cancers, resected with a single operation, we found a different pattern of genetic abnormalities in the two neoplastic foci. The observed discordance involved at least one of the following markers: 3p deletion, loss of heterozygosity (LOH 3p), p53 mutation, and K-*ras* mutation. These data are particularly remarkable since they were obtained in synchronous tumors showing the same histology and occurring in the same pulmonary lobe.

The identification of appropriate intermediate endpoints in another crucial aspect of lung cancer chemoprevention research. Biologic intermediate endpoints will became essential in the near future to monitor the efficacy of preventive strategies, before the actual occurrence of invasive cancer [204]. In order to justify systematic application, intermediate endpoints need to be 1) specific for the process of carcinogenesis under study, 2) quantitatively or qualitatively correlated with the degree of progression, 3) easily measurable on small specimens and tolerable by the subject at repeated intervals, and 4) potentially modulated by the selected preventive agent.

Potential intermediate biomarkers that are under investigation may be grouped into three categories: genetic markers, differentiation markers, and proliferation markers (table 6).

The micronuclei count in exfoliated epithelial cells is the easiest quantitative test of nonspecific DNA damage. In oral leukoplakia, it has been demonstrated that the frequency of micronuclei varies according to the extent of carcinogenic exposure and may be reduced by chemopreventive agents [205]. This marker is now under evaluation in heavy smokers with bronchial metaplasia [206].

Other nonspecific morphologic features, obtained by flow cytometry analysis of the exfoliated epithelium, have been suggested as potential biomarkers of bronchial carcinogenesis. They include quantitative assessment of DNA content, nuclear/cytoplasmic ratio, abnormal DNA profile, and/or aneuploidy. However, a clear relationship to the risk of lung cancer still has to be proven.

As discussed previously, a number of specific genetic changes can be detected in the primary tumor specimen as well as in the microscopically normal bronchial epithelium of patients with early-stage lung cancer. Given the fact that typical deletions, translocations, or polysomies occur with high frequency on specific chromosomes, these sites may now be investigated with the technique of in situ hybridization on tissue blocks, or small bronchial biopsies, without the need for short-term cultures.

At the level of molecular biology, the activation of dominant oncogenes (*myc*, *ras*, *egfr*, *neu*), and inhibition of tumor suppressor genes (*rb*1, p53, RAR-β) on the same target tissues, may represent specific intermediate endpoints in future chemoprevention trials.

Prognostic data on blood group antigens [207], and expression of other tumor-related carbohydrate markers, have increased the interest for monoclonal antibodies in the screening of intermediate biomarkers.

Proliferating Cell Nuclear Antigen (PCNA) is a intranuclear protein related to DNA polymerase-δ that dramatically increases during the S phase of the cell cycle. Antibodies against PCNA work very well on formalin-fixed, paraffin-embedded samples and are then suitable for large-scale retrospective analysis. In premalignant lesions of bronchial epithelium, a remarkable correlation has been found between the frequency of PCNA-positive cells and the degree of histological progression from normal epithelium to squamous metaplasia and dysplasia [204].

Measurement of retinoic acid receptors (RARs) in normal target tissues and premalignant lesions represents another promising way to predict and monitor the efficacy of chemoprevention with retinoids. In fact, since the expression of RARs can be experimentally induced by retinoids, receptor analysis before and during chemoprevention might be used as specific intermediate marker of response to treatment.

Conclusion

In the future of lung cancer research, chemoprevention will hopefully share a larger amount of energy and financial resources. The continuous development of molecular biology and cytogenetics has provided clinicians with extremely powerful techniques to identify high-risk individuals, detect precancerous or noninvasive lesions in the target field, and monitor the results of intervention.

A panel of new preventive agents are ready to be tested in optimal combination schedules, with the aim of counteracting each of the different stages of lung carcinogenesis. From this point of view, it appears justified to incorporate chemopreventive agents in randomized trials testing new adjuvant strategies as well as multimodality treatments.

Through the open window of biology-oriented chemoprevention, rather than morphology-oriented therapy, we can look at the whole problem of lung cancer management with a new perspective.

References

1. National Cancer Institute. Smoking, Tobacco, and Cancer Program 1985–89 Status Report. U.S. Department of Health and Human Services, PHS NIH Publication No. 90-3107.
2. Greenwald P, Stern HR. 1992. Role of biology and prevention in aerodigestive tract cancers. J Natl Cancer Inst Monogr 13:3–14.
3. Parkin DM, Pisani P, Ferlay J. 1993. Estimates of the worldwide incidence of eighteen major cancers in 1985. Int J Cancer 54:594–605.
4. Bjelke E. 1975. Dietary vitamin A and human lung cancer. Int J Cancer 15:561–565.
5. Mettlin C, Saxon G, Swanson M. 1979. Vitamin and lung cancer. J Natl Cancer Inst 62:1435–1438.
6. MacLennan R, Da Costa J, Day NE, Law CH, Ng YK, Shanmugaratnam K. 1977. Risk factors for lung cancer in Singapore Chinese, a population with high female incidence rates. Int J Cancer 20:854–860.
7. Gregor A, Lee PN, Roe FJC, Wilson MJ, Melton A. 1980. Comparison of dietary histories in lung cancer cases and controls with special reference to vitamin A. Nutr Cancer 2:93–97.
8. Hirayama T. 1979. Diet and cancer. Nutr Cancer 1:67–80.
9. Shekelle RB, Lepper M, Liu S, Maliza C, Raynor WJ, et al. 1981. Dietary vitamin A and risk of cancer in the western electric study. Lancet 2:1185–1189.
10. Kvale G, Bjelke E, Gart JJ. 1983. Dietary habits and lung cancer. Int J Cancer 31:397–405.
11. Hinds MW, Kolonel LN, Hankin JH, Lee J. 1984. Dietary vitamin A, carotene, vitamin C and risk of lung cancer in Hawaii. Am J Epidemiol 119:227–236.
12. Ziegler RG, Mason TJ, Stemhagen A, Hoover R, Schoenberg JB, et al. 1984. Dietary carotene and vitamin A and risk of lung cancer among white men in New Jersey. J Natl Cancer Inst 73:1429–1435.
13. Samet JM, Skipper BJ, Humble CG, Pathak DR. 1985. Lung cancer risk and vitamin A consumption in New Mexico. Am Rev Respir Dis 131:198–202.
14. Middleton B, Byers T, Marshall J, Graham S. 1986. Dietary vitamin A and cancer — a multisite case-control study. Nutr Cancer 8:107–116.
15. Pisani P, Berrino F, Macaluso M, Pastorino U, Crosignani P. 1986. Carrots, green vegetables and lung cancer: a case-control study. Int J Epidemiol 15:463–468.
16. Le Marchand L, Yoshizawa CN, Kolonel LN, Hankin JH, Goodman MT. 1989. Vegetable consumption and lung cancer risk: a population-based case-control study in Hawaii. J Natl Cancer Inst 81:1158–1164.
17. Basu TK, Donaldson D, Jenner M, Williams DC, Sakula A. 1976. Plasma vitamin A in patients with bronchial carcinoma. Br J Cancer 33:119–121.
18. Atukorala S, Basu TK, Dickerson JVT, Donaldson D, Sakula A. 1979. Vitamin A, zinc and lung cancer. Br J Cancer 40:927–931.
19. Wald N, Idle M, Boreham J, Bailey A. 1980. Low serum-vitamin A and subsequent risk of cancer: preliminary results of a prospective study. Lancet 2:813–816.

20. Kark J, Smith AH, Switzer BR, Hames CG. 1981. Serum vitamin A (retinol) and cancer incidence in Evans County, Georgia. J Natl Cancer Inst 66:7–15.
21. Peleg I, Heyden S, Knowles M, Hames CG. 1984. Serum retinol and risk of subsequent cancer: extension of the Evans County, Georgia, study. J Natl Cancer Inst 73:1455–1458.
22. Willett WC, Frank Polk B, Underwood BA, Stampfer MJ, Pressel S, Rosner B, Taylor JO, Schneider K, Hames G. 1984. Relations of serum vitamins A and E and carotenoids to the risk of cancer. N Engl J Med 310:430–434.
23. Stahelin HB, Rosel F, Buess E, Brubacher G. 1984. Cancer, vitamins and plasma lipids: prospective Basel study. J Natl Cancer Inst 73:1463–1468.
24. Salonen T, Salonen R, Lappetelainen R, Maenpaa P, Alfthan G, Puska P. 1985. Risk of cancer in relation to serum concentrations of selenium and vitamins A and E: matched case–control analysis of prospective data. Br Med J 290:417–420.
25. Nomura AM, Stemmermann GN, Heilbrun LK, Salked RM, Vuilleumier JP. 1985. Serum vitamin levels and risk of cancer of specific sites in men of Japanese ancestry in Hawaii. Cancer Res 45:2369–2372.
26. Friedman GD, Blaner WS, Goodman DS. 1986. Serum retinol and retinol binding protein levels do not predict subsequent lung cancer. Am J Epidemiol 123:781–789.
27. Menkes MS, Comstock GV, Vuilleumier JP, Helsing KJ, Rider AA, Brookmeyer R. 1986. Serum beta-carotene, vitamins A and E, selenium, and the risk of lung cancer. N Engl J Med 315:1250–1254.
28. Connett JE, Kuller LH, Kjelsberg MO, Polk BF, Collins G, Rider A, Hulley SB. 1989. Relationship between carotenoids and cancer. The Multiple Risk Factor Intervention Trial (MRFIT) Study. Cancer 64:126–134.
29. Kune GA, Kune S, Watson LF, Pierce R, Field B, Vitetta L, Merenstein D, Hayes A, Irving L. 1989. Serum levels of beta-carotene, vitamin A, and zinc in male lung cancer cases and controls. Nutr Cancer 12:169–176.
30. Gridley G, McLaughlin JK, Block G, Blot WJ, Gluch M, Fraumeni JF. 1992. Vitamin supplement use and reduced risk of oral and pharyngeal cancer. Am J Epidemiol 135:1083–1092.
31. Block G, Patterson B, Subar A. 1992. Fruit, vegetables and cancer prevention: a review of the epidemiologic evidence. Nutr Cancer 18:1–29.
32. Bertram JS, Kolonel LN, Meyskens FL. 1987. Rationale and strategies for chemoprevention of cancer in humans. Cancer Res 47:3012–3031.
33. Lippman SM, Kessler JF, Meyskens FL. 1987. Retinoids as preventive and therapeutic anticancer agents (part II). Cancer Treat Rep 71:493–515.
34. Sporn MB, Newton NL. 1979. Chemoprevention of cancer with retinoids. Fed Proc 38:2528–2534.
35. Lotan R. 1980. Effects of vitamin A and its analogs (retinoids) on normal and neoplastic cells. Biochim Biophys Acta 605:33–91.
36. Wolbach SB, Howe PR. 1925. Tissue changes following deprivation of fat soluble A vitamin. J Exp Med 42:753–777.
37. Dowling JE, Wald J. 1960. The biological function of vitamin A acid. Proc Natl Acad Sci USA 46:587–608.
38. Thompson JN, Howell JM, Pitt GAJ. 1964. Vitamin A and reproduction in rats. Proc R Soc Lond 159:510–535.
39. Wong YC, Buck RC. 1971. An electron microscopic study of metaplasia of the rat tracheal epithelium in vitamin A deficiency. Lab Invest 24:55–56.
40. Elias PM, Fritsch P, Lampe MA, Williams ML, Nemanic MK, Grayson S. 1980. Effects of systemic retinoids on epidermal barrier function, proliferation, structure and glycosylation. Clin Res 28:248–253.
41. Moon RC, Mc Cormick DL, Mehta RG. 1983. Inhibition of carcinogenesis by retinoids. Cancer Res 43:2469–2475.
42. Goodman DS. 1984. Vitamin A and retinoids in health and disease. N Engl J Med 310:1023–1031.

43. Jetten AM, Nervi C, Vollberg TM. Control of squamous differentiation in tracheo-bronchial and epidermal epithelial cells: role of retinoids. J Natl Cancer Inst Monogr 13:93–100.

44. Chu EW, Malmgen RA. 1965. An inhibitory effect of vitamin A on the introduction of tumors of forestomach and cervix in the Syrian hamster by carcinogenic policyclic hydro-carbons. Cancer Res 25:884–895.

45. Bollag W. 1972. Prophylaxis of chemically induced benign and malignant epithelial tumors by vitamin A acid (retinoic acid). Eur J Cancer 8:689–693.

46. Nettesheim P, Williams PL. 1976. The influence of vitamin A on the susceptibility of the rat lung to 3-methylcholantrene. Int J Cancer 17:351–357.

47. Sporn MB, Squire RA, Brown CC, Smith GM, Wenk ML, Springer S. 1977. 13-cis-retinoic acid: inhibition of bladder carcinogenesis in the rat. Science 195:487–489.

48. Chopra DP, Wilkoff LJ. 1977. Beta-retinoic acid inhibits and reverses testosterone induced hyperplasia in mouse prostate organ cultures. Nature 265:339–341.

49. Bollag W. 1971. Therapy of chemically induced skin tumour of mice with vitamin A palmitate and vitamin A acid. Experientia 27:90–92.

50. Bollag W. 1975. Prophylaxis of chemically induced epithelial tumors with an aromatic retinoic acid analog. Eur J Cancer 11:721–724.

51. Lotan R, Giotta G, Nork E, Nicolson GL. 1978. Characterization of the inhibitory effects of retinoids on the vitro growth of two malignant murine melanomas. J Natl Cancer Inst 60:1935–1041.

52. Verma AK, Rice HM, Shapas BG, Boutwell RK. 1978. Inhibition of 13-tetradecanoyl-phorbol-13 acetate induced ornithine decarboxylase activity in mouse epidermis by vitamin A analogs (retinoids). Cancer Res 38:793–801.

53. Saffiotti U, Montesano R, Sellakumar AR, Bork SA. 1967. Experimental cancer of the lung, inhibition by vitamin A of the induction of tracheobronchial metaplasia and squamous cell tumor. Cancer 20:857–864.

54. Cone MV, Nettesheim P. 1973. Effects of vitamin A on 3-methylcholanthrene-induced squamous metaplasias and early tumors in the respiratory tract of rats. J Natl Cancer Inst 50:1599–1606.

55. Port CD, Sporn MB, Kauffmann DG. 1975. Prevention of lung cancer in hamsters by 13-cis retinoic acid. Proc Am Assoc Cancer Res 16:21.

56. Smith DM, Rogers AE, Newberne PM. 1975. Vitamin A and benzopyrene carcinogenesis in the respiratory tract of hamsters fed a semisynthetic diet. Cancer Res 35:1485–1488.

57. Trown PW, Buck MJ, Hansen R. 1976. Inhibition of growth and regression of a trans-plantable rat chrondrosarcoma by three retinoids. Cancer Treat Rep 60:1647–1653.

58. Lotan R. 1979. Different susceptibilities of human melanoma and breat carcinoma cell lines to retinoic acid-induced growth inhibition. Cancer Res 39:1014–1019.

59. Todaro GJ, DeLarco JE, Sporn MB. 1978. Retinoid blocks phenotypic cell transformation produced by sarcoma growth factor. Nature 276:272–278.

60. Gensler HL, Matrisian LM, Bowden GT. 1985. Effect of retinoic acid on the late-stage promotion of transformation in JB6 mouse epidermal cells in culture. Cancer Res 45:1922–1925.

61. Tachibana K, Sone S, Tsubura E, Kishino Y. 1984. Stimulatory effect of vitamin A on tumoricidal activity of rat alveolar macrophages. Br J Cancer 49:343–348.

62. Floersheim GL, Bollag W. 1972. Accelerated rejection of skin homografts by vitamin A acid. Transplantation 14:564–567.

63. Dennert G. 1985. Immunostimulation by retinoic acid. In Retinoids, Differentiation and Disease (Ciba Foundation Symposium 113). Pitman: London, pp. 117–131.

64. Evans RM. 1988. The steroid and thyroid hormone receptor superfamily. Science 240:889–895.

65. Parker MG. 1990. Structure and function of nuclear hormone receptors. Semin Cancer Biol 1:81–87.

66. Lotan R, Clifford JL. 1990. Nuclear receptors for retinoids: mediators of retinoid effects on normal and malignant cells. Biomed Pharmacother 45:145–156.
67. Leid M, Kastner P, Chambon P. 1992. Multiplicity generates diversity in the retinoic acid signalling pathways. Trends Biochem Sci 17:427–433.
68. de The H, Marchio A, Tiollais P, Dejean A. 1989. Differential expression and ligand regulation of the retinoic acid receptor a and b genes. EMBO J 8:429–433.
69. Hu L, Gudas LJ. 1990. Cyclic AMP analogs and retinoic acid influence the expression of retinoic acid receptor a, b, and g mRNAs in F9 teratocarcinoma cells. Mol Cell Biol 10:391–396.
70. Clifford J, Petkovich M, Chambon P, Lotan R. 1990. Modulation by retinoids of mRNA levels for nuclear retinoic acid receptors in murine melanoma cells. Mol Endocrinol 4:1546–1555.
71. Mattei MG, Riviere M, Krust A, Ingvarsson S, Vennstrom B, Islam MQ, Levan G, Kautner P, Zelent A, Chambon P, Szpirer J, Szpirer C. 1991. Chromosomal assignment of retinoic acid receptor (RAR) genes in the human, mouse, and rat genomes. Genomics 10:1061–1069.
72. de The H, Vivanco-Ruiz MdM, Tiollais P, Stunnenberg H, Dejean A. 1990. Identification of a retinoic acid responsive element in the retinoic acid receptor β gene. Nature 343:177–180.
73. Lehman JM, Dawson MI, Hobbs PD, Husmann M, Pfahl M. 1991. Identification of retinoids with nuclear receptor subtype-selective activities. Cancer Res 51:4804–4809.
74. De Flora S, Ramel C. 1988. Mechanisms of inhibitors of mutagenesis and carcinogenesis. Classification and overview. Mutat Res 202:285–306.
75. Shamberger RJ. 1976. Relationship of selenium to cancer. I. Inhibitory effect of selenium on carcinogenesis. J Natl Cancer Inst 44:931–936.
76. Horvath PM, Hip C. 1983. Synergistic effect of vitamin E and selenium on the chemoprevention of mammary carcinogenesis in rats. Cancer Res 43:5335–5341.
77. Cerutti PA. 1985. Prooxidant states and tumor promotion. Science 227:375–381.
78. Birt DF, Lawson TA, Julius AD, Runice CE, Salmasi S. 1982. Inhibition by dietary selenium of colon cancer induced in the rat by bis(20xopropyl)nitrosamine. Cancer Res 42:4455–4459.
79. Ip C. 1981. Prophylaxis of mammary neoplasia by selenium supplementation in the initiation and promotion phases of chemical carcinogenesis. Cancer Res 41:4386–4390.
80. Epstein JH. 1977. Effects of beta-carotene on ultraviolet induced cancer formation in the hairless mouse skin. Photochem Photobiol 25:211–213.
81. Mathews-Roth MM. 1982. Antitumor activity of beta-carotene, cathaxanthin and phytoene. Oncology 39:33–37.
82. Rettura G, Stratford F, Levenson SM, Seifter E. 1982. Prophylactic and therapeutic actions of supplemental beta-carotene in mice inoculated with CH3BA adenocarcinoma cells: lack of therapeutic action of supplemental ascorbic acid. J Natl Cancer Inst 69:73–77.
83. Som S, Chatterjee M, Banerjee MR. 1984. Beta-carotene inhibition of 7,12-dimethyl-benzanthracene-induced transformation of murine mammary cells in vitro. Carcinogenesis 5:937–940.
82. De Flora S, Izzotti A, D'Agostini F, Balansky R, Cesarone CF. 1992. Chemopreventive properties of N-acetylcysteine and other thiols. *In* Cancer Chemoprevention, L Wattenberg, M Lipkin, CW Boone, and GJ Kelloff (eds.). CRC Press: Boca Raton, FL, pp. 183–194.
83. De Flora S, Bennicelli C, Camoirano A, Serra D, Romano M, Rossi GA, Morelli A, De Flora A. 1985. In vivo effects of N-acetylcysteine on glutathione metabolism and on the biotransformation of carcinogenic and/or mutagenic compounds. Carcinogenesis 6:1735–1745.
84. Camoirano A, Badolati GS, Zanacchi P, Bagnasco M, De Flora S. 1988. Dual role of

thiols in N-methyl-N'-nitro-N-nitrosoguanidine genotoxicity. Life Sci Adv Exp Oncol 7:21–25.

85. De Flora S, Camoirano A, Izzotti A, Zanacchi P, Bagnasco M, Cesarone CF. 1991. Antimutagenic and anticarcinogenic mechanisms of aminothiols. *In* Anticarcinogenesis and Radiation Protection III, F Nygaard and AC Upton (eds.). Plenum Press: New York, pp. 275–285.

86. Izzotti A, Balansky R, Coscia N, Scatolini L, D'Agostini F, De Flora S. 1992. Chemoprevention of smoke-related DNA adduct formation in rat lung and heart. Carcinogenesis 13:2187–2190.

87. De Flora S, Astengo M, Serra D, Benicelli C. 1986. Prevention of induced lung tumors in mice by dietary N-acetylcysteine. Cancer Lett 32:235–241.

88. Wilpart M, Speder D, Roberfroid M. 1986. Anti-initiation activity of N-acetylcysteine in experimental colonic carcinogenesis. Cancer Lett 31:319–324.

89. Ip C, Ganther HE. 1991. Combination of blocking agents and suppressing agents in cancer prevention. Carcinogenesis 12:365–367.

90. Moon RC, Rao KV, Detrisac CJ, Kelloff GJ. 1992. Animal models for chemoprevention of respiratory cancer. Monogr Natl Cancer Inst (U.S.) 13:45–49.

91. Pastorino U, Soresi E, Clerici M, et al. 1988. Lung cancer chemoprevention with retinol palmitate. Acta Oncol 27:773–782.

92. Bauernfeind JC. 1980. The safe use of vitamin A: a report of the International Vitamin A Consultative Group (IVAG). The Nutrition Foundation, 888 17th St, NW, Washington, DC, 20006.

93. Bendich LL. 1989. Safety of vitamin A. Am J Clin Nutr 49:358–371.

94. Rapaport HG, Herman H, Lehman E. 1942. Treatment of ichtyosis with vitamin A. J Pediatr 21:733–746.

95. Frey JR, Schoch MA. 1952. Therapeutische versuche bei psoriasis mit vitamin A, zugleich ein beitrag zur A-hypervitaminose. Dermatologicala 104:80–86.

96. Schimpf A, Jansen KH. 1972. Hochdosierte vitamin-A-therapie bei psoriasis und mycosis fungoides. Fortschr Ther 90:635–639.

97. Silverman S, Renstrup G, Pindborg J. 1963. Studies in oral leukoplakias: III. Effects of vitamin A comparing clinical, histopathological, cytologic, and hemathologic responses. Acta Odont Scand 21:271–292.

98. Korner WF, Vollm J. 1975. New aspects of the tolerance of retinol in humans. Int J Vit Nutr Res 45:363–372.

99. Pastorino U, Chiesa G, Infante M, et al. 1991. Safety of high-dose vitamin A. Randomized trial on lung cancer chemoprevention. Oncology 48:131–137.

100. Bollag W. 1983. Vitamin A and retinoid: from nutrition to pharmacotherapy in dermatology and oncology. Lancet 1:860–863.

101. Sporn MB, Dunlop NM, Newton DL, Henderson WR. 1976. Relationship between structure and activity of retinoids. Nature 263:110–113.

102. Peck GL, Olsen TG, Butkus D, Pandya M, Arnaud-Battandier J, Yoder F, Levis WR. 1979. Treatment of basal cell carcinomas with 13-cis retinoic acid. Proc Am Assoc Cancer Res 20:56.

103. Kamm JJ, Ashenfelter KO, Emann CW. 1984. Preclinical and clinical toxicology of selected retinoids. *In* The Retinoids, vol. 2, MB Sporn et al. (eds.). Academic Press: Orlando, FL, pp. 287–326.

104. Pennes DR, Ellis CN, Madison KC, Voorhees JJ, Martel W. 1984. Early skeletal hyperostosis secondary to 13-cis-retinoic acid. Am J Radiol 141:979–983.

105. Hong WK, Endicott J, Itri L, et al. 1986. 13-cis-retinoic acid in the treatment of oral leukoplakia. N Engl J Med 315:1501–1505.

106. Sestili MA. 1985. Chemoprevention clinical trials. Problems and solutions. NIH Publication No. 85-2715.

107. Greenwald P, Sondik E, Lynch BS. 1986. Diet and chemoprevention in NCI's research

strategy to achieve national cancer control objectives. Annu Rev Public Health 7:267–291.

108. Sporn MB, Newton DL. 1979. Chemoprevention of cancer with retinoids. Fed Proc 38:2528–2534.

109. Moon RC, Thompson HJ, Becci PL, et al. 1979. N-(4-hydroxyphenyl)retinamide, a new retinoid for prevention of breast cancer. Cancer Res 39:1339–1346.

110. Paulson JD, Oldham JW, Preston RF, et al. 1985. Lack of genotoxicity of the cancer chemopreventive agent N-(4-hydroxyphenyl)retinamide. Fund Appl Toxicol 5:144–150.

111. Formelli F, Carsana R, Costa A, Buranelli F, Campa T, Dossena G, Magni A, Pizzichetta M. 1989. Plasma retinol level reduction by the synthetic retinoid fenretinide: a one year follow-up study of breast cancer patients. Cancer Res 48:6149–6152.

112. Veronesi U, De Palo G, Costa A, et al. 1992. Chemoprevention of breast cancer with retinoids. INCI Monogr 12:93–97.

113. Berni R, Formelli F. 1992. In vitro interaction of fenretinide with plasma retinolbinding protein and its functional consequences. FEBS 308:43–45.

114. Chiesa F, Tradati N, Marazza M, Rossi N, Boracchi P, Mariani L, Clerici M, Formelli F, Barzan L, Carrassi A, Pastorini A, Camerini T, Giardini R, Zurrida S, Minn FL, Costa A, DePalo G, Veronesi U. 1992. Prevention of local relapses and new localisations of oral leukoplachias with the synthetic retinoid fenretinide (4-HPR). Preliminary results. Oral Oncology — Eur J Cancer 28B:97–102.

115. Stich HF, Rosin MP, Hornby AP. 1988. Remission of oral leukoplakias and micronuclei in tobacco/betel quid chewers treated with beta-carotene and with beta-carotene plus vitamin A. Int J Cancer 42:195–199.

116. Garewal HS, Meyskens FL, Killen D. 1990. Response of oral leukoplakia to beta-carotene. J Clin Oncol 8:1715–1720.

117. Lippman SM, Batsakis JG, Toth BB, Weber RS, Lee JJ, Martin JW, Hays GL, Goepfert H, Hong WK. 1993. Comparison of low-dose isotretinoin with beta carotene to prevent oral carcinogenesis. N Engl J Med 328:15–20.

118. Boman G, Bäcker U, Larsson S, Melander B, Wahlander L. 1983. Oral acetylcysteine reduces exacerbation rate in chronic bronchitis: report of a trial organized by the Swedish Society for Pulmonary Diseases. Eur J Respir Dis 64:405–415.

119. Heffner JE, Repine JE. 1989. Pulmonary strategies of antioxidant defense. Am Rev Respir Dis 140:531–554.

120. Flanagan RJ. 1987. The role of acetylcysteine in clinical toxicology. Med Toxicol 2:93–104.

121. Miller LF, Rumack BH. 1983. Clinical safety of high oral doses of acetylcysteine. Semin Oncol 10(suppl 1):76–85.

122. Geenwald P, Stern HR. 1992. Role of biology and prevention in aerodigestive tract cancer. J Natl Cancer Inst Monogr 13:3–14.

123. Kelloff GJ, Boone CW, Malone WF, Steele VE. 1992. Chemoprevention clinical trials. Mutat Res 267:291–295.

124. Dimitrov NV, Bennett JL, McMillan J, Perloff M, Leece CM, Malone W. 1992. Clinical pharmacology studies of oltipraz — a potential chemopreventive agent. Invest New Drugs 10:289–298.

125. Wattenberg LW, Bueding E. 1986. Inhibitory effects of 5-(2-pyrazinyl)-4-methyl-1,2-dithiol-3-thione (Oltipraz) on carcinogenesis induced by benzo(a)pyrene, diethylnitro-samine and uracil mustard. Carcinogenesis 7:1379–1381.

126. Rao CV, Tokomo K, Kelloff G, Reddy BS. 1991. Inhibition by dietary oltipraz of experimental intestinal carcinogenesis induced by azoxymethane in male F344 rats. Carcinogenesis 12:1051–1055.

127. Kensler TW, Groopman JD, Eaton DL, Curphey TJ, Roebuck BD. 1992. Potent inhibition of aflatoxin-induced hepatic tumorigenesis by the monofunctional enzyme inducer 1,2-dithiole-3-thione. Carcinogenesis 13:95–100.

128. Pepin P, Bouchard L, Nicole P, Castonguay A. 1992. Effects of sulindac and oltipraz on the tumorigenicity of 4-(methylnitrosamino)1-(3-pyridyl)-1-butanone in A/J mouse lung. Carcinogenesis 13:341–348.

129. Benson AB III. 1993. Oltipraz: a laboratory and clinical review. J Cell Biochem 17F:278–291.

130. Carper SW, Tome ME, Fuller DJ, Chen JR, Harari PM, Gerner EW. 1991. Polyamine catabolism in rodent and human cells in culture. Biochem J 280:289–294.

131. Rao CV, Tokumo K, Rigotty J, Zang E, Kelloff G, Reddy BS. 1991. Chemoprevention of colon carcinogenesis by dietary administration of piroxicam, alpha-difluoromethylornithine, 16 alpha-fluoro-5-androsten-17-one, and ellagic acid individually and in combination. Cancer Res 51:4528–4534.

132. Kadmon D. 1992. Chemoprevention in prostate cancer: the role of difluoromethylornithine (DFMO). J Cell Biochem Suppl 16H:122–127.

133. Zirvi KA, Atabek U. 1991. In vitro response of a human colon tumor xenograft and a lung adenocarcinoma cell line to alpha-difluoromethylornithine alone and in combination with 5-fluorouracil and doxorubicin. J Surg Oncol 48:34–38.

134. Croghan MK, Aickin MG, Meyskens FL. 1991. Dose-related alpha-difluoromethylornithine ototoxicity. Am J Clin Oncol 14:331–335.

135. Gerrish KE, Fuller DJ, Gerner EW, Gensler HL. 1993. Inhibition of DFMO-induced audiogenic seizures by chlordiazepoxide. Life Sci 52:1101–1108.

136. Doerr-O'Rourke K, Trushin N, Hecht SS, Stoner GD. 1991. Effect of phenethyl isothiocyanate on the metabolism of the tobacco-specific nitrosamine 4-(methylnitrosamino)-1-(3-pyridyl)-1-butanone by cultured rat lung tissue. Carcinogenesis 12:1029–1034.

137. Morse MA, Reinhardt JC, Amin SG, Hecht SS, Stoner GD, Chung FL. 1990. Effect of dietary aromatic isothiocyanates fed subsequent to the administration of 4-(methylnitrosamino)-1-(3-pyridyl)-1-butanone on lung tumorigenicity in mice. Cancer Lett 49:225–230.

138. Boukharta M, Jalbert G, Castonguay A. 1992. Biodistribution of ellagic acid and dose-related inhibition of lung tumorigenesis in A/J mice. Nutr Cancer 18:181–189.

139. Perchellet JP, Gali HU, Perchellet EM, Klish DS, Armbrust AD. 1992. Antitumor-promoting activities of tannic acid, ellagic acid, and several gallic acid derivatives in mouse skin. Basic Life Sci 59:783–801.

140. Stoner GD, Morrissey DT, Heur YH, Daniel EM, Galati AJ, Wagner SA. 1991. Inhibitory effects of phenethyl isothiocyanate on N-nitrosobenzylmethylamine carcinogenesis in the rat esophagus. Cancer Res 51:2063–2068.

141. Albanes D, Virtamo J, Rauthalahti M, et al. 1986. Pilot study: The U.S. Finland lung cancer prevention trial. J Nutr Growth Cancer 3:207–214.

142. Hennekens CH. 1984. Issues in the design and conduct of clinical trials. J Natl Cancer Inst 73:1473–1476.

143. Benner SE, Winn RJ, Lippman SM, Poland J, Hansen KS, Luna MA, Hong WK. 1993. Regression of oral leukoplakia with alpha-tocopherol: a community clinical oncology program chemoprevention study. J Natl Cancer Inst 85:44–47.

144. Lee JS, Benner SE, Lippman SM, Lee JJ, Ro JY, Lukeman JM, Morice RC, Peters EJ, Pang AC, Hittelman HM, Hong WK. 1993. A randomised placebo-controlled chemoprevention trial of 13-cis-retinoic acid (cRA) in bronchial squamous metaplasia. Proc ASCO 13:1117.

145. de Vries N. 1990. The magnitude of the problem. *In* Multiple Primary Tumors in the Head and Neck, N de Vries and JL Glukman (eds.). Thieme: Stuttgard pp. 1–29.

146. Hong WK, Bromer RH, Amato DA. 1985. Paterns of relapse in locally advanced head and neck cancer patients who achieved complete remission after combined modality therapy. Cancer 56:1242–1245.

147. Slaughter DP, Southwick HW, Smejkal W. 1953. 'Field cancerization' in oral stratified squamous epithelium: clinical implications of multicentric origin. Cancer 6:963–968.

148. McDonald S, Haie C, Rubin P, Nelson D, Divers LD. 1989. Second malignant tumors in patients with laryngeal carcinoma: diagnosis, treatment and prevention. Int J Radiat Oncol Biol Phys 17:457–465.

149. de Vries N, van der Waal I, Snow GB. 1986. Multiple primary tumors in oral cancer. Int J Maxillofac Surg 15:85–87.

150. de Vries N, Snow GB. 1986. Multiple primary tumors in laryngeal cancer. J Laryngol Otol 100:915–917.

151. Fontana RS. 1977. Early diagnosis of lung cancer. Am Rev Respir Dis 116:399–402.

152. Pairolero P, Williams DE, Bergstrahl EJ, Piehler JM, Bernatz PE, Payne SP. 1984. Postsurgical stage I bronchogenic carcinoma: morbid implications of recurrent disease. Ann Thorac Surg 38:331–338.

153. Shields TW, Robinette CD. 1973. Long-term survivors after resection of bronchial carcinoma. Surg Gynecol Obstet 136:759–768.

154. Auerbach O, Stout AP, Hammond EC, et al. 1967. Multiple primary bronchial carcinomas. Cancer 20:699.

155. Femeck BK, Flehinger BJ, Martini N. 1984. A retrospective analysis of 10-year survivors from carcinoma of the lung. Cancer 53(6):1405–1408.

156. Hong WK, Lippman JM, Itri L, et al. 1990. Prevention of second primary tumors with isotretinoin in squamous cell carcinoma of the head and neck. N Engl J Med 323:795–801.

157. Benner SE, Lee JS, Goepfert H, Hong WK. 1993. Long term follow up: 13-cis-retinoic acid (cRA) prevention of second primary tumors (SPT) following squamous cell carcinoma of the head and neck (SCCHN). Proc ASCO 12:900.

158. Bolla M, Lefur R, Ton Van J, Domange C, Badet JM, Koskas Y, Laplanche A. 1993. Prevention of second primary with etretinate in squamous cell carcinoma of oral cavity and oropharynx. a randomized double blind study. Proc 2nd Int Cancer Chemo Prevention Conf (CCPC-93). Berlin, April 28–30, p. 76.

159. Pastorino U, Infante I, Maioli M, Chiesa G, Buyse M, Firket P, Rosmentz N, Clerici M, Soresi E, Valente M, Belloni PA, Ravasi G. 1993. Adjuvant treatment of stage I lung cancer with high dose vitamin A. J Clin Oncol 11:1216–1222.

160. De Vries N, Van Zandwijk N, Pastorino U. 1991. The EUROSCAN Study. Br J Cancer 64:985–989.

161. Lippman SM, Benner SE, Hong WK. 1993. Chemoprevention strategies in lung carcinogenesis. Chest 103:15S–19S.

162. Jin Y-S, Mandahl N, Heim S, Schuller H, Mitelman F. 1988. Isochromosomes i(8q) or i(9q) in three adenocarcinomas of the lung. Cancer Genet Cytogenet 33:11–17.

163. Bello MJ, Moreno S, Rey JA. 1989. Involvement of chromosomes 1, 3, and i(8q) in lung adenocarcinoma. Cancer Genet Cytogenet 38:133–135.

164. Lukeis R, Irving L, Garson M, Hasthorpe S. 1990. Cytogenetics of non-small cell lung cancer: Analysis of consistent non-random abnormalities. Genes Chrom Cancer 2:116–124.

165. Sozzi G, Miozzo M, Tagliabue E, Calderone C, Lombardi L, Pilotti S, Pastorino U, Pierotti MA, Della Porta G. 1991. Cytogenetic abnormalities and overexpression of receptors for growth factors in normal bronchial epithelium and tumor samples of lung cancer patients. Cancer Res 51:400–404.

166. Wang Peng J, Knutsen T, Gazdar A, Steinberg SM, Oie H, Linnoila I, Mulshine J, Nau M, Minna JD. 1991. Non random structural and numerical chromosome changes in non-small cell lung cancer. Genes Chrom Cancer 3:168–188.

167. Testa JR, Siegfried JM. 1992. Chromosome abnormalities in human non-small cell lung cancer. Cancer Res 52:2702s–2706s.

168. Hendler FJ, Ozanne BW. 1984. Human squamous cell lung cancers express increased epidermal growth factor receptors. J Clin Invest 74:647–651.

169. Cerny T, Barnes DM, Hasleton P, Barber PV, Healy K, Gullick W, Thatcher N. 1986.

Expression of epidermal growth factor receptor (EGF-R) in human lung tumours. Br J Cancer 54:265–269.

170. Berger MS, Gullick WJ, Greenfield C, Evans S, Addis BJ, Waterfield MD. 1987. Epidermal growth factor receptors in lung tumors. J Pathol 152:297–307.

171. Volm M, Efferth T, Mattern J. 1992. Oncoprotein (c-myc, c-erbB1, c-erbB2, c-fos) and suppressor gene product (p53) expression in squamous cell carcinomas of the lung. Clinical and biological correlations. Anticancer Res 12:11–20.

172. Rodenhuis S, Slebos RJC, Boot AJM, Evers SG, Mooi WJ, Wagenaar SS, Van Bodegom PC, Bos JL. 1988. Incidence and possible clinical significance of K-ras oncogene activation in adenocarcinoma of the lung. Cancer Res 48:5738–5741.

173. Slebos RJC, Kibbelaar RE, Dalesio O, Koolstra A, Stam J, Neifier CJLM, Wagenaar SS, Van der Schueren R, Van Zandwijk N, Mooi WJ, Bos JL, Rodenhuis S. 1990. K-ras oncogene activation as a prognostic marker in adenocarcinoma of the lung. N Engl J Med 323:561–565.

174. Mitsudomi T, Steinberg SM, Oie HK, Mulshine JL, Phelps R, Viallet J, Pass H, Minna JD, Gazdar AF. 1991. ras gene mutations in non-small cell lung cancers are associated with shortened survival irrespective of treatment intent. Cancer Res 51:4999–5002.

175. Rodenhuis S, Slebos RJC. 1992. Clinical significance of ras oncogene activation in human lung cancer. Cancer Res 52:2665s–2669s.

176. Kern JA, Schwartz DA, Nordberg JE, Weiner DB, Greene MI, Torney L, Robinson RA. 1990. p185neu expression in human lung adenocarcinomas predicts shortened survival. Cancer Res 50:5184–5187.

177. Weiner DB, Nordberg J, Robinson R, Nowell PC, Gazdar A, Greene MI, Williams WV, Cohen JA, Kern JA. 1990. Expression of the neu gene-encoded protein (p185neu) in human non-small cell carcinomas of the lung. Cancer Res 50:421–425.

178. Tateishi M, Ishida T, Mitsudomi T, Kaneko S, Sugimachi K. 1991. Prognostic value of c-erbB-2 protein expression in human lung adenocarcinoma and squamous cell carcinoma. Eur J Cancer 27:1372–1375.

179. Shi D, He G, Cao S, Pan W, Zhang HZ, Yu D, Hung MC. 1992. Overexpression of the c-erbB-2/neu-encoded p185 protein in primary lung cancer. Mol Carcinogen 5:213–218.

180. Little CD, Nau MM, Carney DN, Gazdar AF, Minna JD. 1983. Amplification and expression of the c-myc oncogene in human lung cancer cell lines. Nature 306:194–196.

181. Nau MM, Brooks BJ, Battey J, Sausville E, Gazdar AF, Kirsch IR, McBride OW, Bertness V, Hollis GF, Minna JD. 1985. L-myc, a new myc-related gene amplified and expressed in human small cell lung cancer. Nature 318:69–73.

182. Johnson BE, Ihde D, Makuch RW, Gazdar AF, Carney DN, Oie H, Russell E, Nau MM, Minna JD. 1987. myc family oncogene amplification in tumor cell lines established from small cell lung cancer patients and its relationship to clinical status and course. J Clin Invest 79:1629–1634.

183. Shiraishi M, Noguchi M, Shimosato Y, Sekiya T. 1989. Amplification of protooncogenes in surgical specimens of human lung carcinomas. Cancer Res 49:6474–6479.

184. Harbour JW, Lai S-L, Whang-Peng J, Gazdar AD, Minna JD, Kaye FJ. 1988. Abnormalities in structure and expression of the human retinoblastoma gene in SCLC. Science 241:353–357.

185. Horowitz JM, Park SH, Bogenmann E, Cheng J-C, Yandell DW, Daye FJ, Minna JD, Dryja TP, Weinberg RA. 1990. Frequent inactivation of the retinoblastoma anti-oncogene is restricted to a subset of human tumor cells. Proc Natl Acad Sci USA 87:2775–2779.

186. Houle B, Leduc F, Bradley WEC. 1991. Implication of RARB in epidermoid (squamous) lung cancer. Genes Chrom Cancer 3:358–366.

187. Tsuchiya E, Nakamura Y, Weng S-Y, Nakagawa K, Tsuchiya S, Sugano H, Kitagawa T. 1992. Allelotype of non-small cell lung carcinoma — Comparison between loss of heterozygosity in squamous cell carcinoma and adenocarcinoma. Cancer Res 52:2478–2481.

72

188. Hibi K, Takahashi T, Yamakawa K, Ueda R, Sekido Y, Ariyoshi Y, Suyama M, Takagi H, Nakamura Y, Takahashi T. 1992. Three distinct regions involved in 3p deletion in human lung cancer. Oncogene 7:445–449.

189. Gebert JF, Moghal N, Frangioni JV, Sugarbaker DJ, Neel BG. 1991. High frequency of retinoic acid receptor β abnormalities in human lung cancer. Oncogene 6:1859–1868.

190. Iggo R, Gatter K, Bartek J, Lane D, Harris AL. 1990. Increased expression of mutant forms of p53 oncogene in primary lung cancer. Lancet 335:675–679.

191. Chiba I, Takahashi T, Nau M, D'Amico D, Curiel D, Mitsudomi TDB, Carbone D, Piantadosi S, Koga H, Reissmann P, Slamon D, Holmes E, Minna J. 1990. Mutations in the p53 gene are frequent in primary, resected non-small cell lung cancer. Oncogene 5:1603–1610.

192. Takahashi T, Takahashi T, Suzuki H, Hida T, Sekido Y, Ariyoshi Y, Ueda R. 1991. The p53 gene is very frequently mutated in small-cell lung cancer with a distinct nucleotide substitution pattern. Oncogene 6:1775–1778.

193. D'Amico D, Carbone D, Mitsudomi T, Nau M, Fedorko J, Russell E, Johnson B, Buchhagen D, Bodner S, Phelps R, Gazdar A, Minna JD. 1992. High frequency of somatically acquired p53 mutations in small cell lung cancer cell lines and tumors. Oncogene cell 7:339–346.

194. Miller CW, Simon K, Aslo Kok K, Yokota J, Buys CH, Terada M, Koeffler HP. 1992. p53 mutations in human lung tumors. Cancer Res 52:1695–1698.

195. Suzuki H, Takahashi T, Kuroishi T, Suyama M, Ariyoshi Y, Takahashi T, Ueda R. 1992. p53 mutations in non-small cell lung cancer in Japan: association between mutations and smoking. Cancer Res 52:734–736.

196. Kishimoto Y, Murakami Y, Shiraishi M, Hayashi K, Sekiya T. 1992. Aberrations of the p53 tumor suppressor gene in human non-small cell carcinomas of the lung. Cancer Res 52:4799–4804.

197. Hiyoshi H, Matsuno Y, Kato H, Shimosato Y, Hirohashi S. 1992. Clinicopathological significance of nuclear accumulation of tumor suppressor gene p53 product in primary lung cancer. Jpn J Cancer Res 83:101–106.

198. Horio Y, Takahashi T, Kuroishi T, Hibi K, Suyama M, Niimi T, Shimokata K, Yamakawa K, Nakamura Y, Ueda R, Takahashi T. 1993. Prognostic significance of p53 mutations and 3p deletions in primary resected non-small cell lung cancer. Cancer Res 53(1):1–4.

199. Quinlan DC, Davidson AG, Summers CL, Warden HE, Doshi HM. 1992. Accumulation of p53 protein correlates with a poor prognosis in human lung cancer. Cancer Res 52:4828–4831.

200. Sundaresan V, Ganly P, Hasleton P, Rudd R, Sinha G, Bleehen NM, Rabbitts P. 1992. p53 and chromosome 3 abnormalities, characteristic of malignant lung tumours, are detectable in preinvasive lesions of the bronchus. Oncogene 7:1989–1997.

201. Sozzi G, Miozzo M, Donghi R, Pilotti S, Cariani CT, Pastorino U, Della Porta G, Pierotti MA. 1992. Deletions of 17p and p53 mutations in preneoplastic lesions of the lung. Cancer Res 52:6079–6082.

202. Pastorino U, Sozzi G, Miozzo M, Tagliabue E, Pilotti S, Pierotti MA. 1993. Genetic changes in lung cancer. J Cell Biochem 17F:237–248.

203. Chung KY, Mukhopadhyay T, Kim J, Casson A, Ro JY, Goepfert H, Hong WK, Roth JA. 1993. Discordant p53 gene mutations in primary head and neck cancers and corresponding second primary cancers of the upper aerodigestive tract. Cancer Res 53:1676–1683.

204. Lee JS, Lippman SM, Hong WK, Ro JY, Kim SY, Lotan R, Hittelman WN. 1992. Determination of biomarkers for intermediate end points in chemoprevention trials. Cancer Res 52(9)(Suppl):2707s–2710s.

205. Stich HF, Rosin MP, Hornby AP. 1988. Remission of oral leukoplakias and micronuclei in tobacco/betel quid chewers treated with beta-carotene and with beta-carotene plus vitamin A. Int J Cancer 42:195–199.

206. Lippman SM, Peters EJ, Wargovich MJ, et al. 1990. Bronchial micronuclei as a marker of an early stage of carcinogenesis in the human tracheobronchial epithelium. Int J Cancer 45:811–815.
207. Lee JS, Ro JY, Sahin AA, Hong WK, Brown BW, Mountain CF, Hittelman WN. 1991. Expression of blood-group antigen A - a favorable prognostic factor in non-small-cell lung cancer. N Engl J Med 324:1084–1090.

3. Smoking cessation programs

Philip Tønnesen

Introduction

Smoking is the most important single risk factor for lung cancer [1]. Our scientific knowledge about smoking cessation has improved considerable during the last decade, and today we have well-developed, relatively effective treatment modalities for smoking cessation. The cost of smoking cessation (i.e., cost per saved year of life) is several times cheaper than treatment of comparable risk factors such as hypertension and hypercholesterolemia.

The prevalence of smoking varies across countries and time period, and it differs between sexes, social classes, ages, etc. in the same country. The prevalence of smoking in a country can be influenced by many factors, such as legislation, cost of cigarettes, advertisements, public information, etc. Intensive mass media antismoking campaigns in California have been followed by a decline in smoking prevalence to less than 20%; in contrast, the 'laissez faire' attitude in Denmark has resulted in a smoking prevalence of about 44%. Thus, it is possible to influence the smoking habit.

When a physician is confronted with a smoker, he should at least follow the guidelines proposed by the U.S. National Cancer Institute (table 1). To better understand the background for these guidelines, we will focus in this chapter on nicotine addiction and nicotine substitution.

Addiction to smoking (nicotine)

The smoking habit is complex and multifactorial and varies qualitatively and quantitatively between smokers. Social, psychological, habitual, and behavioral factors together with nicotine addiction make up the smoking dependence complex. In 1988, a report from the U.S. Surgeon General concluded that cigarettes are addicting, that nicotine is the drug in tobacco that causes addiction, and that this *nicotine addiction* is similar to heroin and cocaine addiction in its pharmacological and behavioral aspects [2]. This knowledge of nicotine dependence as a major and important factor in the smoking habit has changed our view of how people quit smoking: what was

Heine H. Hansen, (ed), Hansen: Lung Cancer.
© *1994 Kluwer Academic Publishers. ISBN 0-7923-2835-3. All rights reserved.*

Table 1. U.S. National Cancer Institute guidelines to physicians regarding smoking cessation (the four A's)

1. **Ask** all patients about smoking
2. **Advise** smokers to stop
3. **Assist** their efforts with self-help materials, set a quit date, and when indicated use nicotine replacement
4. **Arrange** follow-up

Table 2. Fagerström test for nicotine dependence

Questions	Answers	Points
1. How soon after you wake up do you smoke your first cigarette?	Within 5 min	3
	6–30 min	2
	31–60 min	1
	≥61 min	0
2. Do you find it difficult to refrain from smoking in places where it is forbidden, e.g., in church, at the library, in cinema, etc.?	Yes	1
	No	0
3. Which cigarette would you hate most to give up?	The first one in the morning	1
	All others	0
4. How many cigarettes/days do you smoke?	10 or less	0
	11–20	1
	21–30	2
	31 or more	3
5. Do you smoke more frequently during the first hours after waking than during the rest of the day?	Yes	1
	No	0
6. Do you smoke if you are so ill that you are in bed most of the day?	Yes	1
	No	0

Total score: 0–10. Heavy nicotine addicted: >6.

once only a question of will power is now a matter of treating a dependence disorder with nicotine supplementation. However, this does not mean that all smokers are nicotine addicts! At the extremes are the smoker who only smokes a few cigarettes on Saturdays after a good dinner ('party smoker') and the highly nicotine-addicted subject who smokes 20 to 40 cigarettes daily as well as one or two cigarettes when he wakes up during the night. At present, we have no accurate measure of nicotine dependency. Subjects who smoke less than 5 to 7 cigarettes daily are usually not nicotine addicted, while subjects who smoke more than 10 cigarettes daily usually exhibit varying degrees of nicotine dependence. The Fagerström Questionnaire — a self-completed scale — is the most often used measure of nicotine addiction (table 2) [3]. The first question it asks, namely, 'How soon after you wake up do you smoke your first cigarette?' seems to be the single most important question, perhaps due to low plasma nicotine levels in the morning.

Measurement of plasma nicotine and cotinine (the main metabolite of nicotine) during smoking might further be used to determine the degree of dependency.

Quitting smoking

Quitting smoking is not easy, and most smokers have to try several times before permanent abstinence is achieved. Quitting smoking might be looked upon as a cycle, i.e., smoking – quitting – abstinence – relapsing – smoking [4]. Several cycles are usually needed to stay abstinent permanently. This reality underlines the importance of persistence in this area; a new attempt to quit smoking should be tried after a failure [5]. By explaining to the smoker that failure is not a personal defeat, but rather a learning experience, the physician may increase the self-confidence of the smoker.

The level of motivation to quit smoking is important, although it has not been evaluated systematically in most studies. Four motivational stages have been proposed — precontemplation (contented smoker), contemplation, decision, and action and maintenance [6] — The smoker's stage of motivation is important to the physician's approach to the smoker. In the first two stages, the motivational approach should utilize information about the adverse health effects of smoking; in the second two, when a smoker really tries to quit, he no longer needs health information but rather 'technical' information about the basic skills needed to quit, as well as positive encouragement and support.

When a smoker wants to stop smoking, it is important for the physician to set a quit day, which means that on that specific date the smoker stops smoking completely. This principle is one of the most fundamental in all smoking cessation studies. Subjects who still smoke one or two cigarettes daily after 1 to 2 weeks will almost all return to their usual cigarette consumption in a short period of time. A smoker might try to reduce the number of daily cigarettes in the weeks up to the quit day, although this approach has not been shown to improve outcome; however, from the quit day onward, not even a single cigarette is recommended.

Basic principles

Some 'general rules' and basic principles are fundamental to smoking cessation and smoking cessation programs (some have been mentioned above):
1. Stop smoking completely on the quit day — even 1–2 cigarettes per day may be followed by relapse
2. Use nicotine substitution to double outcome

3. Remember that relapse is highest during the first 3–6 weeks and then gradually declines, similar to other addictions
4. Arrange follow-up to prevent relapse
5. Remember that the one-year success rates in most studies are about 15%–25%
6. Begin the cessation cycle again (after some time) for subjects who failed

Nicotine therapy

The effect of nicotine in the brain is complex and not fully explored. Nicotine binds to cholinergic nicotinic receptors in the brain, the limbic system, and the cortex [7]. The 'positive' effects of nicotine are stimulation of the cortex and stress reduction in the limbic system without any sedation. The 'negative' effect of nicotine is a decrease of withdrawal symptoms [8]. When quitting smoking, the subject will experience several withdrawal symptoms with individual differences for weeks to months, with declining intensity over the first few weeks. These withdrawal symptoms include craving for cigarettes, irritability, anxiety, difficulty concentrating, restlessness, depression, hunger, and increase in weight [9].

The rationale for nicotine substitution is that the administration of nicotine, as gum or patch, decreases withdrawal symptoms in the first months, thus allowing the subject to break the behavioral and psychological habit of smoking. When nicotine products are used instead of smoking, lower nicotine levels are attained and the high plasma peak levels of nicotine during smoking are not reached. After 2 to 6 months, the use of nicotine gum or patch is terminated, usually without recurrence of withdrawal symptoms due to less dependence liability.

Nicotine chewing gum

Since nicotine has a high degree of initial metabolism in the liver, treatment must bypass the gastrointestinal tract.

Nicotine chewing gum or nicotine polacrilex (Nicorette) is available in 2- and 4-mg strengths. Nicotine is bound to a ion-exchange resin in the gum base, and bicarbonate is added to create an alkaline pH in the mouth in order to facilate absorption of nicotine in the mouth.

Patients should be instructed carefully so as to reduce side effects due to swallowed nicotine. Gum users should only chew the gum 5–10 times until they can taste the nicotine; then they should stop chewing for a few minutes, and then chew again to expose a new surface of the gum. The gum can be chewed for about 20–30 minutes. About 0.8 mg of nicotine is absorbed from a 2-mg nicotine gum and about 1.2 mg from a 4-mg piece [10], with a plasma peak concentration of 5–10 ng/ml after approximately 30 minutes, followed by a slow decline to basal levels after 2 to 3 hours. If the gum is used

Table 3. Success rates of double-blind, placebo-controlled trials with 2-mg nicotine chewing gum

Author [ref]	N	Addit. therapy	Time point	Act %	Plac %	Time point	Act %	Plac %
Malcolm [14]	210	Indiv	4 W	34	37	6 M	23	5[b]
Fee [15]	352	Group	5 W	46	33[a]	12 M	13	9
Fagerström [16]	96	Indiv	4 W	89	59[a]	12 M	49	37
Jarvis [17]	116	Group	4 W	62	33[b]	12 M	47	21
Schneider [18]	60	Group	4 W	76	50[a]	12 M	30	20
BTS [19]	802	None	4 W	27	26	12 M	10	14
Christen [20]	208	Group	6 W	34	11[c]			
Hjalmarson [21]	205	Group	6 W	77	52[c]	12 M	29	16[a]
Jamrozik [22]	200	Indiv	4 W	29	24	6 M	10	8
Hall [23]	139	Group	3 W	82	72	12 M	44	21[b]
Fortmann [24]	301	Mail	8 W	35	20[c]	6 M	26	18[a]
Hughes [25]	315	Indiv	4 W	60	47[a]	12 M	10	7
Tønnesen [26]	113	Group	6 W	73	41[c]	12 M	38	22
Median values			4 W	60	37	12 M	23	17

[a] $p < 0.05$.
[b] $p < 0.01$.
[c] $p < 0.001$.
Addit. = additional; Act = active; Plac = placebo; W = week; M = month.

throughout the day, nicotine levels of 7–13 ng/ml for the 2-mg gum and 15–23 ng/ml for the 4-mg gum are attained, compared with a smoking level of 25–30 ng/ml [11–13].

A basic principle of gum use is the ability to self-titrate the dose, as opposed to the patch, which delivers a fixed dose. The advantage of the gum is that it can be used as desired or needed during the day. The disadvantage of the gum is possible underdosing, which might explain the lack of effect in several trials. About 20 pieces of the 2-mg gum provide a dose similar to that delivered by most nicotine patches, but in most studies the mean number of gum pieces consumed daily is around 5–6.

In table 3, the success rates of 13 double-blind, placebo-controlled trials with 2-mg gum are shown [14–26]. In 9 out of 13 trials, a significant improvement was found in short-term outcome in favor of active gum, but only 4 out of 12 trials showed such improvement for long-term outcome. Also, the range of success rate was wide, i.e., 23%–89% for active gum and 11%–59% for placebo for short-term outcome, and 10%–49% for active gum and 5%–37% for placebo after 6 to 12 months. This variability in outcome has many possible explanations, such as subject differences (motivation, dependency), use of adjunctive behavioral and psycological support programs, follow-up procedures, and pharmacological factors, i.e., daily dose of nicotine from the gum and duration of use. The best results were

Table 4. Success rates of double-blind, placebo-controlled trials with 4-mg versus placebo or 2-mg nicotine chewing gum

Author [ref]	N	Addit. therapy	Time point	4-mg %	Plac %	Time point	4-mg %	Plac %
Puska [27]	160	Group	3 W	70	55[a]	6 M	35	28
Blöndal [28]	182	Group	4 W	82	69[a]	12 M	40	27[a]

Ref.	N	Addit. therapy	Time point	4-mg %	2-mg %	Time point	4-mg %	2-mg %
Tønnesen [13]	115	Group	4 W	74	72	12 M	37	33
Kornitzer [29]	199	Work	12 W	45	36	12 M	32	22
Tønnesen [26]	60	Group	6 W	82	55[b]	12 M	44	12[b]

[a] $p < 0.05$.
[b] $p < 0.01$.
Addit. = additional; Act = active; Plac = placebo.

obtained when gum use was combined with 'behavioral' support. In several of the trials, a large proportion of the participants did not use the gum at all. Underdosing might be a plausible explanation for the lack of efficacy in several studies. In most studies, fewer than 50% of subjects still used the gum after six weeks. In our study, the daily consumption of gum after four weeks was about 11 [13–16].

From these observations, it would be logical to try to increase the consumed dose either by a higher number of gum pieces chewed or by using the 4-mg gum. Four studies comparing the 4- and 2-mg gum found that the 4-mg gum was superior to the 2-mg gum for short-term outcome (table 4) [26–29].

Another way to increase the amount of consumed gum might be to administer the gum in fixed dosage schedules. In a study comprising 1218 subjects, Killen et al. [30] compared nicotine gum delivered ad lib or on a fixed regimen with placebo and no gum controls. Use of the active gum resulted in a significant improvement in outcome after 2 and 6 months compared with placebo and no gum; however, in testing the ad lib and the fixed regimen, only the fixed regimen was significantly better than placebo and no gum. The number of pieces of gum consumed was significantly higher in the fixed regimen across the eight treatment weeks — for example, in the first week, 9 pieces versus 5 pieces daily for the fixed regimen and the ad lib regimen, respectivly.

The side effects of gum consist mainly of local symptoms in the mouth, throat, and stomach due to swallowed nicotine. After adequate instruction, most smokers can learn to use the gum properly, i.e., to use correct chewing technique. However, without instructions, many subjects will discontinue use or will underdose. Constant chewing may produce side effects such as oral or throat soreness, aches in mastication muscles, hypertrophy of the masseter muscles, and loss of dental fillings. In addition, nausea, vomiting, indigestion, and hiccups occur with a higher incidence among active gum users. However, in a double-blind study with 0-, 2-, and 4-mg nicotine chewing gum, we reported that only hiccups occurred more frequently among the 4-mg gum users [26].

Overall, side effects from the gum are mild and transient.

Because the gum user can self-titrate the dose, gum use can induce addiction. Long-term gum use can be defined as gum use after 10 to 12 months; from 0% to 25% of successful subjects continue gum use after one year, with an average daily use of less than six pieces [31]. Gradual reduction of gum use seems to be possible in many users without relapse to smoking.

Therefore, long-term use does not seem to be a major problem in smoking cessation. Even among subjects who continue to use the gum for years, the risk of a low dose of nicotine seems negligible compared to the much higher nicotine concentrations during smoking.

We suggest that the smoker be instructed to stop smoking completely, and then to use nicotine gum every hour from early morning onward for at least 8 to 10 hours on a fixed schedule, combined with extra pieces whenever needed. When the smoker returns after 1 to 2 weeks and describes craving and other withdrawal symptoms, it is important to instruct him to increase the daily dosage of gum. The 2-mg gum can be used for low- to medium-dependent smokers (i.e., smokers scoring less than 6 on the Fagerström Scale), while the highly dependent smokers (scoring 6 or higher) should start with the 4-mg gum. When a subject uses more than 15 pieces a day of the 2-mg gum, it may be suitable to switch to the 4-mg gum.

The optimal duration of treatment is not known. However, in most studies the gum has been used for at least 6 to 12 weeks and up to one year. Individualization of treatment duration is recommended.

Nicotine transdermal patch

The nicotine patch is a fixed nicotine delivery system that releases about 1 mg of nicotine per hour for 16 hours (daytime patch) or for 24 hours (24-hour patch). The level of nicotine substitution is about 50% of the smoking level (21-mg patch/24 hours and 15-mg patch/16 hours). It is much easier to administer the patch and use it as compared with the gum, but there is no possibility of self-titration [32].

The total daily nicotine dose absorbed is about 15–21 mg, with a maximal plasma nicotine level of 13–13 µg/1 attained after 4 to 9 hours of use [32]. The morning plasma nicotine concentration is low, i.e., 2–11 µg/1, which is in the same range as that occurring during cigarette consumption.

Short-term outcome is in favor of active patches in almost all the placebo-

Table 5. Success rates from 11 published double-blind, placebo-controlled smoking cessation trials using nicotine skin patch (mean values)

| No. | Percent not smoking | | Weeks | Behavioral component | Author [ref] |
	Active	Placebo			
199	36	23	12	Indiv. Minimal[a]	Abelin [33]
122	39	20	9	Indiv. Minimal	Abelin [34]
85	69	51[b]	9	Group (9 sessions)	Buchkremer [35]
80	40	20	10	Group (10 sessions)	Krumpe [36]
80	48	15	6	Counseling	Mulligan [37]
65	18	06	3	Group (6 sessions)	Rose [38]
70	71	34	6	Group	Hurt [39]
289	53	17	6	Indiv. Moderate	Tønnesen [40]
220	62	38	4	Indiv. Minimal	Sachs [41]
158	39	14	4	Group, Moderate	Daughton [42]
935	61	27	6	Group, Moderate	TN Study Gr [43]

[a] Performed in general practice.
[b] Not significant outcome.

controlled studies reported (10 of 11 studies) [33–43] (table 5). In a multicenter smoking cessation trial from the U.S. that examined the effects of 0-, 7-, 14-, and 21-mg nicotine patches, a dose–response effect of increasing nicotine dosages was reported [43]. In the eight studies examining long-term success, five showed significant outcomes in favor of the active patch.

Side effects are mainly mild local skin irritation occuring in 10% to 20% of subjects. Only in 1.5% to 2% of subjects did patch use have to be terminated due to more persistent and severe skin irritation in the patch area [32].

Two large placebo-controlled trials have recently been published using data from general medical practices [44,45]. In the first study, 600 smokers (smoking more than 14 cigarettes daily) from 30 practices were allocated 15-mg 16-hour daytime nicotine patches or placebo for 18 weeks, combined with minimal support and follow-up after 1, 3, 6, 12, 26, and 52 weeks [44]. The success rate after three weeks was 36% for active patches and 17% for placebo patches, and the one-year continous abstinence rate verified by carbon monoxide was 9.3% for active patches and 5.0% for placebo patches.

In the second study, 1686 smokers from 19 practices received 21-mg 24-hour patches or placebo patches for three months, supported by a nurse and follow-up after 1, 4, 8, and 12 weeks [45]. The three-month success rate was 14.4% for active patches and 8.6% for placebo-treated subjects. Side effects were few, and the treatment was generally well tolerated. Concomitant use of cigarettes and the nicotine patch might increase plasma nicotine to levels higher than during smoking, but only a few subjects reported side effects (nausea). Local skin irritation was reported in about 16% of subjects in the active groups. Sleep disturbances were reported in 20% for active and 8% for placebo-treated subjects using the 24-hour patches, but not in the study with the 16-hour patches. It has been found that nicotine delivery during the night may affect sleep quality [46].

Due to its ease of use, the patch may be the first choice among nicotine delivery systems today. The patch has also been effective when combined only with minimal supportive behavioral therapy, as opposed to the nicotine gum. the findings from the two large trials in general practice are also very encouraging, since they support the findings that nicotine replacement per se (i.e., transdermally) does improve outcome in smoking cessation with minimal adjunctive support. Thus, the patch could also be administered by the busy clinician in most hospitals.

Nicotine vaporizer

Another way to administer nicotine in smoking cessation programs could be through a smoke-free cigarette or an 'inhaler,' in which air is saturated with nicotine before inhalation. We have conducted a controlled trial with a nicohaler to examine the efficacy and safety of the nicohaler in a double-blind clinical smoking trial [47]. The study was a one-year, randomized, double-blind, placebo-controlled trial. Two hundred and eighty-six volunteers who smoked at least 10 cigarettes daily were recuited through a local newspaper, and these subjects were randomly allocated to nicohalers or placebo to be used for three months in a minimal-intervention setup.

Each inhaler contains about 10 mg of nicotine; however, the nicotine concentration in one puff is only approximately one tenth of the concentration in cigarette smoke. After 4 to 8 hours of ad lib use, the maximal plasma nicotine concentration was 8.8 ± 5.9 ng/ml compared to 22.9 ± 8.8 ng/ml after eight hours of smoking. This nicotine level is comparable to the levels found during use of the 2-mg nicotine gum, i.e., relatively low concentrations.

The success rate was significantly higher for the active nicohaler group compared to placebo users. The success rate after six weeks was 28% and 12% ($p < 0.001$) and after one year 15% and 5% ($p < 0.001$), respectively. The mean nicotine substitution based on cotinine determinations after 1 to 2 weeks was 38% to 42% of smoking levels. The treatment was well accepted, and no serious adverse events were reported. In this low-intervention setting, the nicohaler appeared safe to use and improved the outcome in smoking cessation. However, in two similar ongoing studies in the U.S., preliminary results do not show any significant differences in sustained relapse-free outcome. We have to await further analyses of these studies and the results of other ongoing studies before the role of the nicohaler in smoking cessation can be fully determined.

Nicotine nasal spray (NNS)

The NNS consists of a multidose, hand-driven pump spray with nicotine solution. Each puff contains 0.5 mg nicotine; thus, a 1-mg dose is delivered if both nostrils are sprayed as recommended. The NNS is a strong and very fast way to deliver nicotine into the human body, and its pharmacokinetic profile approximates cigarettes very closely. After a single NNS dose of 1 mg nicotine, the peak plasma level is reached within 5 to 10 minutes, with average plasma levels of 16 ng/ml.

Only one study has been published that used the NNS [48]. In this double-blind study, 227 smokers were allocated placebo or active NNS for three months, in combination with six supportive group sessions during the first month. The success rates after three months were 41% for the active and 17% for the placebo NNS and after one year were 26% for the active and 10% for the placebo NNS. Nicotine substitution with the NNS was 40% after one month, but 79% in the long-term users after one year. During use of the NNS, weight gain was reduced as compared with placebo.

This strong spray induces irritative side effects locally, such as sneezing, nasal secretion and irritation, blocked nose, watering eyes, and coughing. Up to 5% of subjects will rate these side effects unacceptable; however, most symptoms will decrease after a few days' use of the spray.

The NNS seems to be effective but difficult to use as a primary tool. Highly nicotine-dependent smokers might be the target goup for this nicotine-delivery method. Also, we have to await further trials with the NNS before its role can be determined.

Nicotine combinations

Laboratory studies have shown that the combination of nicotine gum and patch might affect withdrawal symptoms to the same extent that smoking does [49]. Thus, combinations of different nicotine-delivery methods should be tested in the clinic to see if they improve outcome further.

Use of the nicotine patch as a "basal" nicotine supplier combined with the use of 4 to 6 pieces of nicotine chewing gum during the day whenever needed seems to be safe and effective in daily clinical practice.

Adjunctive therapy

In the above studies, varying degrees of psychological or behavioral therapy have been used as adjunctive therapy. Very few well-controlled studies have examined behavioral therapy per se, and abstinence is not biochemically verified in most of these studies. Aversive procedures (rapid smoking, satiation smoking, nicotine fading) seem to work, with one-year quit rates of 21%–35% (range, 6%–63%).

The U.S. Surgeon General's report [2] concerning nicotine addiction draws the following conclusions about the treatment of tobacco dependence:
1. Tobacco dependence can be treated successfully.
2. Effective interventions include behavioral approaches alone and behavioral approaches with adjunctive pharmacologic treatment (i.e., nicotine).
3. Behavioral interventions are most effective when they include multiple components (procedures such as aversive smoking, skills training, group support, and self-reward). Inclusion of too many treatment procedures can lead to less successful outcomes.
4. Nicotine replacement can reduce tobacco withdrawal symptoms and may enhance the efficacy of behavioral treatment.

Weight gain

A chapter about smoking cessaton would not be complete without a note on weight gain. Many or most smokers gain about 3–5 kg in weight in the first 12 months after quitting.

Nicotine suppresses appetite and increases metabolic rate, probably through release of chatecholamines and other hormones [50,51]. However, nicotine gum, patch, and vaporizer did not prevent weight gain in most studies — which is not unexpected, since cotinine substitution was low and the plasma nicotine curve was flat.

The NNS decreased postcessaton weight gain after one year from 5.8 kg (placebo) to 3.0 kg in 12-month users of active spray [48]. In subjects who stopped using the active spray, the weight gain was 5.5 kg — similar to the placebo group. The high nicotine substitution (i.e., 79% of the smoking level) and the fast and high nicotine peaks in plasma that were reached with the nasal spray might fully explain the preventive effect on weight gain with the nasal spray and the lack of effect with the other modes of administering nicotine.

A two-step approach to weight gain seems to work well for many smokers. First, quit smoking and accept a weight gain. When the smoking habit is broken after 6 to 12 months, then diet and/or exercise as needed to reduce weight.

Recommendations and future goals

When you face a smoker, you have to think of smoking as a disease. As usual, the disease should be classified. How motivated to stop is the smoker? What about his self-confidence and determination? And how dependent is he?

Nicotine dependence should be scored. The most simple method is to

Table 6. Different nicotine delivery systems for smoking cessation

	System			
	Patch	Gum	Vaporizer	Nasal spray
Dosing	Fixed	Ad lib	Ad lib	Ad lib
Dose	Low	Low/medium	Low	High
Fast peak concent.	0	+	+?	+++
Clinical trials	+++	+++	+	+
Abuse potential	Low	Moderate	Low	High (?)
Ease of use	Easy	——Intermittent——		Difficult
First line	Yes	Yes	Yes?	No

determine the number of cigarettes smoked daily and the time to the first cigarette in the morning. The best method is the Fagerström Questionnaire. Carbon monoxide in expired air should be measured, as well as plasma (saliva) nicotine and cotinine. All laboratories should be able to perform nicotine and cotinine analysis; then it would be possible to adjust nicotine substitution on an individual basis.

The four different modes to administer nicotine, i.e., gum, patch, nasal spray, and nebulizer, are compared in table 6.

The nicotine patch seems to be the first choice today due to its ease of use. The more dependent the smoker, the greater is the need for nicotine during the quitting period. The highly dependent smoker should use 4-mg nicotine gum, and others the 2-mg nicotine gum or the nicotine patch. The duration of treatment should be 2 to 3 months, but if neccesary even a year or more. And treatment should include three steps: 1) set a quit day, 2) tell the smoker to quit cigarettes completely at entry, and 3) arrange at least 1 or 2 follow-up visits. Nicotine substitution, the gold standard today, should be prescribed initially.

In the future, many different methods of nicotine administration will probably become available. The results of many clinical trials in the smoking cessation field will be published in the next few years. The pharmacological treatment to be used in smoking cessation might turn out to be more complicated for the physician. However, a more optimal nicotine substitution for smokers might become available, and this might enhance outcome in smoking cessation programs. Smoking should be considered as a chronic disease to be treated by physicians, specialists, general practitioners, and other health workers. The treatment today consists of nicotine substitution; however, it might prove valuable not to consider this substitution as a one-shot treatment, but to try repeated treatments if the smoker fails to quit smoking the first time. We must treat smokers, because even though smoking is a common, treatable epidemic and pandemic disorder, it still kills one person every 13 seconds worldwide.

References

1. U.S. Surgeon General. 1990. The Health Benefits of Smoking Cessation. U.S. Department of Health and Human Services, Rockville, MD.
2. U.S. Surgeon General. 1988. The health consequences of smoking: Nicotine addiction. U.S.Department of Health and Human Services, Rockville, MD.
3. Fagerström KO, Heatherton TF, Kozlowski LT. 1991. Nicotine addiction and its assessment. Ear Nose Throat J 69:763–768.
4. Fisher EB, Bishop DB, Goldmuntz J, Jacobs A. 1988. Implications for the practicing physician of the psychosocial dimensions of smoking. Chest 93(2):69S–78S.
5. Lando HA, McGovern PG, Barrios FX, Etringer BD. 1990. Comparative evaluation of American Cancer Society and American Lung Association smoking cessation clinics. Am J Public Health 80:554–559.
6. Prochaska JO, DiClemente CC. 1983. Stages and processes of self-change of smoking: toward an integrative model of change. J Consult Clin Psych 51:390–395.
7. Corrigall WA. 1991. Understanding brain mechanisms in nicotine reinforcement. Br J Addict 86:507–510.
8. Benowitz NL. 1986. The human pharmacology of nicotine. In Research Advances in Alcohol and Drug Problems, HD Cappel et al. (eds.). Plenum Press: New York, pp. 1–52.
9. American Psychiatric Association. 1987. Diagnostic and Statistical Manual of Mental Disorders (third edition). American Psychiatric Association.
10. Benowitz NL. 1988. Toxicity of nicotine: Implications with regard to nicotine replacement tharapy. In Nicotine Replacement: A Critical Evaluation, Of Pomerleau and CS Pomerleau (eds.). Alan R. Liss: New York, pp. 187–218.
11. McNabb ME, Ebert RV, McCusker K. 1982. Plasma nicotine levels produced by chewing nicotine gum. JAMA 248:865–868.
12. McNabb ME. 1984. Chewing nicotine gum for 3 months: What happens to plasma nicotine levels? Can Med Assoc J 131:589–592.
13. Tønnesen P, Fryd V, Hansen M, Helsted J, Gunnersen AB, Forchammer H, Stockner M. 1988. Two and four mg nicotine chewing gum and group counseling in smoking cessation: An open, randomized, controlled trial with a 22 month follow-up. Addict Behav 13:17–27.
14. Malcolm RE, Sillett RW, Turner JAMcM, Ball KP. 1980. The use of nicotine chewing gum as an aid to stopping smoking. Psychopharmacologia 70:295–296.
15. Fee WM, Stewart MJ. 1982. A controlled trial of nicotine chewing gum in a smoking withdrawal clinic. Practitioner 226:148–151.
16. Fagerström KO. 1982. A comparison of psychological and pharmacological treatment in smoking cessation. J Behav Med 5:343–351.
17. Jarvis MJ, Raw M, Russell MAH, Feyerabend C. 1982. Randomised controlled trial of nicotine chewing-gum. Br Med J 285:537–540.
18. Schneider NG, Jarvik ME, Forsythe AB, Read LL, Elliot ME, Schweiger A. 1983. Nicotine gum in smoking cessation: A placebo-controlled, double-blind trial. Addict Behav 8:253–261.
19. British Thoracic Society. 1983. Comparison of four methods of smoking withdrawal in patients with smoking related diseases. Br J Med 286:595–597.
20. Christen AG, McDonald JL, Olson BL, Drook CA, Stookey GK. 1984. Efficacy of nicotine chewing gum in facilitating smoking cessation. JADA 106:594–597.
21. Hjalmarson AIM. 1984. Effect of nicotine chewing gum in smoking cessation: A randomized, placebo-controlled, double-blind study. JAMA 252:2835–2838.
22. Jamrozik K, Fowler G, Vessey M, Wald N. 1984. Placebo controlled trial of nicotine chewing gum in general medical practice. Br Med J 289:794–797.
23. Hall SM, Tunstall CD, Ginsberg D, Benowitz NL, Jones RT. 1987. Nicotine gum and behavioral treatment: a placebo controlled trial. J Consult Clin Psych 55:603–605.
24. Fortmann SP, Killen JD, Telch MJ, Newmann B. 1988. Minimal contact treatment for smoking cessation. JAMA 260:1575–1580.

25. Hughes JR, Gust SW, Keenan RM, Fenwick JW, Healey ML. 1989. Nicotine vs placebo gum in general medical practice. JAMA 261:1300–1305.

26. Tønnesen P, Fryd V, Hansen M, Helsted J, Gunnersen AB, Forchammer H, Stockner M. 1988. Effect of nicotine chewing gum in combination with group counseling on the cessaption of smoking. N Engl J Med 318:15–18.

27. Puska P, Bjorkqvist S, Koskela K. 1979. Nicotine containing chewing gum in smoking cessation: A double-blind trial with half year follow-up. Addict Behav 4:141–146.

28. Blöndal T. 1989. Controlled trial of nicotine polacrilex gum with supportive measures. Arch Intern Med 149:1818–1821.

29. Kornitzer M, Kittel F, Draimaix M, Bourdoux P. 1987. A double-blind study of 2 mg versus 4 mg nicotine gum in an industrial setting. J Psychosomat Res 31:171–176.

30. Killen JD, Fortmann SP, Newman B, Varady A. 1990. Evaluation of a treatment approach combining nicotine gum with self-guided behavioral treatments for smoking relapse prevention. J Consult Clin Psych 58:85–92.

31. Hughes JR, Gust SW, Keenan R, Fenwick JW, Skoog K, Higgins ST. 1991. Long-term use of nicotine vs placebo gum. Arch Intern Med 151:1993–1998.

32. Fagerström KO, Säwe U, Tønnesen P. 1992. Therapeutic use of nicotine patches: Efficacy and safety. J Smok Rel Dis 3:247–261.

33. Abelin T, Buehler A, Müller P, Vesanen K, Inhof FR. 1989. Controlled trial of transdermal nicotine patch in tobacco withdrawal. Lancet 1:7–10.

34. Abelin T, Ehrsam A, Buhler-Reichert A, et al. 1989. Effectiveness of a transdermal nicotine system in smoking cessation studies. Methods Find Exp Clin Pharmacol 11:205–214.

35. Buchkremer G, Bents M, Horstmann K, Opitz K, Tolle R. 1989. Combination of behavioral smoking cessation with transdermal nicotine substitution. Addict Behav 14:229–238.

36. Krumpe P, Malani N, Adler J, et al. 1989. Efficacy of transdermal nicotine administration as an adjunct for smoking cessation in heavily nicotine addicted smokers (abstract). Am Rev Respir Dis 139(Suppl A):337.

37. Mulligan SC, Masterson JG, Devane JG, Kelly JG. 1990. Clinical and pharmacokinetic properties of a transdermal nicotine patch. Clin Pharmacol Ther 47:331–337.

38. Rose J, Levin ED, Behm FM, Adivi C, Schur C. 1990. Transdermal nicotine facilitates smoking cessation. Clin Pharmacol Ther 47:323–330.

39. Hurt RD, Lauger GG, Offord KP, Kottke TE, Dale LC. 1990. Nicotine-replacement therapy with use of a transdermal nicotine patch — a randomized double-blind placebo-controlled trial. Mayo Clin Proc 65:1529–1537.

40. Tønnesen P, Nørregaard J, Simonsen K, Säwe U. 1991. A double-blind trial of a 16-hour transdermal nicotine patch in smoking cessation. N Engl J Med 325:311–315.

41. Sachs DPL, Sawe U, Simonsen K. 1991. Nicotine transdermal patch, smoking cessation and withdrawal symptoms control. Committee on Problems for Dependence Diseases, Annual Meeting, Florida, June.

42. Daughton DM, Heatley SA, Prendergast JJ, et al. 1991. Effect of transdermal nicotine delivery as an adjunct to low-intervention smoking cessation therapy. Arch Intern Med 151:749–752.

43. Transdermal Nicotine Study Group. 1991. Transdermal nicotine for smoking cessation. JAMA 22:3133–3138.

44. Russell MAH, Stableton JA, Feyerabend C, Wiserman SM, Gustavsson G, Säwe U, Connor P. 1993. Targeting heavy smokers in general practice: randomised controlled trial of transdermal nicotine patches. Br Med J 306:1308–1312.

45. Imperial Cancer Research Fund General Practice Research Group. 1993. Effectiveness of a nicotine patch in helping people to stop smoking: results of a randomised trial in general practice. Br Med J 306:1304–1308.

46. Fagerström KO, Lunnel E, Molander L. 1991. Continuous and intermittent transdermal

delivery of nicotine: blockade of withdrawal symptoms and side effects. J Smok Rel Dis 2:173–180.

47. Tønnesen P, Nørregaard J, Mikkelsen K, Jørgensen S, Nilsson F. 1993. A double-blind trial of a nicotine inhaler for smoking cessation. JAMA 269:1268–1271.

48. Sutherland G, Stapleton JA, Russell MAH, Jarvis MJ, Hajek P, Belcher M, Feyerabend C. 1992. Randomised controlled trial of a nasal nicotine spray in smoking cessation. Lancet 340:324–329.

49. Fagerström KO, Schneider NG, Lunnel E. 1993. Effectiveness of nicotine patch and nicotine gum as individual versus combined treatment for tobacco withdrawal symptoms. Psychopharmacology 110:251–257.

50. Grunberg NE. 1989. Cigarette smoking and body weight. Current perspective and future directions. Ann Behav Med 11(4):154–157.

51. Leisckow SJ, Stitzer ML. 1991. Smoking cessation and weight gain. Br J Addic 86:577–581.

4. Genetics of lung cancer: Implications for early detection and prevention

Sudhir Srivastava and Barnett S. Kramer

Introduction

The development of most cancers is a multistep process involving a series of histopathological, biological, molecular, and genetic changes [1–3]. Not until recently has lung cancer also been shown to be the end result of an accumulated series of molecular, biochemical, and epigenetic changes involving the activation of dominant-acting cellular proto-oncogenes and the inactivation (chromosomal deletion) of recessive or 'tumor suppressor genes. Knowledge of the molecular etiology of human lung cancer has now reached a stage where it may soon have a potential impact on early detection and prevention.

Several environmental and xenobiotic substances have been associated with lung cancer, and smoking has been found to have a significant impact on the cause of human lung cancer [4]. Consequently, current prevention strategies appropriately focus on these agents or factors. Although the cessation of smoking at population levels should be included in prevention strategy, progress in the prevention of lung cancer mortality may additionally require early detection using more refined understanding of genetics and the molecular pathology of lung cancer. In this chapter, we review the genetic basis of lung neoplasia and its potential applications in early detection and prevention of human lung cancer.

Historical perspectives

The biology of preneoplasia has yet to be defined. What constitutes early detection will depend on what is detected. In the past and also today, the accuracy of prediction of biologic behavior has rested upon the pathologist's experience, his or her general judgment, and available detection technology. The limiting factor in this approach is that in most cases patients are brought to a physician's attention when the tumor has already grown in size and has a substantial metastatic potential; therefore, the patient is unlikely to benefit from existing routine methods of detection. What we really need is to detect

Heine H. Hansen, (ed), Hansen: Lung Cancer.
© *1994 Kluwer Academic Publishers. ISBN 0-7923-2835-3. All rights reserved.*

tumors before their clinical manifestations, i.e., early detection should focus on a preclinical stage of the cancer, known by various terminologies discussed below.

The definition of the early lesion has evolved over the years. The term *incipient* refers to morphologic lesions. It is synonymous with *pre-neoplasia*, a term in use for several decades. Precancerous conditions represent clinical states that are associated with a higher risk of cancer than seen on average in the population.

The term *incipient* or *precancer* does not imply that cancer is inevitable. The term, at best, refers to certain well-defined histologic changes that increase the probability or risk for cancer. Although the risk varies in different age groups, in different races, with different lesions, and with other factors, the term alerts us to the fact that cancer can be the final eventuality. The term *precancer* is ambiguous and therefore less appealing than *incipient*. Precancer gives the impression that cancer is surely or extremely likely to follow.

Incipient lesions are part of dynamic and evolving processes, but many of our concepts about early cancer are defined in terms of static histology. Historically, neoplastic diseases have been studied from the end to the beginning, which, according to Foulds [1], has encouraged a backward way of thinking about cancer. It is uncertain at which point the critical neoplastic change is reached or at what point it is no longer reversible [5]. It is generally believed that these lesions follow the sequence from hyperplasia through dysplasia to in situ carcinoma. However, some processes not only deviate from an ordered sequence, but are also reversible — for example, stomach endocrine cell hyperplasia [6].

Incipient neoplasia is conceptually the borderline entity that separates normal tissue from invasive cancer. Invasive cancer has a relatively predictable outcome, whereas the outcome of an incipient lesion is often difficult to predict. Therefore, studies should focus on this stage of the development of cancer to provide a better understanding of its mechanisms of development, mechanisms of progression, and biological manifestations, such as dedifferentiation and genetic instability.

Also falling into this area of incipient neoplasia is the concept of minimal cancer. Originally introduced for small breast cancers less than 0.5 cm, this concept nonetheless expresses uncertainty about the behavior and treatment of small cancers as well as in situ lesions. In the liver, cancers less than 2–3 cm are considered 'small.' In the lung, certain small neoplasms are designated as 'tumorlets.' In the kidney, tumors less than 2–3 cm have been designated as benign adenomas. The term *minimal* as applied to small carcinomas is vague and even misleading because it can refer to either size or behavior or both. It would be ideal to replace vague terms with more precise terminology that clearly refers to the biologic potential and not to appearance, size, or other descriptive characteristics.

A simplistic schematic model of lung carcinoma representing temporal

92

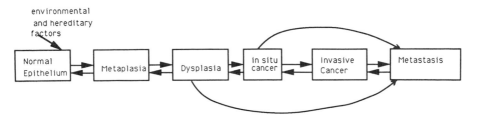

Figure 1. A schematic representation of the pathogenesis in lung cancer. The model is inspired from a comparable model proposed for colon tumorigenesis [38].

changes during progression is presented in figure 1. From a theoretical viewpoint, we propose a pre-neoplastic stage as a potential target for early detection and prevention based on known early molecular and genetic events in lung cancer. In this scheme, each step beginning with metaplasia and ending with cancer represents a hypothetical sequence.

In this model, metaplastic and/or dysplastic cells are considered *precancerous stages*. We define this as a state in which growth is temporally restricted and confined to the anatomic point of origin. The lesion may grow for a while, and then stop or grow slowly, or even regress. For example, during squamous carcinogenesis, metaplasia of squamous cells may represent a precancerous stage. The lesion may or may not grow to become cancerous. It may regress spontaneously. On the other hand, an in situ cancer has greater potential for progression, regresses less frequently, and has the ability to evolve into a fully developed primary cancer acquiring invasive properties.

Genetics of lung cancer

Tumor types

Human lung cancer is a disease of heterogeneous histologies. The World Health Organization groups lung cancers into two major categories: small cell lung cancer (SCLC) and non-small cell lung cancer (NSCLC). SCLC accounts for 20% to 25% of all new cases of lung cancer worldwide. The remaining 75% to 80% fall into the following major types of NSCLC carcinomas: squamous cell carcinoma (SCC), adenocarcinoma, large cell carcinoma (LCC), and infrequently found carcinoids. SCC, also called epidermoid carcinoma, arises from the dysplastic epithelium of the larger, proximal airways. Adenocarcinomas frequently develop in the epithelium of peripheral airways and alveoli. The definition of LCC is sometimes unclear and may include some different types of non-small cell carcinomas, such as poorly differentiated adenocarcinomas, SCCs, or even neuroendocrine

93

tumors. SCLC is an aggressive type of tumor that is nearly always metastatic at the time of clinical presentation. The cells appear to have scant cytoplasm with neuroendocrine properties. Although these types of lung cancers vary in their histology, they appear to share many common genetic events, as described below.

Oncogenes

Two major findings have emerged from the study of the genetic events occurring in human lung cancer: 1) the involvement of dominant cellular proto-oncogenes, and 2) the mutation or chromosomal deletion of recessive or 'anti-oncogenes' or 'tumor suppressor' genes [7–11].

Three well-characterized *ras* genes have been reported: Harvey-ras (H-*ras*), Kirsten-ras (K-*ras*), and neuroblastoma-RAS (N-*ras*). Several articles have appeared in the past on abnormalities of *ras* genes in lung cancer [7,8]. In general, findings reported in literature suggest an important relationship between lung cancer and the following factors: 1) mutations in the K-*ras* oncogene [7] and *p53* tumor suppressor gene [8–11], 2) expression of cell surface tumor antigens shown to be associated with lung cancer [12–15], 3) abnormalities in epidermal growth factor receptors (EGFRs) [16–18], and 4) markers of squamous differentiation in bronchial cells [19].

Frequent mutations in both *p53* and K-*ras* genes occur in lung cancer. The product of the *p53* gene is a 53-kDa phosphoprotein that negatively regulates cell growth and thus inhibits cell proliferation [20]. Somatic *p53* mutations have been frequently found in fresh tissues and cell lines from both SCLC and NSCLC [8,9]. Activating mutations in the *ras* family of proto-oncogenes occur frequently in many types of human cancer. These oncogenes code for 21-kDa guanine nucleotide-binding proteins that are believed to be involved in transduction of growth signals. These proteins have transforming potential when a substitution of amino acid at position 12, 13, or 61 occurs. It has been shown that a point mutation in codon 12 is present in about one third of human lung adenocarcinomas [7]. High incidence of K-*ras* mutations have been seen in other adenocarcinomas, including those of the pancreas and colon [21].

It has been reported recently [7,22] that for both *ras* and *p53* in NSCLC, G:C to T:A transversions are the most common changes. Twelve of 16 (75%) codon 12 or 13 K-*ras* changes in NSCLC were transversions [7,22], and 23 of 30 (77%) *p53* mutations in NSCLC were transversions [7,22]. It is not clear how early in the process of carcinogenesis these mutations occur in bronchial epithelial cells or how many mutations accumulate in one epithelial cell during the process of malignant transformation. The retinoblastoma (*rb*) gene has been found to be deleted in 10% to 20% of NSCLC [23,24] and most SCLCs.

Several types of dominant cellular proto-oncogenes other than *ras* have been found to be mutated and/or deregulated in lung cancer. The c-*jun*

94

proto-oncogene, which is part of the AP-1 complex and thus is intimately involved in the regulation of transcriptional responses to growth stimuli, is deregulated and constitutively expressed in SCLC and NSCLC cell lines [25]. c-*myb* is a nuclear oncogene that has been found to be overexpressed in some lung cancer cell lines [26]. The c-*raf* proto-oncogene, located on the short arm of the chromosome 3p at locus 3p25, encodes a cytoplasmic serine threonine protein kinase involved in the signal transduction of mitogenic pathways and is partially deleted in a majority of SCLC cancers [27]. It is postulated that the terminal deletion of the 3p may activate the c-*raf-1* gene and may cause tumor susceptibility [27]. The specific roles of c-*raf* and c-*myb* genes in tumorigenesis, other than those described above, are not clear. The c-*jun* could, however, cause transformation and/or disrupt signal transduction for differentiation in conjunction with c-*fos* and other proto-oncogenes.

Uncontrolled or poorly controlled proliferation is intimately associated with the genesis of many tumors. Molecular alterations that are associated with this uncontrolled growth may, in part, be mediated through autocrine mechanisms. Several oncogenes encode growth factors or receptors for growth factors. c-*erB-1* encodes the EGFR and c-*erB-2*, also called *Her-2/neu*, encodes a protein homologous with EGF-like receptor function. EGFRs have been found on NSCLC [16]. Overexpression of EGFR has been reported in SCC [17] as have structural alterations of EGFR in NSCLC [18].

In summary, although altered or activated oncogenes are detected in lung cancer, it is unlikely that a single oncogene or factor can cause all lung cancers. It is, therefore, to be noted that the activation of any specific oncogene is but one event in the cascade of tumorigenesis that increases the risk for abnormal cell growth and malignancy. Rather, multiple molecular mechanisms for the activation of oncogenes and inhibition of tumor suppressor genes may generate a complex interplay of regulatory controls of cell growth.

Tumor suppressor genes

Tumor suppressor genes or *anti-oncogenes* exert a negative regulatory role on cell growth, and their mutation may facilitate the development of malignancy. Two major tumor suppressor genes, *p53* and *rb*, described earlier, have been implicated in lung cancer [7,9]. The tumor suppressor genes act in a recessive fashion. The mutant *p53* complexes with the wild-type protein to form an inactive complex causing tumor progression by a dominant negative effect. Further loss of wild-type allele may result in loss of growth control leading to tumor progression, as has been shown in colorectal cancer [9,11]. A germline mutation of one allele could be inherited in a heterozygous Mendelian fashion. The heterozygous carrier could be at higher risk of cancer caused by a mutation in the second normal allele through environmental insult or carcinogens. From a screening and prevention viewpoint, these alleles could be ideal targets because they may allow identification of a particularly high-risk group. Efforts should be made to identify a factor or factors that induce(s) mutations in a second normal allele and to identify germline mutations that predispose to various forms of cancers. We discuss other aspects of genetic predisposition in the following section.

Genetic and environmental interactions

Family studies

The effect of environmental exposure on the incidence of lung cancer has been well described by Doll and Peto [28]. However, risks attributable to environment, mainly tobacco consumption, are also influenced by interindividual differences in susceptibility to environmental exposure [29]. For example, less than 20% of heavy cigarette smokers develop lung cancer [30]. How much of a role a gene, either inherited or somatically mutated, plays in acquired susceptibility was a subject of a recent case–control study conducted in parishes (counties) of Louisiana. Over 50% of the counties in Louisiana rank in the top 10% nationally in terms of lung cancer mortality rates [31]. To investigate the role of genetic predisposition as a contributing factor, 337 case families and 304 control families were recruited in the study. Members of the case families were reported to have a 2.4-fold higher odds ratio of lung cancer than that of the control families [32]. Sellers et al. [33] performed a segregation analysis, using age at onset and the effect of smoking as variables, and found that the pattern of lung cancer in these families could best be explained by Mendelian inheritance of a major autosomal gene that produces earlier age of onset.

There is additional evidence that some of the genetic mutations involved in the pathogenesis of lung cancer may be inherited in a Mendelian fashion [34]. Historically, tumor suppressor genes appear to be good candidates, since the first one discovered, rb, had already been linked to retinoblastoma. Retinoblastoma is a rare childhood cancer that has been the paradigm of inherited neoplasia [35]. The rb has also been found to be associated with SCLC [23,24]. In a recent study, it was reported that the relatives of people with retinoblastoma had a 15-fold increased risk of lung cancer, particularly SCLC [35]. Germline mutations in five families with the Li–Fraumeni familial cancer syndrome, an inherited heterozygous inactivation of the p53 tumor suppressor gene, have been reported. However, the incidence of lung cancer in these patients has not been reported [36,37]. Whether there is a single gene or a cluster of genes disposing patients to cancer is unclear. To date, there has been no report of inherited mutations in dominant oncogenes.

Detection and screening

Compared to colon cancer, a linear array of histopathologic and molecular changes in human lung cancer is less well delineated. The reasons for this have been primarily attributed to dificulty in obtaining tumor samples (biopsy) at varying stages. However, a colorectal model proposed by Fearon and Vogelstein [38] may have relevance to other tumor types, including lung cancer. A comparable multistage sequence of molecular events has been proposed for lung cancer [39]. Broadly, the stages are divided into the following: 1) *Exposure*: A subject is exposed to environmental injury including carcinogens, and, depending on background genotype and metabolic phenotype, the effect of the exposure could be enhanced. 2) *Preproliferative stage*: In response to carcinogen exposure, production of certain growth factors by neuroendocrine cells of the lung is initiated/enhanced. 3) *Proliferative stage*: In this stage, paracrine growth of bronchial epithelial cells is stimulated, and this continued growth could lead to focal cellular proliferation, which is normally benign. 4) *Induction and promotion*: This stage could involve several chromosomal abnormalities occurring in dividing bronchial epithelial cells, abnormalities (developed somatically or inherited) in recessive oncogenes, *p53*, and epigenetic changes, comprising constitutive activation of proto-oncogenes of the *myc* family, the *ras* family, c-*jun*, c-*raf*, and other nuclear-acting genes. Oncogene mutations involving growth factor or growth factor receptors may also occur. Present evidence favors a multistage mechanism in lung cancer as well. It should, however, be noted that present understanding of early events in lung cancer has largely originated from studies on animals [40,41].

The association of these molecular steps with a specific stage of clinical progression in lung tumor is not well delineated. Also, there is no single event that has been shown to account for the development of lung tumors. As Fearon and Vogelstein postulate [38], it may be the accumulation rather

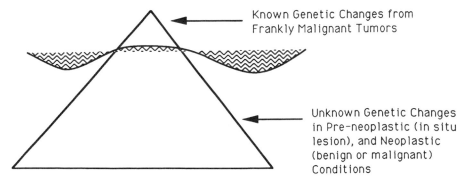

Known Genetic Changes from Frankly Malignant Tumors

Unknown Genetic Changes in Pre-neoplastic (in situ lesion), and Neoplastic (benign or malignant) Conditions

Figure 2. Iceberg of cancer. The pyramid shows the extent of known and unknown genetic events in pathogenesis of lung cancer.

than any fixed order of events that is responsible for tumorigenesis. The study of chronology of events in the molecular paradigm is in its infancy. Looking at many of the known genetic changes arising from studies focusing on the late phase of the cancer is like looking at the tip of an iceberg (figure 2). Studies of frankly malignant and invasive tissues constitute only a small proportion of this iceberg of pathogenesis. Many of the genetic changes represent late events in human lung tumorigenesis and therefore are most appropriate for monitoring the invasiveness and metastatic properties of a tumor. However, the majority of genetic changes (a large portion of the iceberg) occurring in the early phase of the cancerous cells remains unknown. Molecular detection approaches would require studies on the genetic characteristics of tumors before they acquire metastatic potential. Meaningful chemoprevention of lung cancer can only be accomplished if we succeed in identifying a *precursor stage* or premalignant stage, and if we are able to identify a high-risk population for intervention at the cellular level using biologic and molecular markers.

Potential implications for early detection and screening

By documenting molecular and biochemical alterations in a tumorigenesis cascade in human tissues, one could conceivably assess the risk and detect the preclinical stage of a developing tumor. In the following section, we will discuss the biomarkers of early lung cancer, including DNA or protein adducts in assessing risk of lung cancer, and surrogate markers (intermediate endpoints) for measuring the efficacy of prevention interventions.

Biomarkers

In a disease continuum from exposure to premalignant phase, to malignant phase, and finally to a fully developed cancer (figure 3), a biomarker could provide a target for early detection and intervention strategies. This is particularly true in the case of human lung cancer, where a major portion of cases are attributable to environmental factors and many of the early molecular events presumably occur in cells at the epithelial surface and are therefore subject to frequent sampling. In our discussion, a biomarker represents an event that signals an occurrence of one or more biologic processes: 1) *biomarkers of susceptibility*, which measure internal biologic states independent of exposure, e.g., sensitivity of chromosomes to breakage; 2) *biomarkers of exposure*, which measure the presence or concentration of specific environmental agents in a biological sample (blood levels of cotinine, a nicotine metabolite, polycyclic aromatic hydrocarbon–DNA adducts); 3) *biomarkers of biological effects* from exposure, which measure biological changes or damage resulting from exposure, e.g., chromosome breakage resulting from radiation or chemical carcinogen exposure; and 4)

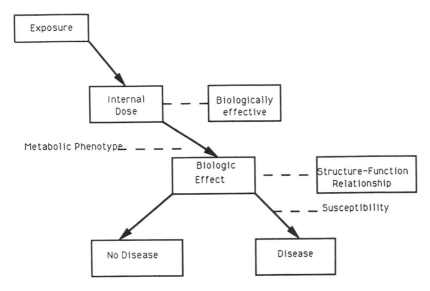

Figure 3. A model for the exposure–disease continuum. The concept is adapted from the work published by Schulte [50].

biomarkers of disease progression, which measure or predict the outcome of interest and reflect the probability of specific clinical outcomes (e.g., invasion, metastasis, recurrence, or death) in the presence of disease. Some markers may function as biomarkers of susceptibility in individuals who have not yet developed a cancer. The distinction between an early cancer detection marker and a cancer risk biomarker is sometimes arbitrary. An effective early detection marker achieves benefit by creating lead time. Lead time is the duration between detection through screening and clinical detection using customary medical practice. A greater lead time may, but does not necessarily, offer the opportunity to favorably impact on mortality. An effective early detection marker must lead to the detection of cancer before the appearance of clinical signs or symptoms. In contrast, a risk or susceptibility biomarker distinguishes individuals at high risk of disease. The amount of lead time produced through its application determines whether a particular biomarker functions more like an early detection marker or a susceptibility marker. Therefore, the uses of such markers in cancer detection and in cancer prevention cannot be separated. Unfortunately, there is no single accurate marker for the earliest phases of lung cancer known to date. However, there are some epigenetic and mutational changes that have potential for use in identifying high-risk populations and early lung cancer. A number of markers listed for various forms of lung cancer (tables 1 and 2) may eventually prove to be of value in the screening and detection of lung cancer.

Table 1. Molecular markers of lung cancer

Tumor type	Marker	Comments
SCLC	*myc* family	Amplification, overexpression
	jun	Expression
	c-*myb*	Amplification, overexpression
	c-*raf-1*	Overexpression, amplification
Adenocarcinoma	K-*ras*	Amplification, point mutation
NSCLC	*myc* family	Amplification, overexpression
	ras family	Frequency of *ras* family
	Erb B-1	involvement is low
	Erb B-2	Expression, amplification
	(Her 2/neu)	Amplification

Table 2. Tumor suppressor genes in lung cancer

Tumor type	Marker	Comments
SCLC	*rb*	Located on chromosome 13q
	p53	Located on chromosome 17p
		Loss of heterozygosity (LOH) frequently reported for short arm (p)
	DCC	Located on chromosome 18, antibodies to a related protein react with SCLC
NSCLC	*p53*	Located on chromosome 17p

Oncogenes and tumor suppressor genes as molecular markers

Increased expression and also structural abnormalities of the *ras* family gene have been detected in a variety of lung cancers. About 30% of adenocarcinomas of the lung have activated *ras* genes. Polymerase chain reaction (PCR) has been used to identify point mutations in K-*ras* in NSCLC [42]. Primary NSCLCs with K-*ras* mutations have been shown to be smaller with a lower metastatic potential than tumors without *ras* mutations [43]. If the presence of K-*ras* can be confirmed as a good prognostic indicator, it may be used to plan prevention strategies in certain groups, such as smokers, where a strong correlation between the incidence of mutations and smoking habits has been reported [43].

Several allelic forms of H-*ras* have been shown to be genetic markers of lung cancer [44]. Using restriction fragment length polymorphism (RFLP) analysis, four common alleles have been identified along with a number of rarer alleles. An abnormal allele distribution is present in aggressive NSCLCs compared to normal lung cells or SCLCs, suggesting a degree of association between the abnormal allele distribution and the aggressive behavior of NSCLCs. RFLP analysis of H-*ras* therefore could be utilized in determining predisposition to the aggressive forms of NSCLC for patient management [44].

The *Her-2/neu* gene has been found to be overexpressed in a subset of NSCLCs [45]. High titered antibody has been used to detect the overexpression in tissues or cells [45]. A systematic study of the overexpression of the *Her-2/neu* in preneoplastic, metaplastic, or dysplastic cells of lung from sputum using the antibody approach may help identify usefulness of the *Her-2/neu* as a genetic marker for lung cancer.

Mutational alterations also involve tumor suppressor genes, *p53* and *rb*, that could have utility in identifying a high-risk population. The *rb* gene has been found mutated in nearly all SCLCs [23,24]. Mutation in the *p53* gene has been reported in the majority of SCLCs and NSCLCs [9–11] and can be detected by using antisera made against the *p53* protein or by PCR amplification of the coding region and analysis by direct sequencing or single-stranded polymorphism analysis. The *p53* may be a better candidate gene for screening for early cancer than the *rb* gene, which is less frequently found in NSCLCs.

Chromosomal abnormalities could also be used as biomarkers of susceptibility. Abnormalities have been reported in chromosome numbers 3, 11, 13 and 17 in lung cancer, most often associated with tumor suppressor genes: *p53* at chromosome 17, *rb* on chromosome 13, and 'deleted in colon cancer' (DCC) on chromosome 18. Losses were found more frequently in SCC than in adenocarcinoma, and chromosome 17 losses were often accompanied by allelic DNA sequence losses on chromosome 11 [46]. Two loci were commonly deleted from chromosome 11 in adenocarcinoma, SCC, and LCC. Chromosome 3p deletions, as well as loss of heterozygosity for chromosomes 13 and 17, have also been reported in SCLC [47,48].

It is, however, to be noted that the use of changes in genes or products resulting from these genetic changes as biomarkers of premalignant or early cancer needs to be validated. A recent retrospective study of the Johns Hopkins Lung Project [12], using monoclonal antibody (Mb) staining of sputum cells collected as part of a randomized screening study of routine cytology, is encouraging. Mb against the SCLC and NSCLC determinants was able to stain 69 specimens that showed atypia in routine cytological examination. The sensitivity and specificity of the stain were 91% and 88%, respectively, for prediction of ultimate diagnosis of cancer an average of 24 months prior to diagnosis. This finding needs to be confirmed prospectively. Ideally, a two-arm randomized study encompassing one group without molecular screening and one with molecular screening would be required to see whether or not these markers are effective in reducing cancer mortality.

Carcinogenic adducts

Although carcinogenic adducts may not lend themselves as markers of early cancer, they could signal the susceptibility of hosts to potential carcinogens, and thereby a predispositin to cancer. In contrast to genetic changes, carcinogen–DNA and –protein adducts appear well before the clinical manifestation of a disease and therefore could provide a lead time suitable for disease prevention.

Carcinogen–DNA adducts have been widely studied in lung cancer and are thought to have implications in the molecular epidemiologic study of lung cancer. Since the majority of lung cancers are caused by cigarette and by environmental factors, adducts of various types are formed. A clear pattern of interaction between heredity and environment emerges from adduct studies. The p-aminohippurate (PAH)–DNA adduct is one of the most widely reported examples of carcinogen–DNA adducts in lung cancer [49]. A variety of markers have been found to be associated with environmental exposure. These include adducts formed by a number of inhaled pollutants, including PAH, nitrosamine, 4-aminobiphenyl, ethylene, oxide, and styrene. It is now possible to detect a single xenobiotic–DNA adduct, such as benzpyrene–DNA, per 10^{10} nucleotide bases [50]. Such biomarkers could potentially be used in epidemiologic studies of lung cancer risk factors to reduce misclassification error of exposed vs. nonexposed study subjects. For example, increased benzpyrene–DNA adducts have been found in individuals who develop cancers at an early age and in first-degree relatives of lung cancer patients [51]. Likewise, smokers with slow acetylator phenotype have higher levels of 4-aminobiphenyl-hemoglobin adducts than smokers with fast acetylator phenotype [52]. There are, however, formidable problems in distinguishing risk at the level of the individual. In order to use these adducts as markers for early diagnosis, the range of normal would have to be known, and the correlation between the number or placement of critical carcinogen adducts and the biological outcomes would have to be defined. At this time, adducts may be useful as a risk biomarker at the population level, but not at the individual level.

Metabolic phenotypes

There has been considerable interest in certain metabolic and detoxifying phenotypes because they provide an opportunity to understand the mechanism of susceptibility at the individual level. It is believed that many carcinogens or mutagens require conversion to active forms before inflicting damage on the host. Individuals differ in their ability to activate potential carcinogens, and thus the extent of biologic effects of carcinogens may vary among individuals. Metabolic phenotypes such as aryl hydrocarbon hydroxylase (AHH) activity, debrisoquine hydroxylation, and glutathione-S-transferase activity have been considered as possible markers of genetic susceptibility to lung cancer [49]. For example, the rapid metabolizer pheno-type for debrisoquine by a P-450 isozyme that also participates in oxidation of the cigarette carcinogens PAH and nitrosamine has been associated with a greater risk of cancer in smokers and in males with a history of workplace exposure to lung carcinogens [52].

All these metabolic studies have identified various phenotypes rather than genotypes. Therefore, these findings cannot yet easily be applied to scre-ening, because the specific marker for the genotype has not yet been charac-terized. There are considerable biases in phenotypic studies, since metabolic effects could be produced by drugs, changes in diet or smoking, or biologic effects of cancer itself [53]. Another type of susceptibility marker is DNA repair capacity, which is known to vary significantly among individuals [54]. A commonly used assay is to measure DNA repair in lymphocytes exposed in vitro to a mutagen or a carcinogen. With recent technology, it has become possible to measure the expression of a DNA repair gene in human tissues. These measurements may shed light on inherent predisposition of a host to cancer and ability to face environmental challenges. Recently, Bondy et at. [55] conducted a study to establish an association between mutagen sensitivity and family history of cancer. The study included 108 patients who registered at the M.D. Anderson Cancer Center with histologically confirmed and previously untreated squamous cell carcinoma of the upper aerodigestive tract. The study revealed that patients who have defective DNA repair capability (measured through mutagen (bleomycin) sensitivity assays) are likely to belong to the families of first-degree relatives affected with cancer. Odds ratios (ORs) for association between the mutagen sensitivity and family history for cancer increased with the increased number of first-degree relatives affected with cancer, e.g., an OR of 2.63 with one first-degree relative and 6.59 with two or more first-degree relatives.

Targets for primary prevention

Proven methods are already available to prevent lung cancer through behavioral interventions aimed at smoking cessation. Prevention at the molecular and genetic levels would require a better understanding of the progression of premalignant state (precursor state). Some approaches would be directed at preventing the premalignant state from developing into cancer and others at reversing the precursor state to the normal state.

Chemopreventive agents have already shown biologic efficacy in preven-ting cancers of the upper aerodigestive tract. There is evidence that these agents reduce some lesions at the precursor state or prevent a second primary cancer [56]. Hong and coworkers [56] reported a randomized con-trolled trial in which patients with completely resected head and neck cancer had a highly significant reduction in their rate of second new cancers after receiving a year of daily oral 13-*cis*-retinoic acid compared to placebo [56].

103

One of the most frequent sites of new primary cancer of head and neck cancer patients is the lung. Despite some problems of toxicity, this randomized trial has demonstrated the effectiveness of a 13-*cis*-retinoic acid as a chemopreventive agent. Preliminary data on the effect of some other chemopreventive agents, such as tamoxifen for breast cancer [57] and 13-*cis*-retinoic acid for upper aerodigestive cancers [58] have been very encouraging. The underlying mechanism for these agents is not clear. It has been hypothesized that the retinoic acid acts by accelerating differentiation and thus preventing progression to cancer of leukemia [59], but multiple possible mechanisms have been proposed [60]. This is an emerging area of research and would require intensive study of the chemopreventive agents in several neoplastic systems: for example, does a chemopreventive agent block initiation, promotion, or progression of a premalignant lesion? One might also look into the effect of these chemopreventive agents on epithelial–mesenchymal interactions. A systematic study of a stage-specific response to chemopreventive agents would open up several avenues for effective prevention strategies.

Lately, there has been growing interest in dietary intervention in cancer incidence and mortality. Vegetables containing beta-carotene are associated with a decreased risk of lung cancer [61]. A protective effect of dietary fiber intake on the risk of colon cancer has also been suggested for other cancers [62]. Similarly, high dietary fat intake has been associated with a increased risk of a variety of cancers including breast, prostate, and colon [63]. How these nutrients and micronutrients prevent cancer is not known, but work is in progress at the National Cancer Institute (NCI) to elucidate their effects on early promotional events.

Future directions in detection and prevention research

It is clear that many human cancers are associated with preneoplastic lesions. Such lesions potentially represent an important target for identifying cellular or molecular changes that might be taking place in the tissue in the course of cancer progression from a premalignant to malignant to metastatic condition. Progression involves a complex pathway of molecular events: e.g., loss of chromosomes, mutation or amplification of certain oncogenes, loss or mutation of cancer suppressor genes, and resulting loss of normal growth control [3]. It has been suggested that the individual steps of this pathway represent 'intermediate endpoints' in the process of tumor progression that can be measured and can serve as biomarkers for this complex process. Although a variety of biomarkers might exist, and although their relationship to each other or to the biologic manifestations of cancer progression are not understood, the concept of biomarkers that could identify and measure early genetic changes is particularly relevant today in view of significant improvements in molecular biology technologies that are capable of detecting these genetic changes. These now permit the detection and mapping of individual point mutations that could be evaluated as possibly sensitive and specific endpoints in early detection studies.

Considerable controversy exists regarding selection and validation of intermediate endpoints and their biologic significance in cancer progression [64]. Thus, the issue of selection of a biomarker as an appropriate intermediate measure of cancer progression has depended, to a large extent, on experiments with animals treated with known carcinogens, high prevalence of a biomarker in populations with a high risk of cancer, or an individual case series in which most cancer patients are found to express a given biomarker. Once selected, a biomarker has to be validated for its role as a cancer surrogate, and this process should proceed through a series of steps involving case–control studies and prospective cohort studies followed by quantification of the marker–cancer association, as has been recently described [65]. The validation process is complex and has been rigorously and consistently applied to very few newly described and promising biomarkers. Some markers may even be specific for particular preventive agents and unhelpful or even misleading for others [64]. Accordingly, validation is necessary if a given biomarker is to be used for early detection or primary prevention of cancer.

The processes of selection and validation of a promising biomarker should include extensive studies with human tissues and body fluids from individuals with well-documented premalignant and early cancer lesions and corresponding tissues from normal subjects or subjects with benign lesions. Newly developed molecular biologic and cellular approaches for identifying early, premalignant changes, e.g., oncogene mutations or a loss or mutation of so-called suppressor oncogenes [9–11], are extremely sensitive, detecting changes as small as a single-base substitution. Although such subtle genetic alterations can now be measured with great precision, the exact biologic consequences of these alterations at specific points in the process of cancer development are not clear. It is not yet established that these alterations are reliable intermediate endpoints, i.e., predictably measure subsequent development or progression of cancer.

The choice of patient populations for early detection or intermediate endpoint studies represents an important and strategically crucial decision. First, availability of sufficient numbers of patients with confirmed and well-documented clinical and histologic diagnoses of premalignant conditions, e.g., with mucosal epithelial cell hyperproliferation [66] for biomarker selection or validation studies, is essential. Second, the relative biologic importance of sequential changes in intermediate endpoints (e.g., if a loss of normal *p53* allele precedes chromosomal changes in chromosomes 17 or 18 in colorectal cancer) could be explored. Third, epidemiologic data, including a documented history of exposure to carcinogens collected at the time of tissue biopsy and correlated with biologic changes occurring in the target tissue, may allow for possible testing of a hypothesis regarding the relationship between an intermediate endpoint and cancer. In this context, not only the size of such high-risk populations but also their availability for serial follow-up specimens might be important practical considerations.

The time span between diagnosis of a premalignant state and cancer may be very long. However, in certain high-risk populations, e.g., patients cured for an initial cancer of the upper aerodigestive tract, the time span for development of squamous cell cancer of the lung may be considerably shorter, making this group particularly well suited for the proposed studies of early detection biomarkers. But attempts to establish any correlations between a biomarker and cancer progression must depend on solid clinical and epidemiologic information.

The development of specific and sensitive biomarkers for early detection of cancer in selected high-risk populations from whom normal, premalignant, and tumor tissues are banked is also dependent on a creative application of novel cellular and molecular biology studies. Specifically, intermediate endpoints need to be sought and correlated with phenotypic alterations in a given target cell or tissue. The difficulty is that gene alterations that occur early in the pathway of colorectal cancer progression are not necessarily the same changes that characterize the early stages of, for example, liver carcinogenesis.

The NCI is addressing some of the issues raised with respect to developing a biorepository of carefully characterized human tissues and body fluids with an associated epidemiologic and clinical information database. The Early Detection Branch of the NCI has established a network of investigators under the Early Detection Research Network (EDRN). Under this program, an awardee institution is to set up a bank of well-characterized premalignant, malignant, and related tissues that are collected, processed, and stored appropriately and uniformly using standard protocols. Medical histories of patients are indexed to correlate with these specimens as well as with information on tumor stage/grade, patient therapies, and clinical outcomes. The initial focus of the EDRN research is on epithelial tumors of the oropharynx, lung, bladder, and prostate, some of which could arise because of field effects. Thus there is a potential for multiple malignant lesions that may develop throughout these organs, and markers could be used to identify early malignant lesions for early treatment and intervention.

Summary

Human lung cancer is a complex disease originating in different cell types. In general, tumorigenesis in the lung appears to involve a complex series of molecular, genetic, and histopathologic events, leading to the transformation of normal cells to malignant cells. It is generally believed that it is the accumulation of biologic changes, not necessarily the order in which they occur, that could best describe the transformation of cells. Our knowledge of genetic changes during tumorigenesis in the lung is limited and comes from studies involving animal models and frankly malignant lung tissues. Such studies can be questioned as to their applicability in primary prevention. A vast majority of genetic changes occurring during the preclinical stage are yet to be documented. Study of these preclinical changes would offer a better opportunity for early detection and prevention. Oncogenes and tumor suppressor genes have potential for use as biomarkers in identifying high-risk groups and in early detection. The interaction between nature and nurture is nowhere as evident as in cancers of the lung, which are influenced by environmental exposure, familial inheritance, and metabolic phenotypes. The gene–environment interaction provides several targets for prevention and early detection. Biomarkers, if validated for specificity, sensitivity, and predictive values, could act as markers of exposure, susceptibility, progression, and disease. Validation of these markers, however, would require well-characterized, prospectively collected samples, representing normal, premalignant, malignant, invasive, and metastatic conditions. The NCI has started an initiative for a tissue bank of prostate, bladder, colorectum, head and neck, and lung cancers. Clinical and epidemiological information are also collected for each sample. Study of genetic and molecular changes in collected samples should shed light on the involvement of these changes in the transformation of normal to malignant tissues.

Acknowledgments

The authors thank Drs. John K. Gohagan and Ron Lubet for their valuable comments, and Ms. Laura Egan for her excellent editorial assistance.

References

1. Foulds L. 1958. The natural history of cancer. J Chronic Dis 8:2–37.
2. Bishop JM. 1987. The molecular genetics of cancer. Science 235:305–311.
3. Weinberg RA. 1989. Oncogenes, antioncogenes, and the molecular basis of multistep carcinogenesis. Cancer Res 49:3713–3721.
4. Surgeon General Office on Smoking and Health. 1984. The health consequences of involuntary smoking. A Report of the Surgeon General. U.S. Public Health Service, Rockville, MD.
5. Bajardi F. 1984. Histogenesis of spontaneous regression of cervical intraepithelial neoplasia. Cancer 54:616–619.
6. Kern SE, Yardley JH, Lazenby AJ, et al. 1984. Reversal by antrectomy of endocrine cell hyperplasia in the gastric body in pernicious anemia: A morphologic study. Mod Pathol 3:561–566.
7. Rodenhuis S, Van De Vater, Mooi W, et al. 1987. Mutational activation of the *K-ras* oncogene. A possible pathogenic factor in adenocarcinoma of the lung. N Engl J Med 317:929–935.
8. Takahashi T, Nau MN, Chiba, et al. 1989. *p53*: A frequent target for genetic abnormalities in lung cancer. Science 246:491–494.

9. Nigro JM, Baker SJ, Preisinger AC, et al. 1989. Mutations in *p53* occur in diverse human tumor types. Nature 342:705–708.
10. Chiba I, Takashi T, Nau MM, et al. 1990. Mutations in the *p53* gene are frequent in primary resected non-small cell lung cancer. Lung Cancer Study Group. Oncogene 5:1603–1610.
11. Hollstein M, Sidransky D, Vogelstein B, Harris CC. 1991. *p53* mutations in human cancers. Science 253:49–53.
12. Memoli VA, Jordan AG, Ball ED. 1984. Monoclonal antibody, SCCL 175, site specificity for small cell carcinoma of lung. Cancer Res 48:7319–7332.
13. Ball ED, Graziano RF, Pettingill OS, et al. 1984. Monoclonal antibodies reactive with small cell carcinoma of lung. J Natl Cancer Inst 72:593–598.
14. Tockman MS, Gupta PK, Myers JD, et al. 1988. Sensitive and specific monoclonal antibody recognition of human lung cancer antigen on preserved sputum cell: A new approach to early lung cancer detection. J Clin Oncol 6:1685–1693.
15. Fargion S, Carney D, Mulshine J, Rosen S, et al. 1986. Cancer Res 46:2633–2638.
16. Serwin S, Minna J, Gazdar A, et al. 1981. Expression of epidermal and nerve growth factor receptors and soft agar growth factor production by lung cancer cells. Cancer Res 41:3538–3542.
17. Yamamoto T, Kamata N, Kawano N, et al. 1986. High incidence of amplification of the epidermal growth factor receptor gene in human squamous carcinoma cell lines. Cancer Res 46:414–416.
18. Veale D, Kerr N, Gibson GJ, Harris AL. 1989. Characterization of epidermal growth factor receptor in primary human non-small cell lung cancer. Cancer Res 49:1313–1317.
19. Mitsudomi T, Steinberg SM, Oie HK, et al. 1991. *ras* gene mutations in non-small cell lung cancers are associated with shortened survival irrespective of treatment intent. Cancer Res 51:4999–5002.
20. Levine A, Momand J, Finlay CA. 1991. The *p53* tumor suppressor gene. Nature 351:453–456.
21. Bos JL, Fearon ER, Hamilton SR, et al. 1987. Prevalence of *ras* gene mutations in human colorectal cancers. Nature 327:293–297.
22. Rodenhuis S, Slebos RJ, Boot AJ, et al. 1988. Incidence and possible clinical significance of *K-ras* oncogene activation in adenocarcinoma of the human lung. Cancer Res 48:5738–5741.
23. Harbour JW, Lai S-L, Whang-Peng J, et al. 1988. Abnormalities in structure and expression of the human retinoblastoma gene in SCLC. Science 241:353–357.
24. Yokata J, Akiyama T, Fung Y-K, et al. 1988. Altered expression of rb gene in SCLC. Oncogene 3:471–475.
25. Schutte J, Nau M, Birrer M, et al. 1988. Constitutive expression of multiple mRNA forms of the *c-jun* oncogene in human lung cancer cell lines. Cancer Res 29:455–459.
26. Grifin C, Baylin S. 1985. Expression of the *c-myb* oncogene in human small cell lung carcinoma. Cancer Res 45:272–275.
27. Rapp U, Heleihel M, Pawson T, et al. 1988. Role of *raf* oncogene in lung carcinogenesis. Lung Cancer 4:162–167.
28. Doll R, Peto R. 1981. The Causes of Cancer. Oxford University Press: Oxford.
29. Parnell RW. 1951. Smoking and cancer. Lancet 1:963.
30. Mattson ME, Pollack ES, Cullen JS. 1987. What are the odds that smoking will kill you. Am J Public Health 77:425–428.
31. Mason TJ, McKay FW, Hoover R, et al. 1975. Atlas of cancer mortality for US counties, 1950–1969 (DHEW Publ. No. 75-780). National Institute of Health: Bethesda, MD.
32. Ooi WL, Elston RC, Chen VW, et al. 1986. Increased familial risk of lung cancer. J Natl Cancer Inst 76:217–221.
33. Sellers RA, Bailey-Wilson JE, Elston RC, et al. 1990. Evidence for Mendelian inheritance in the pathogenesis of lung cancer. J Natl Cancer Inst 82:1272–1276.

108

34. Tokuhata GK, Lilienfeld AM. 1963. Familial aggregation of lung cancer in hospital patients. J Natl Cancer Inst 30:217–222.
35. Knudson AJ, Hethcote HW, Brown BW. 1975. Mutation and childhood cancer. A probabilistic model for the incidence of retinoblastoma. Proc Natl Acad Sci 72:5116–5120.
36. Sanders B, Jay M, Draper G, Roberts E. 1989. Non-ocular cancer in relativies of retinoblastoma patients. Br J Cancer 60:358–365.
37. Carbone DP, Minna JD. 1992. The molecular genetics of lung cancer. In Advances in Internal Medicine, vol. 37, JJ Leonard (ed.). Mosby-Year Book, Inc., vol. 3, pp. 153–171, 1992.
38. Fearon ER, Vogelstein B. 1990. A genetic model for colorectal tumorigenesis. Cell 61:759–767.
39. Minna JD, Battey JF, Brooks BJ, et al. 1986. Molecular genetic analysis reveals chromosomal deletion, gene amplification, and autocrine growth factor production in the pathogenesis of lung cancer. Cold Spring Harbor Symp Quant Biol 51:843–853.
40. Guerrero I, Pellicer A. 1987. Mutational activation of oncogenes in animal model systems of carcinogenesis. Mutat Res 185:2903–2908.
41. You M, Candrian U, Maronpot R, et al. 1989. Activation K-ras protooncogene in spontaneously occurring and chemically induced lung tumors of strain A mice. Proc Natl Acad Sci USA 86:3070–3074.
42. McCormick F. 1989. The polymerase chain reaction and cancer diagnosis. Cancer Cells 1:56–61.
43. Viallet J, Minna JD. 1990. Dominant oncogenes and tumor suppressor genes in the pathogenesis of lung cancer. Am J Respir Cell Mol Biol 2:225–232.
44. Heighway J, Thatcher N, Cerny T, Hasleton PS. 1986. Genetic predisposition to lung cancer. Br J Cancer 53:453–457.
45. Slamon DS, Godolphin W, Jones LA, et al. 1989. Studies on the Her-2/neu protooncogene in human breast and ovarian cancer. Science 244:707–712.
46. Weston A, Willey JC, Modali R, et al. 1989. Differential DNA sequence deletions from chromosomes 3, 11, 13, and 17 in squamous cell carcinoma and adenocarcinoma of the human lung. Proc Natl Acad Sci USA 86:5099–50605.
47. Yokata J, Wada M, Shimosato Y, et al. 1987. Loss of heterozygosity on chromosomes 3, 13, and 17 in small cell carcinoma and on chromosome 3 in adenocarcinoma of the lung Proc Natl Acad Sci USA 84:9252–5257.
48. Mori N, Yokata J, Oshimura M, et al. 1989. Concordant deletions of chromosomes 3p and loss of heterozygosity for chromosome 13 and 17 in small cell carcinoma. Cancer Res 49:5130–5135.
49. Perera FP, Santella R, Brandt-Rauf P, et al. 1991. Molecular epidemiology of lung cancer. In Origins of Human Cancer: A Comprehensive Review, J Brugge, T Curran, E Harlow, and F McCormick (eds.). Cold Spring Harbor Laboratory Press: New York, pp. 219–236.
50. Schulte P. 1987. Methodologic issues in the use of biologic markers in epidemiologic research. Am J Epidemiol 126:1006–1116.
51. Perera F. 1990. Molecular epidemiology: A new tool in assessing risks for environmental carcinogens. CA J Clin 40(5):277–288.
52. Bartsch HN, Caporaso M, Coda M, et al. 1990. Carcinogen hemoglobin adducts, urinary mutagenicity, and metabolic phenotype in active and passive cigarette smokers. J Natl Cancer Inst 82(23):1826–1831.
53. Law MR. 1990. Genetic predisposition to lung cancer. Br J Cancer 61:195–202.
54. Setlow RB. 1983. Varations in DNA repair mechanism among humans. In Human Carcinogenesis, CC Harris and H Autrup (eds.). Academic Press: New York, p. 231.
55. Bondy ML, Spiltz MR, Halabi S, et al. 1993. Association between family history of cancer and mutagen sensitivity in upper aerodigestive tract cancer patients. Cancer Epidemiol Biomarkers Prev 103(2):103–106.
56. Hong WK, Lippman SM, Itri LM, et al. 1990. Prevention of primary tumors in squamous

carcinoma of the head and neck with *13-cis* retinoic acid. N Engl J Med 323:795–801.

57. Love RR. 1990. Commentary: Prospect for antiestrogen chemoprevention of breast cancer. J Natl Cancer Inst 82:18–21.

58. Garewal HS, Sampliner RE, Fennerty MB. 1992. Chemopreventive studies in Barrett's Esophagus: A model premalignant lesion for esophageal adenocarcinoma. J Natl Cancer Inst Monogr 13:51–54.

59. Breitman T, Selonick SB, Collins SJ. 1980. Induction of differentiation of human promyelocytic leukemia by retinoic acid. Proc Natl Acad Sci USA 72:2936–2940.

60. Smith MA, Parkinson DR, Chesoon PD, Friedman LA. 1992. Retinoid in cancer therapy. J Clin Oncol 10:839–864.

61. Peto R, Doll R, Buckley JD, Sporn MD. 1981. Can dietary beta-carotene materially reduce human cancer rates. Nature 290:201.

62. Trock B, Lanza E, Greenwald P. 1990. Dietary fiber, vegetables, and colon cancer: critical review and meta-analysis of the epidemiologic evidence. J Natl Cancer Inst 82:650–657.

63. Willett WC. 1991. Diet and human cancer. In Origins of Human Cancer: A Comprehesive Revies, J Brugge, T Curran, E Harlow, and F McCormick (eds.). Cold Spring Harbor Laboratory Press: Cold Spring Harbor, NY, pp. 191–197.

64. Schatzkin A, Freedman LS, Schiffman MH, Dawsey SM. 1990. Validation of intermediate end points in cancer research. J Natl Cancer Inst 82:1746–1752.

65. Kellof GJ, Malone WF, Boone CW, Sigman CC, Fay JR. 1990. Progress in applied chemoprevention research. Semin Oncol 17(4):438–455.

66. Lipkin M. 1988. Biomarkers of increased susceptibility to gastrointestinal cancer. New applications to studies of cancer prevention in human subjects. Cancer Res 48:235–245.

5. Growth factors and lung cancer

Tariq Sethi and Penella J. Woll

Introduction

Lung cancer is the principal cause of cancer deaths in the Western world. New approaches to its treatment are urgently needed. It is likely that these will arise from a better understanding of the extracellular factors and intracellular molecular events that are responsible for sustaining its growth.

Small cell lung cancer

Small cell lung cancer (SCLC), which constitutes 25% of all pulmonary malignancies, follows an aggressive clinical course despite initial sensitivity to chemotherapy and radiation [1]. SCLCs are characterized by the presence of small dense cytoplasmic granules that secrete a variety of hormones and neuropeptides [2–8]. Peptide production has attracted clinical interest because it provides useful markers for the pathologic diagnosis of SCLC and because it causes endocrine abnormalities, such as the syndrome of inappropriate secretion of vasopressin. Neuropeptides produced by SCLC include bombesin-like peptides, neurotensin, and vasopressin [2,3]. Of these, the bombesin-like peptides were the first suggested to act as autocrine growth factors for SCLC [8].

Bombesin/gastrin-releasing peptide

Bombesin is one of a family of naturally occurring peptides that share a carboxyl-terminal heptapeptide (table 1). Mammalian gastrin-releasing peptide (GRP) has 9/10 C-terminal amino acids identical to bombesin. Studies with synthetic bombesin-like peptides have demonstrated that full biological activity requires more than seven but no more than nine C-terminal amino acids [9].

Bombesin and GRP are potent mitogens for murine Swiss 3T3 cells [10]. Chronic bombesin administration to rodents leads to antral gastric cell proliferation and pancreatic hypertrophy [11,12]. The latter effect is partly

Heine H. Hansen, (ed), Hansen: Lung Cancer.
© 1994 Kluwer Academic Publishers. ISBN 0-7923-2835-3. All rights reserved.

Table 1. Amino-acid sequence of bombesinlike peptides

Amphibian														
Bombesin	pGlu	Gln	Arg	Leu	Gly	Asn	Gln	Trp	Ala	Val	Gly	His	Leu	Met	NH₂
Ranatensin				pGlu	Val	Pro	Gln	Trp	Ala	Val	Gly	His	Leu	Met	NH₂
Litorin						pGlu	Gln	Trp	Ala	Val	Gly	His	Leu	Met	NH₂
Mammalian														
GRP(1–27) Human	Val	Pro	Leu	Pro	Ala	Gly	Gly	Gly	Thr	Val	Leu	Thr	Lys–		
	–Met	Tyr	Pro	Arg	Gly	Asn	His	Trp	Ala	Val	Gly	His	Leu	Met	NH₂
GRP(1–27) Procine	Ala	Pro	Val	Ser	Val	Gly	Gly	Gly	Thr	Val	Leu	Ala	Lys–		
	–Met	Tyr	Pro	Arg	Gly	Asn	His	Trp	Ala	Val	Gly	His	Leu	Met	
GRP10 (Neuromedin C)					Gly	Asn	His	Trp	Ala	Val	Gly	His	Leu	Met	NH₂
Neuromedin B					Gly	Asn	Leu	Trp	Ala	Thr	Gly	His	Leu	Met	NH₂

direct and partly mediated by cholecystokinin [13]. Bombesin/GRP is increasingly implicated in the growth of many human tumors in addition to lung cancers. GRP has recently been shown to stimulate the growth of a human gastrinoma xenograft [14] and breast cancer cells [15]. Some breast cancer cells also express the GRP gene and peptide [16,17].

Bombesin-like peptides are sparsely present in the neuroendocrine cells lining the bronchi of the human adult lung. In contrast, they are abundant in the fetal lung [18]. Pro-GRP mRNA and GRP-associated peptides are also present, indicating that the GRP is synthesized there [19,20]. GRP mRNAs are first detectable in the fetal lung at 9 to 10 weeks gestation, becoming maximal (25-fold adult levels) between 16 and 30 weeks, and declining to adult levels by 34 weeks [19,20]. In neonates with acute respiratory distress syndrome, bombesin levels throughout the lungs are significantly lower than normal [21]. Willey et al. [22] reported that bombesin and GRP acted as growth factors for explants of normal human bronchial epithelium cells. These findings have led to the intriguing suggestion that GRP could act as an important growth factor for the fetal lung.

In the normal lung, secretion of GRP by pulmonary neuroendocrine cells occurs in response to alterations in pulmonary oxygenation, such as those associated with birth (increased oxygenation) or with chronic obstructive airways disease (decreased oxygenation) [23]. Elevated levels of GRP have been found in bronchoalveolar lavages of normal smokers compared to nonsmokers [24]. This finding may indicate a role for GRP and abnormal oxygenation in the initiation of smoking-related tumors.

Bombesin-like peptides were first detected in lung cancer in the early 1980s [4,25]. Although present in the greatest amounts in SCLC, small quantities were detected in some lung adenocarcinomas. Plasma GRP is elevated in patients with extensive metastic SCLC, but is not suitable as a tumor marker for early detection of SCLC because of low serum levels and its rapid metabolism in the blood (it has a plasma half life of 2.8 minutes [26]). Demonstration of prepro-GRP mRNA, pro-bombesin C-terminal peptide, and multiple GRP gene-associated peptides in SCLC confirm that the peptides originate in these tumors [20,27,28]. In addition to secreting bombesin-like peptides, SCLC also exhibits receptors for them, as demonstrated by specific binding of $[^{125}I\text{-Tyr}^4]$ bombesin to SCLC [29,30]. Estimates of receptor number are in the range of $1-3 \times 10^3$ per cell. This suggests that GRP could act as an autocrine growth factor for SCLC.

The GRP receptor and neuromedin B receptors have been cloned from SCLC cells and murine Swiss 3T3 cells. These receptors are G-protein linked with seven transmembrane domains. Two consensus protein kinase C (PKC) phosphorylation sites are conserved in these receptors [31]. Because fewer cell lines appear to express receptors for GRP than to secrete it, autocrine stimulation probably only occurs in a subset of SCLC [32].

The signal transduction pathways stimulated by bombesin/GRP have been extensively studied in Swiss 3T3 cells [33]. The demonstration that similar signals are elicited in SCLC confirms that the effects of bombesin/GRP in these cells are specific and receptor mediated. Because nonhydrolyzable GTP analogues could modulate phospholipase C (PLC) activation in response to GRP [34,35], it was concluded that the GRP receptor in SCLC was coupled to PLC by a G-protein. This activation is accompanied by a rapid and transient elevation of intracellular calcium concentration ($[Ca^{2+}]_i$) [36]. GRP stimulation of Inositol(1,4,5) trisphosphate (InsP$_3$) and increase in $[Ca^{2+}]_i$ were inhibited by prior treatment with phorbol 12-myristate 13-acetate, suggesting that protein kinase C might exert negative feedback regulation on this response.

GRP and bombesin have been shown to act as growth factors in SCLC both in vitro and in vivo: Weber et al. [37] reported that GRP enhanced DNA synthesis in two SCLC cell lines, but not in two NSCLC cell lines. In another study, colony formation in 9/10 SCLC cell lines was stimulated up to 150-fold by GRP, with maximal effects at 50 nM [38]. However, there was no correlation between amounts of GRP secreted, response to exogenous GRP, and the number of binding sites in individual cell lines. Growth of SCLC xenografts (NCI-H69) was reported to be increased 77% above control in nude mice treated thrice daily with intraperitoneal injections of bombesin 20 µg/kg [39].

The hypothesis of autocrine growth stimulation by GRP in SCLC was tested by Cuttita et al. [8], who used a monoclonal antibody to [Lys^3] bombesin (2A11). It inhibited the clonal growth of two SCLC cell lines in serum-free medium, and retarded the growth of one cell line growing as xenografts in nude mice. The recent demonstration of a complete clinical response in an SCLC patient treated with 2A11 antibody adds further support to the hypothesis that GRP is an autocrine growth factor for at least some SCLCs [40].

Other neuropeptides

The neuroendocrine nature of SCLC has long been recognized. The number of peptide hormones and growth factors secreted continues to expand (see table 2). They have been detected by measuring plasma levels and immunohistochemistry of tumor samples and cell lines. Most of these products are present in only a minority of tumors, although some SCLCs appear capable of synthesizing many ectopic hormones. Some of these products have also been found in NSCLCs [41]. Many of these bioactive peptides can also be produced by the normal lung [64]. Most are synthesized as prohormones that acquire biological activity only after specific posttranslational modifications, e.g., carboxy-terminal alpha-amidation [65].

We now propose that many of these peptides can act as autocrine growth factors for SCLC. This requires the presence of functional receptors for these peptides on SCLC cells. Intracellular calcium ion concentrations can be monitored in a luminescence fluorimeter after incubating the cells with

Table 2. Peptides and hormones secreted by SCLC

Peptide hormone	Ref.
Adrenocorticotrophic hormone	[42]
Atrial natriuretic peptide	[43,44]
Calcitonin	[2,45]
Calcitonin gene-related peptide	[45]
Cholecystokinin	[46,47]
Chorionic gonadotrophin	[2,48]
Endothelin	[2]
Estradiol	[2]
Follicle-stimulating hormone	[2]
Gastrin	[47,48]
Glucagon	[2,45]
Granulocyte colony-stimulating factor	[50]
Growth hormone	[2]
GRP/bombesin	[25,49]
Insulin-like growth factor-I	[51,52]
Insulin-like growth factor-I binding protein	[53,54]
Lipotropin	[2,50]
Neuromedin B	[55,56]
Neurotensin	[45,57]
Opioid peptides	[58]
Oxytocin	[2,3,7]
Parathyroid hormone	[2,59]
Physalaemin	[60]
Prolactin	[2]
Serotonin	[2]
Somatostatin	[4]
Stem cell factor	[61]
Substance K	[45]
Substance P	[25]
Transferrin	[62]
Vasoactive intestinal peptide	[50,63]
Vasopressin	[5,44]

the fluorescent Ca^{2+} indicator fura-2. Studies with SCLC (described above) have shown that GRP stimulates mobilization of intracellular Ca^{2+} and inositol phosphate turnover [35,36]. We have demonstrated that bradykinin, cholecystokinin (CCK), galanin, neurotensin, and vasopressin induce a rapid and transient increase in $[Ca^{2+}]_i$ in SCLC cell lines [66]. The Ca^{2+}-mobilizing effects are mediated by distinct receptors, as shown by the use of specific antagonists and by the induction of homologous desensitization. Each of the five cell lines studied responded to at least two different agents, but the expression of individual receptors was heterogeneous among the lines [66,67]. Studies from other laboratories are in agreement with these findings [68–70].

The observation that galanin, a 29-amino acid neuropeptide, causes Ca^{2+}

mobilization in SCLC is of special interest. In pancreatic cells, galanin activates an ATP-sensitive K^+ channel, hyperpolarizes the plasma membrane, and inhibits the activity of voltage-dependent Ca^{2+} channels [71]. In this manner it reduces Ca^{2+} influx and blocks the activity of various agents that increase the intracellular concentration of Ca^{2+}. Surprisingly, in SCLC cell lines galanin caused a rapid and transient increase in $[Ca^{2+}]_i$ [66]. Subsequent studies showed that galanin induced rapid mobilization of Ca^{2+} from internal stores and stimulated early production of inositol phosphates, particularly $Ins(1,4,5)P_3$ [67]. In contrast to the pancreatic cells, addition of galanin to SCLC cell lines did not alter membrane potential. Thus, these studies suggest that SCLC express a novel type of galanin receptor that is coupled to Ca^{2+} mobilization.

The finding that CCK induces rapid mobilization of Ca^{2+} from internal stores in SCLC cell lines prompted the characterization of the receptors involved. Gastrin and CCK share a C-terminal pentapeptide and bind to common cell surface receptors. The CCK_A receptors have a 500-fold higher affinity for CCK than for gastrin. In contrast, CCK_B receptors bind CCK and gastrin with approximately equal affinities [72]. We demonstrated that gastrin and CCK induce rapid Ca^{2+} mobilization in the SCLC cell line NCIH510, at comparable concentrations. Furthermore, selective CCK_B antagonists blocked the increase in $[Ca^{2+}]_i$ induced by either gastrin or CCK. Thus, the effects of gastrin and CCK in SCLC NCIH510 are mediated by CCK_B receptors [73].

Collectively, these studies indicate that SCLCs exhibit receptors for multiple neuropeptides and that the expression of these receptors is heterogeneous among SCLC cell lines.

Multiple neuropeptides stimulate clonal growth in SCLC

Because SCLCs secrete a wide variety of peptides and exhibit receptors for many of them, it has been proposed that SCLC growth is regulated by multiple autocrine and/or paracrine circuits [66,67,74,75]. The demonstration that these peptides can promote SCLC growth was necessary to support this hypothesis. The growth of SCLC cell lines in serum-free liquid culture is exponential and is not increased by the addition of mitogens. Tumor and transformed cells are able to form colonies in soft agar. There is a positive correlation between cloning efficiency of the cells and the aggressive clinical behavior of SCLC tumors. Under the stringent conditions of the clonogenic assay, the effects of mitogens can be studied. We examined the ability of Ca^{2+}-mobilizing neuropeptides to promote growth in SCLC cells. The results demonstrated that, at nanomolar concentrations, bradykinin, neurotensin, vasopressin, CCK, galanin, and GRP induce similar increases (250%−350%) in SCLC clonal growth. The effects of the peptides bradykinin, cholecystokinin, galanin, GRP, neurotensin, and vasopressin are dose dependent. The stimulatory effect was less at concentrations above those

116

required to induce an optimal response [67,74], presumably due to homologous desensitization in this long-term assay. Time-dependent mitogenic desensitization has been reported in other cellular systems [67,74,76,77].

Collectively, these findings support the hypothesis that SCLC growth is sustained by an extensive network of autocrine and paracrine interactions involving multiple neuropeptides. Approaches designed to block SCLC growth must take into account this mitogenic complexity.

Other factors

Insulin-like growth factor-I (IGF-I)

IGF-I (also known as somatomedin C) is a 70-amino-acid polypeptide closely related to insulin [78], but with distinct high-affinity receptors. IGF-I binds to a receptor with intrinsic tyrosine kinase activity [79]. It has been shown to be mitogenic in a variety of cell types, including fibroblast and erythroid progenitor cells and breast and thyroid tumor cells [78,80,81]. Although insulin is necessary for serum-free culture of SCLC [82], supraphysiological concentrations are required for optimal growth, suggesting that insulin binds with low affinity to the IGF-I receptor. IGF-I is secreted by SCLC and NSCLC cell lines and tumors [53,83,84]. High-affinity binding sites have been shown for IGF-I, and IGF-I receptor mRNA were detected on SCLC cell lines [51,84–86].

The growth of SCLC cell lines was also stimulated by exogenous IGF-I [87]. Preliminary clinical data showed that serum IGF-I levels were significantly higher in patients with lung cancer than in controls, and patients with metastases showed significantly higher levels of IGF-I than patients without. However, no significant difference in IGF-I mean values were seen before and after surgical removal of tumors. Furthermore, a monoclonal antibody to the IGF-I receptor inhibited IGF-I and insulin-stimulated cell growth in four SCLC cell lines [87]. Hence, IGF-I acts as an autocrine growth factor in SCLC. Since bombesin and insulin act synergistically to stimulate mitogenesis in Swiss 3T3 cells [10], this may also occur in SCLC. IGF-II receptors have also been characterized on SCLC cell lines [88].

The production of IGF-binding proteins by lung cancer cell lines modifies the autocrine/paracrine model for IGFs, since these proteins can either enhance or inhibit the effects of IGFs on tumor growth [52–54].

Transferrin

Transferrin is an 80-kDa β-globulin that is synthesized in the liver and transports iron in the plasma. It is required for the serum-free growth of SCLC [82]. The SCLC cell lines NCI-H345 and NCI-H510 secrete immunoreactive transferrin and have a transferrin requirement for growth [62].

Gallium salts, which block iron uptake, inhibited SCLC growth in vitro [89]. Thus, there is preliminary evidence for an autocrine growth loop involving transferrin in SCLC. Transferrin has also been identified as a lung-derived growth factor that stimulates the growth of lung-metastasizing tumor cells [90].

Hemopoietic growth factors

Hemopoietic growth factors are increasingly used to circumvent the myelo-suppressive effects of cytotoxic chemotherapy. There is concern that these growth factors could stimulate the growth of SCLC cells. Various solid tumors and cell lines have receptors for granulocyte stimulating factor (G-CSF) as well as granulocyte-macrophage colony-stimulating factor (GM-CSF), but their significance is uncertain. Some lung tumors appear to secrete G-CSF, but it does not seem to act as an autocrine growth factor [50,91] Although G-CSF and GM-CSF have been shown to stimulate the clonal growth of a few lung cancer cell lines [92–94], growth inhibition has also been described [95,96]. The most comprehensive studies, including panels of 10 and 11 cell lines, found no evidence of growth stimulation with G-CSF or GM-CSF [97–99]. It seems unlikely that these hemopoietic growth factors will have any important effect on lung tumor growth, but it is essential that long-term follow-up be performed in randomized clinical trials in order to determine whether relapse or second malignacy rates differ in patients receiving these growth factors.

Stem cell factor

Stem cell factor (SCF) is a pluripotent growth factor that has been suggested to play an important role in proliferation and differentiation in various types of fetal and adult tissues as the ligand for a transmembrane tyrosine kinase receptor encoded by the c-*kit* oncogene. Expression of the ligand and the receptor is seen in SCLCs [100]. The human SCF gene is transcribed into two major forms of alternatively spliced mRNAs with different molar ratio in fetal, adult, and malignant tissues [61]. This aberrant expression is seen almost exclusively in SCLCs. c-*kit* is autophosphorylated in response to SCF, resulting in significant chemotaxis and moderate proliferation of SCLC cells in vitro. Molecular analysis of the c-*kit* gene also revealed an amino acid substitution within the transmembrane domain in an SCLC cell line [101]. It is not known whether exogenous SCF will stimulate the proliferation of SCLC in vivo or act as an autocrine growth factor.

Opioids

Endogenous opiate peptides including the enkephalins, endorphins, and dynorphins are widely distributed in the mammalian nervous system.

118

Multiple subtypes of receptors have been identified using a variety of agonists and antagonists. Because of its central role in pain transmission, opiate pharmacology has been studied in detail [102]. β-endorphins have been shown to stimulate lymphocyte proliferation in vitro [103], although this effect may not be mediated directly through opiate receptors, since it was not blocked by naloxone. Dynorphins and enkephalins appear to be involved with vasopressin in the proliferative response of the marrow to hemorrhage [104].

Opioid peptides, β-endorphin, enkephalin, and dynorphin are secreted by SCLC cells. Some NSCLCs secrete the pentapeptide neo-kyotorphin [105], but whether this substance can stimulate tumor or stromal growth is unknown. The detection of opioid receptors on the same cells postulated the existence of an opiod autocrine loop [58,106]. It appears that opioids can have a stimulatory and inhibitory effects on SCLC growth depending on the ligand and receptor subtype present [103,107]. Methadone has been found to significantly inhibit the in vitro and in vivo growth of human lung cancer cells. The in vitro growth inhibition (occurring at 1–100 nM methadone) was associated with changes in cell morphology and viability detected within one hour and was irreversible after 24-hour exposure to the drug. These effects of methadone could be reversed in the first six hours by naltrexone, actinomycin D, and cycloheximide, suggesting the involvement of opioid-like receptors and a requirement for de novo mRNA protein synthesis. The inhibitory effects of methadone could also be achieved with the less addictive (+) isomer of methadone. The binding sites were high affinity (nM), but the binding characteristics appeared to be different from methadone sites present in rat brain. Methadone decreases cAMP levels in lung cancer cells, but the receptors are not coupled to a pertussis-sensitive guanine nucleotide-binding regulatory protein [107]. These receptors have been further characterized and are found to be nonconventional opioid receptors that are not antagonized by naloxone. Neuroblastoma xenograft growth has been inhibited by naltrexone, an opiate antagonist [108], suggesting a possible role for these drugs in treating some cancers.

Tachykinins

A recent study reported that tachykinins were able to mobilise Ca^{2+} in SCLC cells but not to stimulate growth in liquid culture [109]. Physalaemin, an amphibian tachykinin, is detectable in some SCLCs [60] and has been shown to inhibit clonal and mass culture of SCLC in vitro at picomolar concentrations [45].

Somatostatin

Somatostatin and its analogues inhibit the endogenous production of IGF-I and insulin [110] and have been shown to inhibit breast cancer growth in vitro [111]. They also inhibit the growth of experimental prostate tumors [112,113]. Somatostatin receptors are present on many tumors [114,115], and somatostatin analogues are useful in the treatment of hormone-secreting tumors, including apudomas and carcinoids [116]. It is therefore interesting to note that a somatostatin analogue administered twice daily as a perilesional infusion was cytostatic in SCLC xenografts [117]. Two active octapeptide analogues of somatostatin inhibited clonal growth of SCLC cells and VIP-stimulated cAMP formation [117,118]. More recent studies showed that somatostatin receptors were present on 3/4 SCLC cell lines but not in two NSCLC cell lines. The growth of 1/3 somatostatin-receptor-positive SCLC cell lines was significantly inhibited by the long-acting somatostatin analogue octreotide (10^{-9} M). Twenty SCLC patients were treated with octreotide 250 mg three times per day, before chemotherapy (6 patients) and after chemotherapy (14 patients). Octreotide was well tolerated, and serum levels of IGF-I were suppressed to 62% $\pm$ 7% of pretreatment levels, but there was no evidence of antitumor activity in these patients [119].

Non-small cell lung cancer

Bronchogenic carcinomas arise from the mucosa of the tracheobronchial tree. They include squamous cell carcinomas, which demonstrate upregulation of EGF receptor expression and markers characteristic of squamous differentiation (involucrin, transglutaminase activity, higher molecular weight keratins and cornified envelope formation) [120,121]. Adenocarcinomas are mucin-containing or mucin-secreting tumors [120,121]. They often demonstrate morphological features of lepidic and papillary growth and include the subtypes bronchioloalveolar and papillary. Large cell carcinomas are predominantly undifferentiated tumors. Bronchial carcinoids are a minor category of lung cancers that have neuroendocrine features. These tumors are thought to arise from submucosal glands and are not highly malignant. Neuroendocrine features can be found in some NSCLC tumors, including about 25% of adenocarcinomas. Such tumors are associated with increased sensitivity to chemotherapy and radiotherapy. They are faster growing and have a worse prognosis compared to NSCLC without neuroendocrine features [122].

Epidermal growth factor

Epidermal growth factor (EGF) is a polypeptide hormone that has both growth-stimulatory and growth-inhibitory effects on normal and tumor cells in vitro [123]. EGF and transforming growth factor-α (TGF-α) both act through the EGF receptor. Examination of EGF receptors from binding studies and by Northern blot analysis of mRNA indicated that they were present on both NSCLCs (1300–2700 fmol/mg protein) and SCLCs

120

(10–120 fmol/mg protein) [124]. Although EGF receptor expression is generally elevated in human lung squamous carcinoma, the biological significance of this phenomenon and the role of EGF and TGF-α in this disease are poorly understood. In one study, three human squamous lung carcinoma cell lines have been shown to express EGF receptors; addition of EGF or TGF-α resulted in growth inhibition. mRNA for TGF-α was detected in all three cell lines [125]. In contrast, several other studies have reported that EGF and TGF-α at nanomolar concentrations increase [^{3}H] thymidine incorporation in squamous and adenocarcinoma cell lines [126–129]. This stimulating effect can be blocked by suramin, an antihelminthic, which competitively blocked the binding of [^{125}I]TGF-α to the EGF receptor [130]. EGF and TGF-α can also stimulate NSCLC cell clonal growth in soft agarose and growth in nude mice. A monoclonal antibody (Ab 108) to the EGF receptor inhibited this growth stimulation in vitro and in vivo [131].

Therapeutic implications

Neuropeptides are increasingly implicated in the control of cell proliferation, and their mechanisms of action are attracting intense interest. These peptides may also act as autocrine growth factors for certain SCLC cells. The results discussed here strongly suggest that the autocrine growth loop of bombesin-like peptides may be only a part of an extensive network of autocrine and paracrine interactions involving a variety of Ca^{2+}-mobilizing neuropeptides in SCLC, including bradykinin, cholecystokinin, galanin, neurotensin, and vasopressin.

As understanding of the effects of growth factors in cancer increases, it has become possible to plan rational therapeutic interventions. If an autocrine growth loop is considered, in which cells synthesize, secrete, bind, and respond to the same growth factor, it is evident that interruption of this cycle at any point will block mitogenesis. Paracrine growth stimulation could be blocked in the same way. Because SCLC growth appears driven, at least in part, by multiple autocrine and paracrine circuits involving Ca^{2+}-mobilizing neuropeptides, antagonists capable of blocking the biological effects of multiple neuropeptides (i.e., broad-spectrum neuropeptide antagonists) could provide an effective approach in the treatment of SCLC.

The first such antagonist to be studied was an analogue of substance P, [DArg^1,DPro^2,DTrp^{7,9},Leu^{11}] substance P (antagonist A). Substance P is structurally unrelated to bombesin, but antagonist A was found to block the secretory effects of bombesin on a pancreatic cell preparation [132]. It was subsequently found to block ^{125}I-GRP binding and bombesin-stimulated early signaling events and mitogenesis in Swiss 3T3 cells [133–135]. Further substance P analogues were therefore studied [75,136].

Two interesting compounds were [DArg^1,DPhe^5,DTrp^{7,9},Leu^{11}] substance P and [Arg^6,DTrp^{7,9},MePhe^8] substance P(6–11) (antagonists D and G).

Both were shown to inhibit signal transduction and DNA synthesis stimulated by bombesin, GRP, bradykinin, and vasopressin by reversibly preventing ligand binding [75,136]. It is important to note that the antagonists neither block DNA synthesis by platelet-derived growth factor, which stimulates Ca^{2+} mobilization through a different mechanism from neuropeptides (i.e., mediated by tyrosine phosphorylation rather than by a G protein), nor inhibit mitogenesis stimulated by vasoactive intestinal peptide, which induces cyclic AMP accumulation without Ca^{2+} mobilization via a G-protein linked receptor [75,136]. Thus, the substance P antagonist showed broad-spectrum specificity against the neuropeptide mitogens bombesin/GRP, vasopressin, bradykinin, and endothelin, which act through distinct G-protein linked receptors in Swiss 3T3 cells but activate common signal transduction pathways. The molecular mechanism by which these antagonists interfere with the action of Ca^{2+}-mobilizing neuropeptides remains to be defined.

The compounds characterized as broad-spectrum antagonists in Swiss 3T3 cells were tested as inhibitors of neuropeptide-mediated signals and growth in SCLC cell lines. Because SCLC is a heterogeneous group of tumors, each compound was tested in several cell lines. The broad-spectrum antagonists inhibited Ca^{2+} mobilization stimulated by GRP, vasopressin, bradykinin, CCK, and galanin in diverse cell lines [67,75] and inhibited the growth of SCLC cell lines in liquid and semisolid media [67,75,137,138]. Antagonists D and G were equipotent, with half-maximal effect at about $20\,\mu M$, whereas antagonist A was fivefold less potent.

The broad-spectrum antagonists (D and G) caused a dramatic reduction in the cloning efficiency of these cells in the absence and presence of exogenous peptide [67,75,137]. The striking finding that broad-spectrum antagonists inhibit the basal and stimulated clonal growth of many cell lines, regardless of positivity for bombesin receptors, suggests that broad-spectrum antagonists could be more useful anticancer drugs than ligand-specific growth factor antagonists.

As a first step to test this possibility, the effect of broad-spectrum antagonist on the growth of SCLC xenografts was examined. The antagonists inhibited the growth of the tumor, as compared with the control group [138]. The inhibitory effect was clearly maintained beyond the duration of administration. These results demonstrate that broad-spectrum antagonists can inhibit SCLC growth in vivo as well as in vitro.

Additional strategies to block growth factor action include the use of growth inhibitory factors, monoclonal antibodies to clear secreted factors, and drugs designed to interrupt intracellular signaling pathways. Because multiple growth factors are implicated in the growth of lung cancers, antibodies and antagonists to specific factors are unlikely to be clinically useful except in a minority of cases. Cocktails of antibodies or specific antagonists would be complicated and expensive to administer. They would also carry a high risk of immune reactions. The development of antibodies to EGF and antagonists to PDGF make these approaches possible for NSCLC in addition to SCLC [139,140]. The broad-spectrum antagonists circumvent these problems and retain the advantage of small size with potentially good tumor penetration. The development of orally bioavailable nonpeptide antagonists promises to provide interesting new compounds for clinical study. Growth-inhibitory factors, such as the somatostatin analogues, have shown considerable activity in vitro, but more potent compounds are awaited for clinical use [119]. Drugs that affect intracellular signal transduction pathways include the protein kinase C activator bryostatin [141] and tyrosine kinase inhibitors such as tyrphostins [142].

A detailed understanding of the receptors and mitogenic action of neuropeptides will serve to identify novel targets for therapeutic intervention. Exciting advances have already been made. We anticipate that these will soon be translated into new treatments for lung cancer.

References

1. Smyth JF, Fowlie SM, Gregor A, Crompton GK, Busutill A, Leonard RCF, Grant IWB. 1986. The impact of chemotherapy on small cell carcinoma of the bronchus. QJ Med 61:969–976.
2. Sorenson GD, Pettengill OS, Brinck-Johnsen T, Cate CC, Maurer LH. 1981. Hormone production by cultures of small-cell carcinoma of the lung. Cancer 47:1289–1296.
3. Maurer LH. 1985. Ectopic hormone syndrome in small cell carcinoma of the lung. Clin Oncol 4:1289–1296.
4. Wood SM, Wood JR, Ghatei MA, Lee YC, O'Shaughnessy D, Bloom SR. 1981. Bombesin, somatostatin and neurotensin-like immunoreactivity in bronchial carcinoma. J Clin Endocrinol Metab 53:1310–1312.
5. North WG, Maurer LH, Valtin H, O'Donnell JF. 1980. Human neurophysins as potential tumor markers for small cell carcinoma of the lung: application of specific radioimmunoassays. J Clin Endocrinol Metab 51: 892–896.
6. Goedert M, Reeve JG, Emson PC, Bleehen NM. 1984. Neurotensin in human small cell lung carcinoma. Br J Cancer 50:179–183.
7. Sausville E, Carney D, Battey J. 1985. The human vasopressin gene is linked to the oxytocin gene and is selectively expressed in a cultured lung cancer cell line. J Biol Chem 260(18):10236–10241.
8. Cuttitta F, Carney DN, Mulshine J, Moody TW, Fedorko F, Fischler A, Minna JD. 1985. Bombesin-like peptides can function as autocrine growth factors in human small-cell lung cancer. Nature 316(6031):823–826.
9. Heimbrook DC, Boyer ME, Garsky VM, Balishin NL, Kiefer DM, Oliff A, Riemen MW. 1988. Minimal ligand analysis of gastrin releasing peptide. Receptor binding and mitogenesis. J Biol Chem 263(15):7016–7019.
10. Rozengurt E, Sinnett-Smith J. 1983. Bombesin stimulation of DNA synthesis and cell division in cultures of Swiss 3T3 cells. Proc Natl Acad Sci USA 80:2936–2940.
11. Lhoste EF, Longnecker DS. 1987. Effect of bombesin and caerulein on early stages of carcinogenesis induced by azaserine in the rat pancreas. Cancer Res 47(12):3273–3277.
12. Lehy T, Accary JP, Labeille D, Dubrasquet M. 1983. Chronic administration of bombesin stimulates antral gastrin cell proliferation in rat. Gastroenterology 84:914–919.
13. Douglas BR, Woutersen RA, Jansen JB, Rovati LC, Lamers CB. 1989. Study into the role of cholecystokinin in bombesin-stimulated pancreatic growth in rats and hamsters. Eur J Pharmacol 161(2–3):209–214.

14. Chung DH, Evers BM, Beauchamp RD, Upp JR, Rajaraman S, Townsend CM, Thompson JC. 1992. Bombesin stimulates growth of human gastrinoma. Surgery 112: 1059–1065.

15. Yano T, Pinski J, Groot K, Schally AV. 1992. Stimulation by bombesin and inhibition by bombesin/gastrin-releasing peptide antagonist RC-3095 of growth of human breast cancer cell lines. Cancer Res 52:4545–4547.

16. Vangsted AJ, Andersen EV, Nedergaard L, Zeuthen J. 1991. Gastrin releasing peptide GRP(14–27) in human breast cancer cells and in small cell lung cancer. Breast Cancer Res Treat 19(2):119–128.

17. Pagani A, Papotti M, Sanfilippo B, Bussolati G. 1991. Expression of the gastrin-releasing peptide gene in carcinomas of the breast. Int J Cancer 47(3):371–375.

18. Moody TW. 1984. Bombesin-like peptides in the normal and malignant lung. In The Endocrine Lung in Health and Disease, KL Becker and AF Gazdar (eds.). W.B. Saunders: Philadelphia, pp. 328–335.

19. Spindel ER, Sunday ME, Hofler H, Wolfe HJ, Habener JF, Chin WW. 1987. Transient elevation of messenger RNA encoding gastrin-releasing peptide, a putative pulmonary growth factor in human fetal lung. J Clin Invest 80(4):1172–1179.

20. Cuttitta F, Fedorko J, Gu JA, Lebacq VA, Linnoila RI, Battey JF. 1988. Gastrin-releasing peptide gene-associated peptides are expressed in normal human fetal lung and small cell lung cancer: a novel peptide family found in man. J Clin Endocrinol Metab 67(3):576–583.

21. Ghatei MA, Sheppard MN, Henzen-Logman S, Blank MA, Polak JM, Bloom SR. 1983. Bombesin and vasoactive intestinal peptide in the developing lung: marked changes in the respiratory distress syndrome. J Clin Endocrinol Metab 57:1226–1232.

22. Willey JC, Lechner JF, Harris CC. 1984. Bombesin and the C-terminal tetradecapeptide of gastrin-releasing peptide are growth factors for normal human bronchial epithelial cells. Exp Cell Res 153:245–248.

23. Schuller H. 1991. Receptor-mediated mitogenic signals and lung cancer. Cancer Cells 3:496–503.

24. Aguayo SM, King TJ, Waldron JJ, Sherritt KM, Kane MA, Miller YE. 1990. Increased pulmonary neuroendocrine cells with bombesin-like immunoreactivity in adult patients with eosinophilic granuloma. J Clin Invest 86(3):838–844.

25. Moody TW, Pert CB, Gazdar AF, Carney DN, Minna JD. 1981. High levels of intracellular bombesin characterize human small-cell lung carcinoma. Science 214:1246–1248.

26. Bork E, Hansen M, Urdal P, Paus E, Holst JJ, Schifter S, Fenger M, Engbaek F. 1988. Early detection of response in small cell bronchogenic carcinoma by changes in serum concentrations of creatine kinase, neuron specific enolase, calcitonin, ACTH, serotonin and gastrin releasing peptide. Eur J Cancer Clin Oncol 24(6):1033–1038.

27. Sunday ME, Choi N, Spindel ER, Chin WW, Mark EJ. 1991. Gastrin-releasing peptide gene expression in small cell and large cell undifferentiated lung carcinomas. Hum Pathol 22(10):1030–1039.

28. Sausville EA, Lebacq-Verheyden AM, Spindel ER, Cuttitta F, Gazdar AF, Battey JF. 1986. Expression of the gastrin-releasing peptide gene in human small cell lung cancer. Evidence for alternative processing resulting in three distinct mRNAs. J Biol Chem 261(5):2451–2457.

29. Moody TW, Carney DN, Cuttitta F, Quattrocchi K, Minna JD. 1985. High affinity receptors for bombesin/GRP-like peptides on human small cell lung cancer. Life Sci 37(2):105–113.

30. Layton JE, Scanlon DB, Soveny C, Morstyn G. 1988. Effects of bombesin antagonists on the growth of small cell lung cancer cells in vitro. Cancer Res 48(17):4783–4789.

31. Corjay MH, Dobrzanski DJ, Way JM, Viallet J, Shapira H, Worland P, Sausville EA, Battey JF. 1991. Two distinct bombesin receptor subtypes are expressed and functional in human lung carcinoma cells. J Biol Chem 266(28):18771–18779.

32. Kado-Fong H, Malfroy B. 1989. Effects of bombesin on human small cell lung cancer

cells: Evidence for a subset of bombesin non-responsive cell lines. J Cell Biochem 40(4): 431–437.

33. Rozengurt E. 1991. Neuropeptides as cellular growth factors: role of multiple signalling pathways. Eur J Clin Invest 21:123–134.

34. Sharoni Y, Viallet J, Trepel JB, Sausville EA. 1990. Effect of guanine and adenine nucleotides on bombesin-stimulated phospholipase C activity in membranes from Swiss 3T3 and small cell lung carcinoma cells. Cancer Res 50(17):5257–5262.

35. Trepel JB, Moyer JD, Heikkila R, Sausville EA. 1988. Modulation of bombesin-induced phosphatidylinositol hydrolysis in a small-cell lung-cancer cell line. Biochem J 255(2): 403–410.

36. Heikkila R, Trepel JB, Cuttitta F, Neckers LM, Sausville EA. 1987. Bombesin-related peptides induce calcium mobilization in a subset of human small cell lung cancer cell lines. J Biol Chem 262:16456–16460.

37. Weber S, Zuckerman JE, Bostwick DG, Bensch KG, Sikic BI, Raffin TA. 1985. Gastrin releasing peptide is a selective mitogen for small cell lung carcinoma in vitro. J Clin Invest 75(1):306–309.

38. Carney DN, Cuttitta F, Moody TW, Minna JD. 1987. Selective stimulation of small cell lung cancer clonal growth by bombesin and gastrin-releasing peptide. Cancer Res 47(3): 821–825.

39. Alexander RW, Upp JJ, Poston GJ, Gupta V, Townsend CJ, Thompson JC. 1988. Effects of bombesin on growth of human small cell lung carcinoma in vivo. Cancer Res 48(6): 1439–1441.

40. Kelley MJ, Avis I, Linnoila RI, Richardson G, Snider R, Phares J, et al. 1993. Complete response in a patient with small cell lung cancer (SCLC) treated on a phase II trial using a murine monoclonal antibody (2A11) directed against gastrin releasing peptide. Proc Am Soc Clin Oncol 12:339.

41. Luster W, Gropp C, Kern HF, Havemann K. 1985. Lung tumour cell lines synthesizing peptide hormones established from tumours of four histological types: Characterization of the cell lines and analysis of their peptide hormone production. Br J Cancer 51(6): 865–875.

42. Becker KL, Silva OL, Gazdar AF, Snider RH, Moore CF. 1984. Calcitonin and small cell cancer of the lung. In The Endocrine Lung in Health and Disease, KL Becker and AF Gazdar (eds.). W.B. Saunders: Philadelphia, pp. 528–548.

43. Bliss De, Battey JF, Linnoila RI, Birrer MJ, Gazdar AF, Johnson BE. 1990. Expression of the atrial natriuretic factor gene in small cell lung cancer tumors and tumor cell lines. Jr Natl Cancer Inst 82(4):305–310.

44. Gross AJ, Steinberg SM, Reilly JG, Bliss DP, Brennan J, Tram Le P, Simmons A, Phelps R, Mulshine JL, Ihde DC, Johnson BE. 1993. Atrial natriuretic factor and arginine vasopressin production in tumor cell lines from patients with lung cancer and their relationship to serum sodium. Cancer Res 53:67–74.

45. Bepler G, Rotsch M, Jaques G, Haeder M, Heymanns J, Hartogh G, Kiefer P, Havemann K. 1988. Peptides and growth factors in small cell lung cancer: production, binding sites, and growth effects. J Cancer Res Clin Oncol 114(3):235–244.

46. Moody TW. 1988. Neuropeptide receptors on small cell lung cancer cells. Lung Cancer 4:186.

47. Rehfeld JF, Bardram L, Hilsted L. 1989. Gastrin in human bronchogenic carcinomas: Constant expression but variable processing of progastrin. Cancer Res 49(11):2840–2843.

48. Gazdar AF, Carney DN. 1984. Endocrine properties of small cell carcinoma of the lung. In The Endocrine Lung in Health and Disease, KL Becker and AF Gazdar (eds.). W.B. Saunders: Philadelphia, pp. 501–508.

49. Erisman MD, Linnoila RI, Hernandez O, DiAugustine RP, Lazarus LH. 1982. Human lung small-cell carcinoma contains bombesin. Proc Natl Acad Sci USA 79:2379–2383.

50. Abe K, Kameya T, Yamaguchi K, Kikuchi K, Adachi I, Tanaka M, Kimura S, Kodama T, Shimosato Y, Ishikawa S. 1984. Hormone-producing lung cancers: endocrinologic and

morphologic studies. In The Endocrine Lung in Health and Disease, KL Becker and AF Gazdar (eds.). W.B. Saunders Philadelphia, pp. 549–595.

51. Macaulay VM, Everard MJ, Teale JD, Trott PA, Van-Wyk JJ, Smith IE, Millar JL. 1990. Autocrine function for insulin-like growth factor I in human small cell lung cancer cell lines and fresh tumor cells. Cancer Res 50(8):2511–2517.

52. Reeve JG. 1991. Expression of insulin-like growth factor (IGF) and IGF binding protein genes in human lung tumor cell lines (meeting abstract). Br J Cancer ●●.

53. Jaques G, Kiefer P, Rotsch M, Hennig C, Goke R, Richter G, Havemann K. 1989. Production of insulin-like growth factor binding proteins by small-cell lung cancer cell lines. Exp Cell Res 184(2):396–406.

54. Kiefer P, Jaques G, Schoneberger J, Heinrich G, Havemann K. 1991. Insulin-like growth factor binding protein expression in human small cell lung cancer cell lines. Exp Cell Res 192(2):414–417.

55. Giaccone G, Battey J, Gazdar AF, Oie H, Draoui M, Moody TW. 1992. Neuromedin B is present in lung cancer cell lines. Cancer Res 52:52732–52736.

56. Cardona C, Rabbitts PH, Spindel ER, Ghatei MA, Bleehen NM, Bloom SR, Reeve JG. 1991. Production of neuromedin B and neuromedin B gene expression in human lung tumor cell lines. Cancer Res 51(19):5205–5211.

57. Moody TW, Carney DN, Korman LY, Gazdar AF, Minna JD. 1985. Neurotensin is produced by and secreted from classic small cell lung cancer cells. Life Sci 36(18): 1727–1732.

58. Roth KA, Barchas JD. 1986. Small cell carcinoma cell lines contain opioid peptides and receptors. Cancer 57:769–773.

59. Yoshimoto K, Yamasaki R, Sakai H, Tezuka U, Takahashi M, Iizuka M, Sekiya T, Saito S. 1989. Ectopic production of parathyroid hormone by small cell lung cancer in a patient with hypercalcemia. J Clin Endocrinol Metab 68(5):976–981.

60. Lazarus LH, Hernandez O. 1985. Physalaemin-like immunoreactivity from human lung small cell carcinoma: isocratic reversed-phase hplc analysis of the chemically modified peptide. Recent Results Cancer Res 99(56):56–66.

61. Hibi K, Takahashi T, Sekido Y, Ueda R, Hida T, Ariyoshi Y, Takagi H, Takahashi T. 1991. Coexpression of the stem cell factor and the c-*kit* genes in small-cell lung cancer. Oncogene 6(12):2291–2296.

62. Nakanishi Y, Cuttitta F, Kasprzyk PG, Avis I, Steinberg SM, Gazdar AF, Mulshine JL. 1988. Growth factor effects on small cell lung cancer cells using a colorimetric assay: can a transferrin-like factor mediate autocrine growth? Exp Cell Biol 56(1–2):74–85.

63. Gozes I, Nakai H, Byers M, Avidor R, Weinstein Y, Shani Y, Shows TB. 1987. Sequential expression in the nervous system of c-myb and VIP genes, located in human chromosomal region 6q24. Somat Cell Mol Genet 13(4):305–313.

64. Becker KL, Gazdar AF. 1985. What can the biology of small cell cancer of the lung teach us about the endocrine lung? Biochem Pharmacol 34(2):155–159.

65. Quinn KA, Treston AM, Scott FM, Kasprzyk PG, Avis I, Siegfried JM, Mulshine JL, Cuttitta F. 1991. Alpha-amidation of peptide hormones in lung cancer. Cancer Cells 3(12):504–510.

66. Woll PJ, Rozengurt E. 1989. Multiple neuropeptides mobilise calcium in small cell lung cancer: Effects of vasopressin, bradykinin, cholecystokinin, galanin and neurotensin. Biochem Biophys Res Commun 164(1):66–73.

67. Sethi T, Rozengurt E. 1991. Galanin stimulates Ca^{2+} mobilization, inositol phosphate accumulation, and clonal growth in small cell lung cancer cells. Cancer Res 51(6): 1674–1679.

68. Staley J, Fiskum G, Moody TW. 1989. Cholecystokimn elevates cytosolic calcium in small cell lung cancer cells. Biochem Biophys Res Commun 163:605–610.

69. Staley J, Fiskum G, Davis TP, Moody TW. 1989. Neurotensin elevates cytosolic calcium in small cell lung cancer cells. Peptides 10:1217–1221.

70. Bunn PA, Dienhart DG, Chan D, Puck TT, Tagawa M, Jewett PB, Braunschweiger E.

126

1990. Neuropeptide stimulation of calcium flux in human lung cancer cells: Delineation of alternative pathways. Proc Natl Acad Sci USA 87(6):2162–2166.

71. Dunne MJ, Bullett MJ, Li GD, Wollheim CB, Petersen OH. 1989. Galanin activates nucleotide-dependent K$^+$ channels in insulin-secreting cells via a pertussis toxin-sensitive G-protein. EMBO J 8:413–420.

72. Jensen RT, Wank SA, Rowley WH, Sato S, Gardner JD. 1989. Interaction of CCK with pancreatic acinar cells. Trends Pharmacol Sci 10:418–423.

73. Sethi T, Rozengurt E. 1992. Gastrin stimulates Ca(2+) mobilization and clonal growth in small cell lung cancer cells. Cancer Res 52(21):6031–6035.

74. Sethi T, Rozengurt E. 1991. Multiple neuropeptides stimulate clonal growth of small cell lung cancer: effects of bradykinin, vasopressin, cholecystokinin, galanin, and neurotensin. Cancer Res 52(13):3621–3623.

75. Woll PJ, Rozengurt E. 1990. A neuropeptide antagonist that inhibits the growth of small cell lung cancer in vitro. Cancer Res 50(13):3968–3973.

76. Millar JBA, Rozengurt E. 1989. Heterologous desensitization of bombesin-induced mitogenesis by prolonged exposure to vasopressin: a post-receptor signal transduction block. Proc Natl Acad Sci USA 86(9):3204–3208.

77. Millar JBA, Rozengurt E. 1990. Chronic desensitization to bombesin by progressive down-regulation of bombesin receptors in Swiss 3T3 cells. Distinction from acute desensitization. J Biol Chem 265(20):12052–12058.

78. Clemmons DR. 1989. Structural and functional analysis of insulin-like growth factors. Br Med Bull 45:465–480.

79. Czech MP. 1989. Signal transmission by the insulin-like growth factors. Cell 59:235–238.

80. Rosen N, Yee D, Lippman ME, Paik S, Cullen KJ. 1991. Insulin-like growth factors in human breast cancer. Breast Cancer Res Treat 18:51.

81. Williams DW, Williams ED, Wynford-Thomas D. 1989. Evidence for autocrine production of IGF-I in human thyroid adenomas. Mol Cell Endocrinol 61(1):139–143●●.

82. Simms E, Gazdar AF, Abrams PG, Minna JD. 1980. Growth of human small cell (oat cell) carcinoma of the lung in serum-free growth factor-supplemented medium. Cancer Res 40:4356–4363.

83. Minuto F, Del MP, Barreca A, Alama A, Cariola G, Giordano G. 1988. Evidence for autocrine mitogenic stimulation by somatomedin-c/insulin-like growth factor I on an established human lung cancer cell line. Cancer Res 48(13):3716–3719.

84. Macauly VM, Teale JD, Everard MJ, Joshi GP, Smith IE, Millar JL. 1988. Somatomedin-C/insulin-like growth factor-I is a mitogen for human small cell lung cancer. Br J Cancer 57(1):91–93.

85. Jaques G, Rotsch M, Wegmann C, Worsch U, Maasberg M, Havemann K. 1988. Production of immunoreactive insulin-like growth factor I and response to exogenous IGF-I in small cell lung cancer cell lines. Exp Cell Res 176(2):336–343.

86. Havemann K, Rotsch M, Schoneberger HJ, Erbil C, Hennig C, Jaques G. 1990. Growth regulation by insulin-like growth factors in lung cancer. J Steroid Biochem Mol Biol 37(6):877–882.

87. Nakanishi Y, Mulshine JL, Kasprzyk PG, Natale, RB, Maneckjee R, Avis I, Treston AM, Gazdar AF, Minna JD, Cuttitta F. 1988. Insulin-like growth factor-I can mediate autocrine proliferation of human small cell lung cancer cell lines in vitro. J Clin Invest 82(1):354–359.

88. Schardt C, Rotsch M, Erbil C, Goke R, Richter G, Havemann K. 1993. Characterization of insulin-like growth factor II receptors in human small cell lung cancer cell lines. Exp Cell Res 204(1):22–29.

89. Vostrejs M, Moran PL, Seligman PA. 1988. Transferrin synthesis by small cell lung cancer cells acts as an autocrine regulator of cellular proliferation. J Clin Invest 82(1):331–339.

90. Cavanaugh PG, Nicolson GL. 1991. Lung-derived growth factor that stimulates the growth of lung-metastasizing tumor cells: Identification as transferrin. J Cell Biochem 47(3):261–271.

91. Nakamura H, Sayami P, Hayata Y. 1992. Analysis of G-CSF-producing lung cancer cell lines and non-growth stimulatory effects of rhG-CSF on lung cancer cells in vitro and in vivo. Lung Cancer 8:141–152.
92. Foulke RS, Marshall MH, Trotta PP, van Hoff DD. 1990. In vitro assessment of the effects of granulocyte-macrophage colony-stimulating factor on primary human tumors and cell lines. Cancer Res 50:6264–6267.
93. Baldwin GC, Gasson JC, Kaufman SE, et al. 1989. Nonhematopoietic tumor cells express functional GM-CSF receptors. Blood 73:1033–1037.
94. Avalos BR, Gasson JC, Hedrat C, et al. 1990. Human granulocyte colony-stimulating factor: biologic activities and receptor characterization on hematopoietic cells and small cell lung cancer cell lines. Blood 75:851–859.
95. Yamashita Y, Nara N, Aoki N. 1989. Antiproliferative and differentiative effect of granulocyte-macrophage colony-stimulating factor on a variant human small cell lung cancer cell line. Cancer Res 49:5334–5338.
96. Ruff MR, Farrar WL, Pert CB. 1986. Interferon gamma and granulocyte/macrophage colony-stimulating factor inhibit growth and induce antigens characteristic of myeloid differentiation in small-cell lung cancer cell lines. Proc Natl Acad Sci USA 83(17): 6613–6617.
97. Twentyman PR, Wright KA. 1991. Failure of GM-CSF to influence the growth of small cell and non-small cell lung cancer cell lines in vitro. Eur J Cancer 27:6–8.
98. Vellenga E, Biesma B, Meyer C, Wagteveld L, Esselink M, de VE. 1991. The effects of five hematopoietic growth factors on human small cell lung carcinoma cell lines: Interleukin 3 enhances the proliferation in one of the eleven cell lines. Cancer Res 51(1):73–76.
99. Nemunaitis J, Singer JW. 1989. The effect of recombinant human granulocyte macrophage-colony stimulating factor (rhGM-CSF) and recombinant human interleukin-1 (rhIL-1) on proliferation of human tumor cell lines. Cancer J 2(11):369–372.
100. Rygaard K, Nakamura T, Spang TM. 1993. Expression of the proto-oncogenes c-*met* and c-*kit* and their ligands, hepatocyte growth factor/scatter factor and stem cell factor, in SCLC cell lines and xenografts. Br J Cancer 67(1):37–46.
101. Sekido Y, Takahashi T, Ueda R, Takahashi M, Suzuki H, Nishida K, Tsukamoto T, Hida T, Shimokata K, Zsebo KM, Takahashi T. 1993. Recombinant human stem cell factor mediates chemotaxis of small cell lung cancer cell lines aberrantly expressing the c-*kit* protooncogene. Cancer Res 53:1709–1714.
102. Snyder SH. 1980. Brain peptides as neurotransmitters. Science 209:976–983.
103. Davis TP, Burgess HS, Crowell S, Moody TW, Culling BA, Liu RH. 1989. Beta-endorphin and neurotensin stimulate in vitro clonal growth of human SCLC cells. Eur J Pharmacol 161(2–3):283–285.
104. Feuerstein G, Molineaux CJ, Rosenberger JG, Zerbe RL, Cox BM, Faden AI. 1985. Hemorrhagic shock and the central vasopressin and opioid peptide system of rats. Am J Physiol 249:E244–E250.
105. Zhu YX, Hsi KL, Chen ZG, Zhang HL, Wu SX, Zhang SY, Fang PF, Guo SY, Kao YS, Tsou K. 1986. Neo-kyotorphin, an analgesic peptide isolated from human lung carcinoma. FEBS Lett 208(2):253–257.
106. Maneckjee R, Minna JD. 1990. Opioid and nicotine receptors affect growth regulation of human lung cancer cell lines. Proc Natl Acad Sci USA 87(9):3294–3298.
107. Maneckjee R, Minna JD. 1992. Nonconventional opioid binding sites mediate growth inhibitory effects of methadone on human lung cancer cells. Proc Natl Acad Sci USA 89(4):1169–1173.
108. Zagon IS, McLaughlin PJ. 1987. Modulation of murine neuroblastoma in nude mice by opioid antagonists. J Natl Cancer Inst 78(1):141–147.
109. Takuwa N, Takuwa Y, Ohue Y, Mukai H, Endoh K, Yamashita K, Kumada M, Munekata E. 1990. Stimulation of calcium mobilization but not proliferation by bombesin

and tachykinin neuropeptides in human small cell lung cancer cells. Cancer Res 50(2): 240–244.

110. Nilsson T, Arkhammar P, Rorsman P, Berggren PO. 1989. Suppression of insulin release by galanin and somatostatin is mediated by a G-protein. An effect involving repolarization and reduction in cytoplasmic free Ca^{2+} concentration. J Biol Chem 264:973–980.

111. Scambia G, Panici PB, Baiocchi G, Perrone L, Iacobelli S, Mancuso S. 1988. Antiproliferative effects of somatostatin and the somatostatin analog SMS 201-995 on three human breast cancer cell lines. J Cancer Res Clin Oncol 114(3):306–308.

112. Schally AV. 1988. Oncological applications of somatostatin analogues. Cancer Res 48: 6977–6985.

113. Murphy WA, Lance VA, Moreau S, Moreau JP, Coy DH. 1987. Inhibition of rat prostate tumor growth by an octapeptide analog of somatostatin. Life Sci 40(26):2515–2522.

114. Reubi JC, Laissue J, Krenning E, Lamberts SW. 1992. Somatostatin receptors in human cancer: Incidence, characteristics, functional correlates and clinical implications. J Steroid Biochem Mol Biol 43(1–3):27–35.

115. Reubi JC, Waser B, Sheppard M, Macaulay V. 1990. Somatostatin receptors are present in small-cell but not in non-small-cell primary lung carcinomas: Relationship to EGF-receptors. Int J Cancer 45(2):269–274.

116. Gorden P, Comi RJ, Maton PN, Go VL. 1989. Somatostatin and somatostatin analogue (SMS 201-995) in treatment of hormone-secreting tumors of the pituitary and gastrointestinal tract and non-neoplastic diseases of the gut. Ann Intern Med 110(1):35–50.

117. Taylor JE, Bogden AE, Moreau JP, Coy DH. 1988. In vitro and in vivo inhibition of human small cell lung carcinoma (NCI-H69) growth by a somatostatin analogue. Biochem Biophys Res Commun 153(1):81–86.

118. Taylor JE, Moreau JP, Baptiste L, Moody TW. 1991. Octapeptide analogues of somatostatin inhibit the clonal growth and vasoactive intestinal peptide-stimulated cyclic amp formation in human small cell lung cancer cells. Peptides 12(4):839–843.

119. Macaulay VM, Smith IE, Everard MJ, Teale JD, Reubi JC, Millar JL. 1991. Experimental and clinical studies with somatostatin analogue octreotide in small cell lung cancer. Br J Cancer 64(3):451–456.

120. Gazdar AF, Bunn P Jr, Minna JD, Baylin SB. 1985. Origin of human small cell lung cancer. Science 229(4714):679–680.

121. World Health Organization. 1982. The World Health Organization. Histological typing of lung tumours. Neoplasma 29(1):111–123.

122. Graziano SL, Mazid R, Newman N, Tatum A, Oler A, Mortimer JA, et al. 1989. The use of neuroendocrine immunoperoxidase markers to predict chemotherapy response in patients with non small cell lung cancer. J Clin Oncol 7:1398–1406.

123. Kamata N, Chida K, Rikimaru K, Horikoshi M, Enomoto S, Kuroki T. 1986. Growth-inhibitory effects of epidermal growth factor and overexpression of its receptors on human squamous cell carcinomas in culture. Cancer Res 46(4, Pt 1):1648–1653.

124. Damstrup L, Rygaard K, Spang TM, Poulsen HS. 1992. Expression of the epidermal growth factor receptor in human small cell lung cancer cell lines. Cancer Res 52(11): 3089–3093.

125. Rabiasz GL, Langdon SP, Bartlett JM, Crew AJ, Miller EP, Scott WN, Smyth JF, Miller WR. 1992. Growth control by epidermal growth factor and transforming growth factor-alpha in human lung squamous carcinoma cells. Br J Cancer 66:254–259.

126. Haeder M, Rotsch M, Bepler G, Hennig C, Havemann K, Heimann B, Moelling K. 1988. Epidermal growth factor receptor expression in human lung cancer cell lines. Cancer Res 48(5):1132–1136.

127. Söderdahl G, Betsholtz C, Johansson A, Nilsson K, Bergh J. 1988. Differential expression of platelet-derived growth factor and transforming growth factor genes in small- and non-small-cell lung carcinoma cell lines. Int J Cancer 41:636–641.

128. Veale D, Kerr N, Gibson GJ, Harris AL. 1989. Characterization of epidermal growth

factor receptor in primary human non-small cell lung cancer. Cancer Res 49:1313–1317.

129. Fang K, Li L, Jansen J, Fidler I, Roth JA. 1991. Brain metastatic variants of human lung cancer cells acquire independence from autocrine growth stimulation by TGF alpha. Proc Am Soc Clin Oncol 32:A302.

130. Putnam EA, Yen N, Gallick GE, Steck PA, Fang K, Akpakip B, Gazdar AF, Roth JA. 1992. Autocrine growth stimulation by transforming growth factor-alpha in human non-small cell lung cancer. Surg Oncol 1(1):49–60.

131. Lee M, Draoui M, Zia F, Gazdar A, Oie H, Bepler G, Bellot F, Tarr C, Kris R, Moody TW. 1992. Epidermal growth factor receptor monoclonal antibodies inhibit the growth of lung cancer cell lines. Monogr Natl Cancer Inst 13:112–123.

132. Jensen RT, Jones SW, Folkers K, Gardner JD. 1984. A synthetic peptide that is a bombesin receptor antagonist. Nature 309:61–63.

133. Zachary I, Rozengurt E. 1985. High-affinity receptors for peptides of the bombesin family in Swiss 3T3 cells. Proc Natl Acad Sci USA 82(22):7616–7620.

134. Sinnett-Smith J, Lehmann W, Rozengurt E. 1990. Bombesin receptor in membranes from Swiss 3T3 cells. Binding characteristics, affinity labelling and modulation by guanine nucleotides. Biochem J 265:485–493.

135. Zachary I, Rozengurt E. 1986. A substance P antagonist also inhibits the specific binding and mitogenic effects of vasopressin and bombesin-related peptides in Swiss 3T3 cells. Biochem Biophys Res Commun 137:135–141.

136. Woll PJ, Rozengurt E. 1988. [D-Arg^1,D-Phe^5,D-Trp^{7,9},Leu^{11}] substance P, a potent bombesin antagonist in murine Swiss 3T3 cells, inhibits the growth of human small cell lung cancer cells in vitro. Proc Natl Acad Sci USA 85(6):1859–1863.

137. Sethi T, Langdon S, Smyth J, Rozengurt E. 1992. Growth of small cell lung cancer cells: Stimulation by multiple neuropeptides and inhibition by broad spectrum antagonists in vitro and in vivo. Cancer Res 52:s2737–s2742.

138. Langdon S, Sethi T, Ritchie A, Muir M, Smyth J, Rozengurt E. 1992. Broad spectrum neuropeptide antagonists inhibit the growth of small cell lung cancer in vivo. Cancer Res 52(16):4554–4557.

139. Modjtahedi H, Styles JM, Dean CJ. 1993. The human EGF receptor as a target for cancer therapy: six new rat mAbs against the receptor on the breast carcinoma MDA-MB 468. Br J Cancer 67:247–253.

140. Engström U, Engström A, Ernlund A, Westermark B, Heldin C-H. 1992. Identification of a peptide antagonist for platelet derived growth factor. J Biol Chem 267:16581–16587.

141. Prendiville J, Crowther D, Thatcher N, et al. 1993. A phase I study of intravenous bryostatin 1 in patients with advanced cancer. Br J Cancer 68:418–424.

142. Levitzki A. 1992. Tyrphostins: tyrosine kinase blockers as novel antiproliferative agents and dissectors of signal transduction. FASEB J 6:3275–3282.

6. The development and progression of adenocarcinoma of the lung

Masayuki Noguchi and Yukio Shimosato

Introduction

Adenocarcinoma is the most common lung cancer in Japan and is said to be increasing in some other countries. Etiologically, it is less strongly associated with cigarette smoking than either squamous cell carcinoma or small cell carcinoma, and the mechanism of carcinogenesis of adenocarcinoma is not well understood.

Histologically and cytologically, adenocarcinoma is divided into many subtypes. The relationship between the histologic subtypes used by the World Health Organization (WHO) for diagnosing lung adenocarcinoma and the cytological subtypes of lung adenocarcinoma proposed by Shimosato et al. [1] is shown in table 1. Shimosato et al. subdivided pulmonary adeno-carcinomas cytologically into five subtypes: 1) cells resembling bronchial surface epithelial (BSE) cells with no or little mucin production, 2) goblet cells, 3) bronchial gland cells (BGC), 4) nonciliated bronchiolar epithelial cells (Clara cells), and 5) type II pneumocytes. Each cell type has its normal counterpart in the lung and possesses a biological identity that constitutes heterogeneity of lung adenocarcinomas ranging from fast-growing malignant tumors with massive distant metastases to slow-growing, locally spreading malignant tumors without extrathoracic metastasis, such as mucus-producing bronchioloalveolar carcinoma [2,3]. For example, goblet-cell-type adeno-carcinomas showed a better outcome than Clara-cell- and BSE-type adeno-carcinomas [4]. However, when reevaluated according to TNM parameters, the outcome of those two groups became similar. This means that the favorable outcome of goblet-cell-type adenocarcinomas is due to their characteristic distribution in the TNM staging system, that is, localized growth within the lung but frequent, and probably transbronchial, intrapul-monary metastasis [4]. On the other hand, BGC-type adenocarcinoma, which has a tendency to arise from larger bronchi, may show endobronchial growth and occurs more frequently in younger patients (mean age, 50.5 years) than in patients with other types of adenocarcinoma (mean age, 60.1 years). However, there is no difference in disease stage based on TNM factors and outcome between BGC-type adenocarcinoma and

Heine H. Hansen, (ed), Hansen: Lung Cancer.

Table 1. Relationship between histological classification of WHO and cytological subtypes of lung adenocarcinoma

Histological classification (WHO)	Cytological subtypes
Acinar adenocarcinoma	Bronchial gland cell type
Papillary adenocarcinoma	Bronchial surface epithelial
Bronchioloalveolai carcinoma	cell type without mucus
	Goblet cell type
Solid carcinoma with mucus formation	Nonciliated bronchiolar cell (Clara cell) type
	Type II alveolar epithelial cell type

peripheral-type (either Clara or type II pneumocyte) adenocarcinoma [5].

Although there is obvious histologic and biological heterogeneity among the lung adenocarcinomas as described above, this chapter will focus on the development and progression of the major types of peripheral-type adeno-carcinoma (Clara cell type, BSE type, type II pneumocyte type) from the morphological, biological, and molecular points of view [1].

Development

Denial of scar cancer concept

A majority of adenocarcinomas of the lung develop in the peripheral airway, that is, the bronchioloalveolar region. Most peripheral adenocarcinomas contain a central or subpleural anthracotic and fibrotic focus, which is often associated with a pleural indentation. This characteristic feature is the basis of the concept of scar cancer, which has been believed to be common in the lung for many years. However, Shimosato, Suzuki, and their associates verified that in most adenocarcinomas seen in routine practice, the central fibrosis or fibrotic focus with anthracosis forms not before, but after the development of carcinoma [1,6,7]. Much of the fibrotic focus is formed by the collapse of alveoli that had been lined by cancer cells, and is composed of aggregates of elastic fibers of alveolar septal origin. Denial of the scar cancer concept in lung adenocarcinoma is supported by the fact that in early-stage adenocarcinoma a fibrotic focus is often absent, as are fibro-blastic proliferation and collagenization in areas with dense aggregates of elastic fibers. Convergence of bronchi and pulmonary vessels toward the tumor, which is often associated with pleural indentation, is observed fre-quently on chest x-ray films and provides evidence supporting the morpho-logical events [7]. Therefore, scar cancers are considered to be very rare in the lung except for carcinomas arising from diffuse pulmonary fibrosis [6].

132

So-called atypical adenomatous hyperplasia (probably adenoma)

Another concept to consider is multistep carcinogenesis. We have not in-frequently encountered papillary or bronchioloalveolar lesions, which suggest the development of adenocarcinoma, in a focus of atypical adenomatous hyperplasia (AAH), or adenoma (figures 1a and 1b). In the National Cancer Center Hospital, Tokyo, from 1965 to 1989, 108 cases with atypical adenomatous lesions (5%) were found out of 2098 cases of resected primary lung carcinoma (table 2). Papillary or bronchioloalveolar adenomatous lesions are usually less than 1 cm in diameter, are often multiple, and are composed of atypical cuboidal cells with an increased nuclear cytoplasmic ratio replacing the lining of the alveoli. They resemble either Clara cells or type II pneumocytes. Mitotic figures are rarely seen. Within such a lesion, an area may be seen with increased cellularity and cell atypia suficient for it to be called well-differentiated adenocarcinoma. Such atypical adenomatous lesions are not infrequently seen at the periphery of advanced papillary adeno-carcinoma (figures 2a, 2b, and 2c), suggesting a late stage of the adenoma–carcinoma sequence, which is well known in the colon.

Recently, these lesions have been examined extensively. For example, Miller et al. [8,9] examined the detailed histology of resected specimens with lung adenocarcinomas and proposed an adenoma–carcinoma sequence, analogous to that of colonic tumors.

Kodama et al. [10] morphometrically examined well differentiated adeno-carcinomas and adenomatous cuboidal cell hyperplastic lesions with and

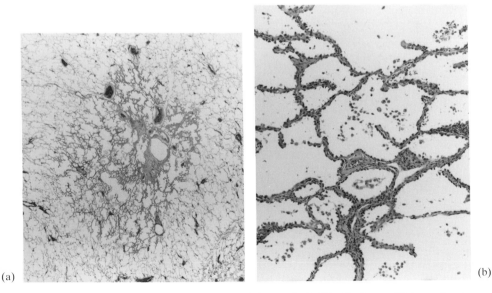

(a)   (b)

Figure 1. (a,b) Histological sections of AAH (adenoma). AAH cells show mild to moderate nuclear atypia.

Table 2. Atypical adenomatous hyperplasia (AAH) (bronchio-loalveolar adenoma) of the lung in surgical cases

Histologic type of tumor	Total	Carcinoma associated with AAH (adenoma)
Adenocarcinoma	1,118	87 (7.8%)
Squamous cell carcinoma	766	7 (1.0%)
Large cell carcinoma	152	10 (6.6%)
Small cell carcinom	62	4 (6.5%)
Total	2,098	108 (5.1%)

Source: National Cancer Center Hospital, Tokyo, 1965–1989.

without atypia and found that many cases of AAH could be distinguished from well-differentiated adenocarcinoma by means of the nuclear areas and the standard deviation of the mean nuclear area.

A few years later, Nakayama et al. [11] measured the nuclear DNA content of AAH by cytofluorometry and compared it with that of adeno-carcinomas and reactive type II pneumocyte hyperplasia, and indicated that AAH showed clonal proliferation, was closely related to small-sized well-

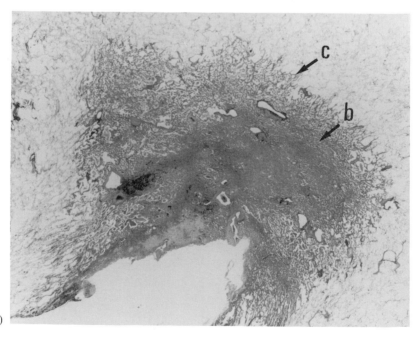

(a)

Figure 2. (a,b,c) Histological sections of adenocarcinoma associated with AAH (adenoma). Adenocarcinoma cells (b) show more nuclear pleomorphism and hyperchromasia than AAH cells (c).

134

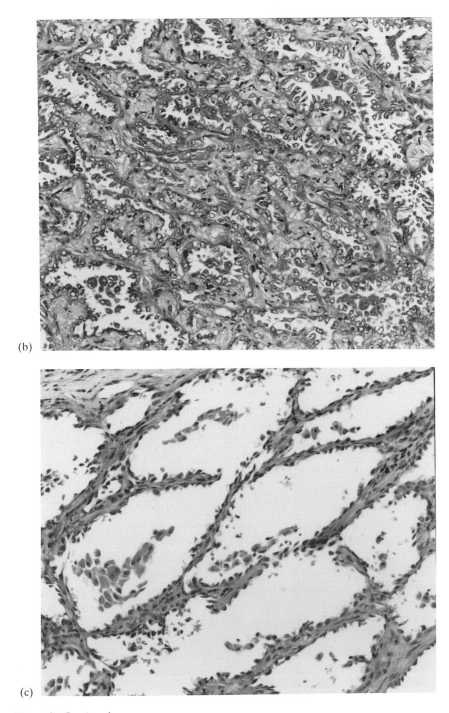

(b)

(c)

Figure 2. Continued

135

differentiated papillary adenocarcinoma, and was either adenoma or very well-differentiated adenocarcinoma.

These findings indicate that AAH may be either the most important precancerous lesion of the peripheral type adenocarcinoma or already a neoplastic growth — that is, adenoma or low-grade malignant adenocarcinoma, which possesses the potential to progress to become the more malignant carcinoma. Although there may be adenocarcinomas that show de novo development, some peripheral-type adenocarcinomas undoubtedly develop through AAH or adenoma [12,13]. Eighty percent of peripheral adenocarcinomas less than 2 cm in diameter with no lymph node metastasis showed such neoplastic progression [14].

Progression

Phenotypic progression

Clayton [2] subdivided peripheral-type adenocarcinoma into three subtypes: mucinous, nonmucinous, and sclerosing bronchioloalveolar carcinomas. Sclerosing bronchioloalveolar carcinomas are composed of tumor cells that are cytologically and ultrastructurally similar to those of nonmucinous bronchioloalveolar carcinomas, but that also contain a central area of dense sclerosis with entrapped, distorted acini of tumor cells. He proposed a possible etiology for such fibrosis: the tumor evolves, developing a mechanism to induce fibrin deposition, which results in both angiogenesis and, ultimately, fibrosis. This may explain the poor prognosis of sclerosing bronchioloalveolar carcinoma relative to nonmucinous bronchioloalveolar carcinoma. In addition, the evolution is thought to be the most typical example of malignant progression of nonmucinous bronchioloalveolar carcinoma.

Adenosquamous carcinoma of the lung is a relatively rare subtype of lung carcinoma. Clinicopathologically, the outcome of adenosquamous carcinoma is poorer than that of adenocarcinoma and squamous cell carcinoma, particularly in stages I and II [15]. The histogenesis of adenosquamous carcinoma is unclear; there are many possibilities, including adenocarcinoma with squamous metaplasia, collision tumor, high-grade mucoepidermoid carcinoma, and bipotential undifferentiated cell origin. But many adenosquamous carcinomas are considered to be the result of malignant progression of adenocarcinoma, since squamous components are not seen in the area of adenocarcinoma with slight cell atypia but are almost always seen in the area with moderate to marked cell atypia.

Similar to the process of development of adenocarcinoma in adenoma, histologically and cytologically more atypical or more malignant-appearing areas develop within carcinoma. Such morphological progression can be confirmed not only by cytological and histological examination of hematoxylin and eosin-stained sections but also by other means of determining phenotypes, such as immunohistochemical staining for carcinoembryonic antigen (CEA) and examination for markers of proliferative activity. The appearance of mucin-producing or mucin-containing cells within nonmucin-producing Clara-cell-type and type II pneumocyte-type bronchioloalveolar carcinoma is considered to be a feature of malignant progression, since those cells are almost always found not in areas with in situ bronchioloalveolar growth but in areas of invasive growth in the mid- or central portion of tumors, and show increased nuclear atypia [1].

With reference to CEA immunostaining, sclerosing bronchioloalveolar carcinoma displaying stepwise progression from AAH (or adenoma) in the periphery to a papillary arrangement in the midzone and solid nests in the central portion may disclose negative, weak to moderate, and marked staining of CEA, respectively, as nuclear atypia increases [13].

Growth properties

The growth properties of tumors can be evaluated by the frequency of mitotic figures, but to obtain mitotic indices by counting the mitotic figures is not only time consuming but also inaccurate. Greater accuracy is obtained by counting the DNA-synthesizing (S phase) cells by labeling the cell with ^{3}H-thymidine followed by autoradiography, or labeling them with bromo-deoxyuridine followed by immunohistochemical examination. With this method, Yoshida et al. [16] demonstrated that the labeling index was around 19% and 11% in small cell carcinoma and squamous cell carcinoma, respectively. In adenocarcinoma, the labeling index ranged widely from less than 11% to 19%, to being 3% or less in two thirds of the cases, indicating that adenocarcinomas are a very heterogenous group of tumors with respect to their growth properties. The bromodeoxyuridine-labeling index of brain metastases of adenocarcinoma of the lung was higher than 5% [17], indicating that adenocarcinoma with a labeling index of 3% or less may be unable to form hematogenous metastases.

More recently, proliferating cells have been identified by immunohistochemical examination for proliferating cell nuclear antigen and proliferation-associated nuclear antigen Ki-67 [18,19]. By that method, areas in adenocarcinoma with more atypical cells were found to show an increased number of positive cells — that is, increased growth properties — compared to areas of the tumor with fewer atypical cells. Therefore, malignant progression in adenocarcinoma can be verified by evaluating the growth properties of various parts of the tumor.

Nuclear DNA content and aneuploidy

The mean nuclear DNA content has been shown to increase in less differentiated adenocarcinoma in the advanced stage, and is significantly greater in stage I adenocarcinomas with recurrence within five years after surgery than in those without recurrence [20,21]. Within a primary tumor, the mean nuclear DNA content of tumor cells is significantly greater in areas with an increased amount of stroma in alveolar septae [22]. Comparison of the mean nuclear DNA content of primary tumors and metastatic foci in the lymph noted, brain, and liver disclosed that hematogenous metastases were frequently composed of tumor cells with greater mean nuclear DNA content than that in the primary tumor, whereas the mean nuclear DNA content of lymph node metastases, particularly metastases in the hilar lymph nodes, was almost equal to that of the primary tumor, although cells with greater DNA content were noted in mediastinal node metastases. Furthermore, analysis of the histogram patterns of hematogenous metastases suggested that a small focus with greater DNA content, which had been undetected, developed in some primary tumors and was the source of metastasis [23]. However, histogram patterns in other cases suggested the presence of abnormal cell lines with increased DNA content in foci of hematogenous metastases. From these observations, the nuclear DNA content is considered to be a parameter of malignancy, at least in adenocarcinoma of the lung, that can be used to prove stepwise progression in malignancy.

Genetic changes

In adenocarcinoma, several oncogenes and their protein products, including c-Ki-*ras*, c-*myc*, c-*erbB2*, and p53, have been found to be amplified, rearranged, or overexpressed [24,25]. On the other hand, loss of heterozygosity of 3p, 11p, 13q, and 17p has also been detected [26,27].

Point mutation in the c-Ki-*ras* gene is seen in 15% to 30% of lung adenocarcinomas [28,29], and clinicopathologically point mutation of c-Ki-*ras* codon 12 was reported to be correlated with the T factors and N factors of the TNM system and with smoking history, but not with the degree of histological differentiation. Our study, however, suggested that point mutational activation of the c-Ki-*ras* gene at codon 12 occurs frequently in goblet-cell-type adenocarcinomas followed by the BSE type, and very rarely, if ever, in the pure Clara cell type [28].

Amplification of *myc* family genes has not been seen in the primary adenocarcinoma of the lung (0/18), but is frequently seen in brain metastases (13/17) (Nakajima et al., unpublished data).

Forty percent to 50% of adenocarcinomas overexpress p185*neu* (product of c-*erbB2*) relative to levels of expression seen in the uninvolved bronchiolar epithelium [30] (figure. 3a). The overexpression of p185*neu* is strongly associated with tumorigenicity of human bronchial epithelial cells [31]. For adenocarcinomas, p185*neu* expression was reported to be associated with older age and short survival. Using Cox's multivariate survival analysis, p185*neu* expression was found to be a significant determinant of survival even after accounting for the effect of the tumor stage [30].

Nuclear staining as the result of nuclear accumulation of the p53 gene

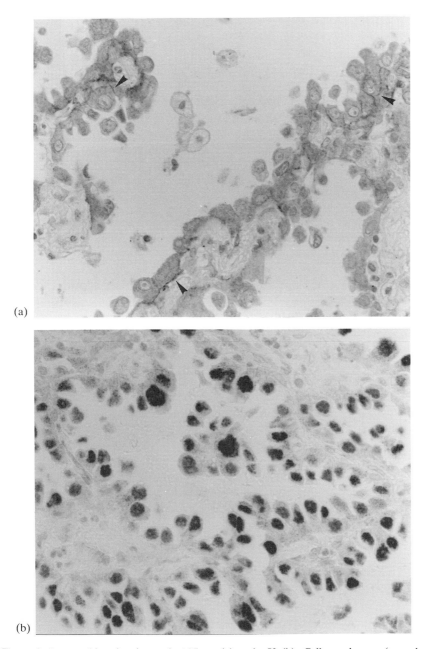

(a)

(b)

Figure 3. Immunohistochemistry of p185*neu* (a) and p53 (b). Cell membranes (arrowheads) and nuclei are stained by anti-p185*neu* and anti-p53 antibodies, respectively.

product is said to be closely associated with point mutation of the gene [32,33] (figure 3b). In single tumors, positive immunostaining was statistically significantly associated with lymph node and distant organ metastases and with the stage of the disease in adenocarcinoma, although such an association was not seen in squamous cell carcinoma and small cell carcinoma [34]. Positive nuclear staining was seen more frequently in nuclei showing increased atypia. In addition to nuclear atypia, the cell type may also be important, since both of two cases of goblet-cell-type bronchioloalveolar carcinoma of the lung examined so far showed entirely negative immunostaining.

Some of the findings described here may indicate multistep malignant progression of the adenocarcinoma due to genetic abnormalities.

Summary

This chapter has briefly reviewed the development and progression of peripheral-type adenocarcinoma of the lung, focusing particularly on bronchioloalveolar carcinoma consisting of the nonmucus-producing cell type with or without sclerosis.

Histoloical examination reveals that scar cancers are rare except in cases of diffuse pulmonary fibrosis and that many nonmucus-producing bronchioloalveolar carcinomas appear to develop from atypical adenomatous hyperplasia, which can be called adenoma or very well-differentiated adenocarcinoma, and to progress stepwise.

Stepwise progresssion in malignancy can be disclosed not only by cytological and histological examination but also by proliferative activity of the tumor, such as mitotic activity, the percentage of DNA-synthesizing cells and the frequency of proliferating cell nuclear antigen-positive cells, the mean nuclear DNA content of tumor cells and occurrence of aneuploid cell lines, and abnormalities of oncogenes (c-Ki-*ras*, *myc* family, and c-*erbB2*), such as point mutation, rearrangement, amplification, and tumor suppressor genes (point mutation and deletion) such as p53.

References

1. Shimosato Y, Kodama T, Kameya T. 1982. Morphogenesis of peripheral type adenocarcinoma of the lung. In Morphogenesis of Lung Cancer, Y Shimosato, MR Melamed, and P Nettesheim (eds.). CRC Press: Boca Raton, FL, pp. 65–89.
2. Clayton F. 1988. The spectrum and significance of bronchioloalveolar carcinomas. Pathol Annu 23(part 2):361–394.
3. Nomori H, Matsuno Y, Noguchi M, Tsugane S, Shimosato Y, Hirohashi S. 1992. Adenocarcinoma of the lung with selective metastasis to the lung: Clinical, histologic and DNA-cytofluorometric analyses. Jpn J Cancer Res 83:93–100.
4. Gemma A, Noguchi M, Hirohashi S, Tsugane S, Tsuchiya R, Niitani H, Shimosato Y.

1991. Clinicopathologic and immunohistochemical characteristics of goblet cell type adenocarcinoma of the lung. Acta Pathol Jpn 41:737–743.

5. Hirata H, Noguchi M, Shimosato Y, Uei Y, Goya T. 1990. Clinicopathological and immunohistochemical characteristics of bronchial gland cell type adenocarcinoma of the lung. Am J Clin Pathol 93:20–25.

6. Shimosato Y, Hashimoto T, Kodama T, et al. 1979. Prognostic implications of fibrotic focus (scar) in small peripheral lung cancer. Am J Surg Pathol 4:365–373.

7. Suzuki A. 1982. Growth characterictics of peripheral type adenocarcinoma of the lung in terms of roentgenologic findings. In Morphogenesis of Lung Cancer, Y Shimosato, MR Melamed, and P Nettesheim (eds.). CRC Press: Boca Raton, FL, pp. 91–110.

8. Miller RR. 1990. Bronchioloalveolar cell adenomas. Am J Surg Pathol 14:904–912.

9. Miller RR, Nelems B, Evans KG, Muller NL, Ostrow DN. 1988. Glandular neoplasia of the lung. A proposed analogy to colonic tumors. Cancer 61:1009–1014.

10. Kodama T, Biyajima S, Watanabe S, Shimosato Y. 1986. Morphometric study of adenocarcinomas and hyperplastic epithelial lesions in the peripheral lung. Am J Clin Pathol 85:146–151.

11. Nakayama H, Noguchi M, Tsuchiya R, Kodama T, Shimosato Y. 1990. Clonal growth of atypical adenomatous hyperplasia of the lung: cytofluorometric analysis of nuclear DNA content. Modern Pathol 3:314–320.

12. Shimosato Y. 1989. Pulmonary neoplasms. In Diagnostic Surgical Pathology, vol. 1, SS Sternberg (ed.). Raven Press: New York, pp. 758–827.

13. Shimosato Y, Noguchi M, Matsuno Y. 1993. Adenocarcinoma of the lung: its development and malignant progression. Lung Cancer 9:99–108.

14. Kurakawa T, Matsuno Y, Noguchi M, Mizuno S, Shimosato Y. 1994. Surgically curable "early" adenocarcinoma in the periphery of the lung. Am J Surg Pathol 18(5):431–438.

15. Takamori S, Noguchi M, Morinaga S, Goya T, Tsugane S, Kakegawa T, Shimosato Y. 1991. Clinicopathologic characteristics of adenosquamous carcinoma of the lung. Cancer 67:649–654.

16. Yoshida K, Morinaga S, Shimosato Y, Hayata Y. 1989. A cell kinetic study of pulmonary adenocarcinoma by an immunoperoxidase procedure after bromodeoxyuridine labeling. Cancer 64:2284–2291.

17. Cho KG, Hoshino T, Pitts LH, Nomura K, Shimosato Y. 1988. Proliferative potential of brain metastases. Cancer 62:512–515.

18. Brown DC, Gatter KG. 1990. Monoclonal antibody Ki-67: its use in histopathology. Histopathology 17:489–503.

19. Matsuno Y, Hirohashi S, Furuya S, Sakamoto M, Mukai K, Shimosato Y. 1990. Heterogeneity of proliferative activity in nodule-in-nodule lesions of small hepatocellular carcinoma. Jpn J Cancer Res 81:1137–1140.

20. Asamura H, Nakajima T, Mukai K, Noguchi M, Shimosato Y. 1989. DNA cytofluorometric and nuclear morphometric analyses of lung adenocarcinoma. Cancer 64:1657–1664.

21. Asamura H, Nakajima T, Mukai K, Shimosato Y. 1989. Nuclear DNA content by cytofluorometry of stage I adenocarcinoma of the lung in relation to postoperative recurrence. Chest 96:312–318.

22. Nomori H, Hirohashi S, Noguchi M, Matsuno Y, Shimosato Y. 1991. Tumor cell heterogeneity and subpopulations with metastatic ability in differentiated adenocarcinoma of the lung. Histologic and cytofluorometric DNA analyses. Chest 99:934–940.

23. Nomori H, Nakajima T, Noguchi M, Iga R, Shimosato Y. 1991. Cytofluorometric analysis of metastases from lung adenocarcinoma with special reference to the difference between hematogenous and lymphatic metastases. Cancer 67:2941–2947.

24. Kishimoto Y, Murakami Y, Shiraishi M, Hayashi K, Sekiya T. 1992. Aberrations of the p53 tumor suppressor gene in human non-small cell carcinomas of the lung. Cancer Res 52:4799–4804.

25. Shiraishi M, Noguchi M, Shimosato Y, Sekiya T. 1989. Amplification of protooncogenes in

surgical specimens of human lung carcinomas. Cancer Res 49:6474–6479.

26. Shiraishi M, Morinaga S, Noguchi M, Shimosato Y, Sekiya T. 1987. Loss of genes on the short arm of chromosome 11 in human lung carcinomas. Jpn J Cancer Res 78:1302–1308.

27. Yokota J, Wada M, Shimosato Y, Terada M, Sugimura T. 1987. Loss of heterozygosity on chromosomes, 3, 13, 17 in small cell carcinoma and on chromosome 3 in adenocarcinoma of the lung. Proc Natl Acad Sci USA 84:9252–9256.

28. Kobayashi T, Tsuda H, Noguchi M, Hirohashi S, Shimosato Y, Goya T, Hayata Y. 1990. Association of point mutation in c-Ki-ras oncogene in lung adenocarcinoma with particular reference to cytologic subtypes. Cancer 66:289–294.

29. Rosenhuis S, Slebos RJC, Boot AJM, et al. 1988. Incidence and possible clinical significance of K-ras oncogene activation in adenocarcinoma of the human lung. Cancer Res 48:5738–5741.

30. Kern JA, Schwartz DA, Nordberg JE, Weiner DB, Greene MI, Torney L, Robinson RA. 1990. p185*neu* expression in human lung adenocarcinomas predicts shortened survival. Cancer Res 50:5184–5191.

31. Noguchi M, Murakami M, Bennett W, Lupu R, Hui F Jr, Harris CC, Gerwin BI. 1993. Biological consequence of overexpression of a transfected c-*erbB*-2 gene in immortalized human bronchial epithelial cells. Cancer Res 53:2035–2043.

32. Noguchi M, Maezawa N, Nakanishi Y, Matsuno Y, Shimosato Y, Hirohashi S. 1993. Application of the p53 gene mutation pattern for differential diagnosis of primary versus metastatic lung carcinomas. Diagn Mol Pathol 2:29–35.

33. Rodrigues NR, Rowan A, Smith MEF, et al. 1990. p53 mutations in colorectal cancer. Proc Natl Acad Sci USA 87:7555–7559.

34. Hiyoshi H, Matsuno Y, Kato H, Shimosato Y, Hirohashi S. 1992. Clinicopathological significance of nuclear accumulation of tumor suppressor gene p53 product in primary lung cancer. Jpn J Cancer Res 83:101–106.

7. Neuroendocrine characteristics in malignant lung tumors: Implications for diagnosis, treatment, and prognosis

Thomas Senderovitz, Birgit G. Skov, and Fred R. Hirsch

Introduction

Twenty years ago, Pearse identified a group of endocrine cells sharing multiple morphological and biochemical features. He named them APUD cells (Amine Precurser Uptake and Decarboxylation) because of their amine-handling properties, one of their main functions being their ability to take up and decarboxylate relatively simple amino precursor substances, such as dihydroxyphenylanaline (DOPA) and 5-hydroxytryptamine (5-HT), thus producing biogenic amines [1]. Today, these cells are known as neuro-endocrine (NE) cells and the APUD system as the Dispersed Neuroendocrine System (DNS), currently consisting of more than 40 different cell types.

Neuroendocrine cells can thus be defined as cells with secretory granules and the capability of producing polypeptide hormones or biogenic amines. They occur in various locations, including the islets of Langerhans in the pancreas, the crypts of Liberkuhn in the small intestine and the appendix, the C-cells of the thyroid gland, the adrenal medulla, and the granular basal layer of the bronchial epithelium. Traditionally, the neuroendocrine tumors of the lung include the carcinoid tumors (typical and atypical) and the small cell lung carcinomas [2]. They are characterized by the presence of the above-mentioned granules (which in the electron microscope are seen as dense-core granules) and high concentrations of the key amine-handling enzyme aromatic-L-amino acid decarboxylase (refered to as L-dopa decarboxylase), and they produce various hormones and neuro-peptides [3–6].

In order to demonstrate neuroendocrine differentiation, various markers have been identified. The presence of one or more of these markers indicates a neuroendocrine origin of the tumor. Unfortunately, no interna-tional standards exist regarding which markers and how many of them are needed to identify a tumor as neuroendocrine. Furthermore, different methods, different antibodies, and so forth are often used to demonstrate these markers, which makes comparison of results from clinical studies difficult.

Neuroendocrine markers in the histopathologic diagnosis

General neuroendocrine markers

Neuron-specific enolase (NSE). NSE is a gamma–gamma isoenzyme of the glycolytic enzyme 2-phospho-D-glycerate hydrolase. It was first believed that the gene coding for this isomer was restricted to neurons. However, NSE has been detected in APUD cells of the central and peripheral neuroendocrine system [7,8]. Several studies have studied the expression of NSE in lung carcinomas, especially SCLC but also adenocarcinoma of the lung. In one of the first studies, Sheppard et al. [9] were unable to detect immunoreactivity in 10 adenocarcinomas, while 18 of 31 SCLCs were positive. Thus, this antibody was thought to be a good marker for SCLC. However, more recently, many NSCLC tumors including adenocarcinomas have shown positive reactions for anti-NSE, with a range of 12%–57% [6,10–13]. In a study from Grazianno et al. [12], a polyclonal antibody against NSE was positive in pretreatment biopsies of NSCLC in 14 of 26 (54%) patients who responded to chemotherapy compared to 7 of 26 (27%) in nonresponding patients. Twelve of these 14 responding patients had adenocarcinoma. In a study by Skov et al. [13], a monoclonal antibody to NSE was applied and 18 of 114 patients (16%) with adenocarcinoma of the lung had positive staining reactions.

From the literature, it can be concluded that immunohistochemical staining for NSE in adenocarcinoma (and in other NSCLC) show positive reactions in 0% to 60% of tumors. In most of the studies, polyclonal antibodies were applied, and these sera are difficult to control in terms of specificity.

Immunohistochemical studies using monoclonal antibodies to NSE are needed to evaluate the usefulness of these antibodies as a specific marker for neuroendocrine-derived neoplasms.

Chromogranin A (ChrA). Several studies have described ChrA as a marker for endocrine cells containing dense-core granules, but only a small number of studies have looked at adenocarcinoma of the lung. In the study by Linnoila et al. [6], 4 of 39 patients (10%) with adenocarcinoma had positive tumors using a monoclonal antibody, and the positive reactions were associated with the presence of other neuroendocrine markers. Skov et al. [13] found a positive ChrA reaction in 22 of 114 patients (19%) with stage III and IV adenocarcinoma of the lung. By using Northern blot hybridizations, Gazdar et al. [14] detected ChrA (mRNA) in 6/25 NSCLC (without further subtyping), and found a 100% concordance between the expression of ChrA and the presence of dense-core granules [14].

Thus, antibodies against ChrA are a specific but not very sensitive marker for neuroendocrine cells. This marker is useful in a panel with other neuroendocrine markers for the classification of lung cancer.

Leu 7. Leu 7 is an antigen expressed by a subpopulation of lymphocytes as well as nerves, most NE cells, and their neoplasms throughout the body [6,15]. Antibodies to the Leu 7 antigen recognize a neural cell adhesion molecule (see below). Eleven out of 39 surgically resected lung adenocarcinomas (28%) were positive in the study by Linnoila et al. [6], and Graziano et al. [12] obtained positivity in 12 of 51 adenocarcinomas (24%). Leu 7 may be a good marker for NE cells, but more studies are needed to determine the specificity and sensitivity of this marker.

Synaptophysin (SY 38). An integral membrane glycoprotein (MW 38,000), SY 38 has been identified in presynaptic vesicles in neurons, but also in some epithelial cells. Very few studies have looked at its presence in adenocarcinoma of the lung. Kayser et al. [11] found expression of SY 38 in only 2 of 25 adenocarcinomas. In order to evaluate the diagnostic use of this marker, more studies are required.

Specific neuroendocrine products

A large number of neuropeptides and hormones have been demonstrated in malignant lung tumors, especially in bronchial carcinoids and in SCLC. In one of the previously cited studies, hormones and neuropeptides were found in lung adenocarcinomas as follows: bombesin (7/39), calcitonin (1/39), serotonin (1/39), ACTH (7/39), vasopressin (7/39), and neurotensin (0/39) [6]. Hamid et al. [16] were unable to detect bombesin and pro-bombesin in 57 adenocarcinomas.

Because of the great diversity of these NE products and their variable expression, the use of these markers as broad spectrum markers for NE neoplasms is limited.

Neural cell adhesion molecules (NCAMs). This group of surface glycoproteins is involved in direct cell–cell adhesion; they play an important role in cell proliferation, migration and differentiation [17]. NCAMs were originally considered to be mainly restricted to neurons, but recently it has been shown that NCAMs are also expressed in some non-neural tissues, including some endocrine cell. The antibodies against NCAM were characterized and clustered (cluster 1) in the International Workshops on SCLC antigens [18]. NCAM are also expressed on natural killer cells and have been termed CD 56 in the Leucocyte Antigen Workshop. It has been demonstrated that NCAM expression in lung tumor cell lines is associated with the expression of neuroendocrine markers of differentiation, independent of the histological type of lung cancer [19]. In a study using three NCAM antibodies (SL 11.14, MOC 1, and NE 25), a homogeneous reaction in 2 of 5 adenocarcinomas and 11 of 34 squamous cell carcinomas was demonstrated, as compared to 7 of 7 SCLC and 2 of 3 carcinoids. For all the NSCLC tumors, the reactivity of the three antibodies was significantly higher in stage III as compared to stage I and II, and poorly differentiated

145

tumors had significantly more positive reactions than well-differentiated tumors [20].

In another study using MOC 1, 1 of 39 adenocarcinomas had positive reactions compared to 19 of 19 SCLC and 20 of 102 squamous cell carcinomas [21]. Mooi et al. [22] demonstrated NCAMs (123C3) in 4 of 68 adenocarcinomas and in 38 of 185 squamous cell carcinomas. By the use of four MOC antibodies, NE differentiation was demonstrated in 43% of patients with lung adenocarcinomas in a study by Berendsen et al., and in about half of these tumors more than 50% positive cells were detected [23]. Komminoth and co-workers [24] have immunohistochemically examined the expression af sialyated NCAM in a small number of small cell lung carcinomas and bronchial and gastrointestinal carcinoids. They described its differential expression in small cell lung cancer, but not on carcinoids, and suggested polysialyated NCAM to be a useful marker to distinguish between these tumors.

In conclusion, antibodies recognizing epitopes on NCAM seem to be useful as markers of NE differentiation. Unfortunately, unfixed tissue is necessary for the use of the present available antibodies.

Combination of NE markers in the histopathologic diagnosis

From the literature it seems clear that one single NE marker is not useful in categorizing malignant lung tumors as carcinoids, SCLC, and NSCLC. However, by applying a panel of NE markers, a better subclassification of malignant lung tumors seems to be possible. Linnoila et al. [6] used a statistical model in an immunohistochemical multimarker study. Seven of 77 NSCLC tumors had a staining pattern indistinguishable from SCLC, and 95% of the tumors were correctly classified by application of a statistical model created from staining indices of three general NE markers (ChrA, Leu-7, NSE) and three other markers [6]. Thus, ChrA, Leu-7, and NSE together make a suitable panel for screening lung tumors with NE features. If one considers the expression of two or more of these markers as a definition for a neuroendocrine phenotype, about 75% of the SCLC and 25% of the NSCLC have this phenotype. From this, it is obvious that the demonstration of NE differentiation in lung carcinomas cannot be used as a tool to differentiate between histological subtypes (especially the differentiation between SCLC and NSCLC). Patients with NE-positive tumors may have different clinical characteristics than other patients with NSCLC tumors, including responsiveness to chemotherapy, and this is discussed below.

Neuroendocrine properties and chemotherapy sensitivity in NSCLC

During recent years, several investigators have reported the demonstration of neuroendocrine features in NSCLC. It has been difficult to compare the results of the clinical studies due to the different methods used for identification of NE features and differences in the treatment regimens. Furthermore, the group has mostly been studied as a whole, without taking into consideration the possibility of a difference in survival and response in the different subgroups (i.e., adenocarcinoma, squamous cell carcinoma, and large cell carcinoma).

In vitro studies

In a study by Gazdar et al. [25], 55 lung cancer cell lines (including 32 NSCLC cell lines, 4 carcinoid cell lines, and 19 SCLC cell lines) were investigated for the presence of common NE markers (L-dopa decarboxylase, dense-core granules, ChrA, and synaptophysin) by immunohistochemical methods in order to determine the association between morphological type and NE differentiation with the in vitro chemosensitivity. Chemosensitivity was determined for five cytotoxic drugs (VP-16, cisplatin, doxorubicin, melphalan, and carmustine). Cell lines expressing two or more markers were defined as having a neuroendocrine phenotype. Of the 32 cell lines examined, 5 expressed the NE phenotype (16%). The group of NSCLC having the NE phenotype was found to be as chemosensitive as SCLC cell lines, while NSCLC lacking NE markers were found to be relatively chemoresistant. The bronchial carcinoids were found to be highly chemoresistant [25].

Clinical studies

Until recently, the therapies of choice in NSCLC have been surgery whenever possible (stage I, II, and selected stage III patients) or just palliative care. Chemotherapy in NSCLC has been quite disapointing. Even though the platinum agents alone or in combination with other drugs may result in a marginal improvement of the survival time, no studies have so far been able to demonstrate any real advantage compared to the best palliative care; nor have the same good response rates as in SCLC been achieved. No studies so far have explained these facts. It is tempting to hypothesize that the subset of the NSCLC tumors expressing NE markers would have the same biologic characteristics as SCLC (or at least a SCLC-like behavior) and therefore would respond much better to chemotherapy, with a prolongation of the survival time. This hypothesis has been supported by the in vitro data. Another question would be whether the use of adjuvant chemotherapy in the subset of the NE–NSCLC group of patients who are radically operated would result in a prolongation of the survival time.

Berendsen et al. [23] investigated 141 biopsies from untreated NSCLC patients, and a panel of monoclonal antibodies (MOC-1, MOC-21, MOC-32, MOC-51, and MOC-52) against SCLC-associated antigens was used to detect neuroendocrine markers. Thirty-one percent of the specimens contained cells expressing one or more of the assessed NE markers (50%–100% positive staining cells), and they were found more often in adenocarcinoma (44%) than in squamous cell carcinoma or large cell carcinoma. A multivariate analysis for prognostic factors was performed, and among these factors tumors with more than 50% positive-staining cells with the MOC-1 antibody were shown to be a negative prognostic factor. This finding could be compatible with the hypothesis of biologic similarities between these NE-NSCLC and SCLC tumors.

In a retrospective study by Kibbelaar et al. [26], 308 surgically resected lung carcinomas of various histological subtypes were studied. A panel of monoclonal antibodies recognizing different NCAM epitopes was used. These included MAb 123C3, which is a monoclonal antibody raised against a membrane preparation of SCLC [22], and the antigen recognized is present mainly in neuroendocrine cells as the polypeptide backbone of NCAM [27]. Tumors positive for MAb 123C3 were found in 53 out of 278 NSCLC patients (19%), but material from only 91 NSCLC patients was available for additional immunostaining with the other antibodies. Of these tumors, 42 (46%) were positive for MAb 123C3. Patients having NSCLC tumors positive for MAb 123C3 had a postoperative overall and disease-free survival times significantly shorter than 123C3-negative NSCLC tumors.

Sundaresan et al. [28] presented a study in which 317 patients with NSCLC were evaluated retrospectively and 44 patients were evaluated prospectively by immunohistochemical methods. The specimens were examined for the presence of NSE, CK-BB, bombesin, neurotensin, ChrA, synaptophysin, and UJ.13A. Two or more markers were found in 30% of the tumors. While a significant correlation between degree of metastases and NE differentiation was found, no correlation between NE differentiation and survival could be detected.

The prognostic significance of NE differentiation in surgically resected NSCLC is not quite clear. The above-mentioned studies were retrospectively designed, and different neuroendocrine markers have been used. However, a certain trend towards a more SCLC-like behavior of the NE-positive NSCLC can be seen (higher degree of metastases and shorter postoperative survival).

Further investigations, preferably designed as prospective randomized trials, are needed to solve the role of chemotherapy in resectable NE-NSCLC.

The problem of whether inoperable NE-NSCLC patients should be treated with or without chemotherapy is still also an open question.

In a retrospective immunohistochemical study (NSE, Leu 7, and ChrA) in chemotherapy-treated NSCLC patients, Graziano et al. [12] evaluated 52 patients for the presence of neuroendocrine markers. Twenty-six patients with advanced NSCLC who had responded (completely or partially) to chemotherapy were compared to 26 patients who did not respond to cytotoxic chemotherapy. The two groups were balanced in terms of major prognostic features. Of the 52 patients, 40 had adenocarcinomas, 5 squamous cell carcinomas, 2 large cell carcinomas, and 5 adenosquamous cell carcinomas. Ten of 26 responding patients (38%) had tumor positive for two markers, whereas none of the nonresponders showed this feature ($p < 0.01$). Furthermore, responders with two or more positive markers had significantly longer survival (median 79 weeks) compared to responders with less than two positive markers (median 51 weeks) and nonresponders (median 27 weeks) [12]. It should be noted that this retrospective study included material from only 52 patients, and the patients were selected. Furthermore, NSE was detected by polyclonal antiserum with a lower specificity than monoclonal antibodies.

Skov et al. [13] investigated 114 patients with inoperable bronchogenic adenocarcinoma, all of whom received chemotherapy according to a prospective randomized trial. Specimens obtained prior to chemotherapy were examined immunohistochemically using monoclonal antibodies against NSE and ChrA in order to determine the frequency and prognostic impact of such marker expression. The evaluated specimens were divided into three groups depending on the number of positive staining cells, namely, no reaction, 1%–10% positive cells, and more than 10% positive cells. NSE was expressed in more than 10% of the cells in 18 patients (16%). ChrA was expressed in 22 patients (19%) with tumors having more than 10% positive cells. The response rate to chemotherapy was 44% (complete or partial response) in patients with tumors containing more than 10% NSE-positive cells compared to 17% of the patients with less than 10% positive cells ($p < 0.025$). Corresponding values for ChrA were 30% versus 19% responding patients (not statistically significant). Although no statistically significant difference was found in median survival times between the groups, a trend could be seen, since the highly NE-positive group of patients had a median survival time of 262 days compared to 159 days for the nonstaining group of patients [13].

In a more recent study by van Zandwijk et al. [29], 42 patients with locally advanced or metastatic NSCLC were prospectively evaluated for serum levels of NSE and LDH in order determine the prognostic value of these tumor markers. Elevated NSE levels were significantly more common in patients with extensive disease than in locally diseased patients. A strong positive correlation factor was found between serum levels of NSE and LDH, while no correlation was found between serum enzyme levels and either age, sex, performance status, or histology. Patients with high levels of serum NSE and LDH were found to have a better response (complete or partial) to chemotherapy than patients with lower levels. In a univariate analysis, high pretreatment levels of NSE and LDH were found to be associated with shorter survival, as was extensive disease, but when adjustment for extent of disease was made, no significant association between tumor marker levels and survival could be demonstrated [29].

Linnoila et al. [6] evaluated the clinical outcome of 113 patients with

NSCLC to determine whether NSCLC tumors with neuroendocrine differentiation (NE-NSCLC) behaved more like SCLC. NE-NSCLC were
defined as NSCLC with positive reactivity of at least 2 out of 3 well-defined
NE markers (ChrA, Leu-7, and NSE) as determined by immunohistochemical methods. Neuroendocrine differentiation was found in 19/111 patients
(17%); 8 of these had chemotherapy (42%), and 4 out of 8 (50%) obtained
a complete or partial response, versus 6/38 (16%) of the other chemotherapy-
treated NSCLC patients. Unfortunately, the number of patients in the
groups was small, and no significant difference in survival between NE-
positive and NE-negative NSCLC patients was seen. The NE-NSCLC
patients developed metastases more often than the other groups ($p \leq 0.05$).
The authors conclude that NE-NSCLC had a biological behavior intermediate between NSCLC and SCLC [6].

Two recently published preliminary reports have presented the relation
between NE markers and chemotherapy response and survival. Carles et al.
[30] examined 97 patients with NSCLC who were treated with cisplatin-
based chemotherapy in order to assess the significance of pretreatment and
treatment characteristics. NSE, synaptophysin, ChrA, and Leu-7 were
determined by immunohistochemical methods. NSE was found in 43 of 92
patients (44%), synaptophysin in 2 of 97 (2%), ChrA in 21 of 92 (22%), and
Leu-7 in 4 of 92 (4%). NSE was a better predictor of survival in the NE-
positive NSCLC patients (survival 11 months) than in patients with NE-
negative tumors (survival 7.4 months) [30].

Ruckdeschel et al. [31] studied 237 ressected NSCLC patients and 219
patients with extensive NSCLC or SCLC in a retrospective study. Immunohistochemical methods were used to detect the neuroendocrine markers NSE, ChrA, Leu-7, and bombesin. The presence of NSE in patients
with extensive disease was associated with an increased response to chemotherapy, but not with survival, while the presence of CEA was associated
with a longer survival. However, in the operable patients, the presence of
NE markers had no influence on either response or survival [31].

Neuroendocrine peptides as growth factors

In the past decade, over 1000 continous human cell lines have been established from lung cancer biopsy specimens, and many growth factors and
receptors have been identified in SCLC cell lines [32]. SCLC is a NE tumor
that contains numerous peptides, including bombesin/gastrin releasing
peptide (BN/GRP), and receptors. High levels of BN/GRP were detected in
many SCLC cell lines and biopsy specimens [33], and the growth of SCLC is
inhibited by a monoclonal antibody (2A11) against BN/GRP [34]. Clinical
trials have begun using this antibody, which neutralizes GRP [35].

GRP is also present in the plasma of SCLC patients, but due to the rapid
metabolism of GRP in the blood (it has a half-life of approximately

150

five minutes), it is not suitable as a marker for SCLC. GRP secretion is increased by vasoactive intestinal peptide (VIP) [36]. Current efforts have focused on developing GRP receptor antagonists, which bind to the receptor with high affinity and are not readily degraded by serum proteases.

High level of another peptide, neurotensin (NT), have been found in many classic SCLC cell lines examined [37]. NT has also been found to stimulate clonal growth of SCLC cell lines [38], but unfortunately NT antagonists are not currently available.

In contrast to SCLC adenocarcinomas, large cell carcinomas and squamous cell carcinomas do not have immunoreactive GRP or NT, and GRP antagonists did not inhibit the growth of NSCLC cell lines [39].

Conclusions and future perspectives

Pulmonary neuroendocrine cells are the first cells to diffentiate from the primitive respiratory epithelium during lung development. The cells produce a variety of hormones, and some of them have been shown to be growth factors for bronchial epithelial cells.

Neuroendocrine hyperplasia and increased release of bombesin-like (BN) peptides occur in several diseases of the airways, including chronic obstructive pulmonary disease (COPD) and bronchopulmonary dysplasia. In addition, extremely high levels of immunorcactive BN were observed in the bronchial lavage fluid and urine of SCLC patients and smokers [40], and it has been suggested that bombesin/GRP acts as a mitogen in the lung and may be important in the development of malignant lung tumors of the SCLC- and non-SCLC type. The hypothesis that bombesin-like peptide are a marker for lung injury that identifies a subset of smokers at increased risk for the development of lung cancer is presently being tested [41]. BN and GRP have been demonstrated to stimulate the clonal growth of SCLC. Thus, BN/GRP receptor antagonists not only may be useful in the treatment of SCLC but also may function as chemopreventive agents.

Identification of NE markers in both SCLC and non-SCLC tumors supports the unitarian theory of a common origin for the malignant lung tumors [42]. There is a continuum between typical SCLC and NSCLC tumors that was recognized by M. Matthews [43] in 1975 through traditional light microscopy and that was later added to the IASLC classification of malignant lung tumors [44]. Therefore, today we know that there is a 'grey zone' between the SCLC and NSCLC types, and there is a subset of NSCLC tumors (about 20%–30%) that shares NE features with the SCLC tumors (NE-NSCLC). Based on in vitro data and several retrospective clinical studies, these NE-NSCLC tumors seems to be chemosensitive. However, we still do not have any good prospective clinical data showing whether patients with NE-NSCLC tumors should be offered chemotherapy or not, and it would be of particularly great interest to elucidate whether adjuvant chemotherapy after 'radical' surgery in patients with NE-NSCLC tumors would have any significant effect on survival.

It can be concluded that by identification of NE markers in 'normal' and neoplastic lung tissue, we have learned more about the biology of lung tumors, and NE peptides might play an important role in the carcinogenesis of lung cancer. However, whether or not these markers can be used in future screening or in early detection of lung cancer is a question to be answered in prospective studies. Furthermore, prospective studies must answer the question of whether or not patients with NE-NSCLC tumors will have any significant benefit from being treated with chemotherapy. Taking into consideration the relatively large absolute number of NE-NSCLC tumors per year (in the U.S., about 13,000 per year) and the possible benefits of chemotherapy for these patients, the answer to this question seems to be of utmost importance.

References

1. Pearse AGE. 1969. The cytochemistry and ultrastructure of polypeptide hormone producing cells of the APUD series, and the embryologic, physiologic and pathologic implications of the concept. J Histochem Cytochem 17:303–313.
2. Gould VE, Warren WH, Memoli VA. 1984. Neuroendocrine neoplasms of the lung. In The Endocrine Lung in Health and Disease, KL Becker and AF Gazdar (eds.). W.B. Saunders Company: Philadelphia, pp. 406–445.
3. Baylin SB, Abeloff MD, Goodwin G, et al. 1980. Activities of L-Dopa decarboxylase and diamine oxidase (histaminase) in human lung cancers and decarboxylase as a marker for small (oat) cell cancer in cell culture. Cancer Res 40:1990–1994.
4. Bensch KG, Corrin B, Pariente R, Spencer H. 1968. Oat cell carcinoma of the lung: its origin and relationship to bronchial carcinoid. Cancer 22:1163–1172.
5. Gould VE, Linnoila RI, Memoli VA, Warren WH. 1983. Neuroendocrine components of the bronchopulmonary tect: hyperplasias, dysplasias and neoplasms. Lab Invest 49:519–537.
6. Linnoila RI, Mulshine JL, Steinberg SM, et al. 1988. Neuroendocrine differentiation in endocrine and nonendocrine lung carcinomas. Am J Clin Pathol 90:641–652.
7. Schmedchel D, Marangos PJ, Brightman M. 1987. Neuron specific enolase in a molecular marker for peripheral and central neuroendocrine cells. Nature 276:834–836.
8. Tapia FJ, Barbosa AJA, Marangos PJ. 1981. Neuron-specific enolase is produced by neuroendocrine tumours. Lancet 1:808–811.
9. Sheppard MN, Corrin B, Bennett MH, et al. 1984. Immunohistochemical location of neuron specific enolase in small-cell carcinoma and carcinoid tumours of the lung. Histopathology 8:171–181.
10. Bergh J, Escher T, Steinholtz LM, et al. 1985. Immunohistochemical demonstration of Neuron-Specific Enolase (NSE) in human lung cancer. Am J Clin Pathol 84:1–7.
11. Kayser K, Schmid W, Ebert W, Wiedenmann B. 1988. Expression of neuroendocrine markers (Neuron Specific Enolase, synaptophysin and bombesin) in carcinoma of the lung. Pathol Res Pract 183:412–417.
12. Graziano SL, Mazid R, Newman N, et al. 1989. The use of neuroendocrine immunoperoxidase markers to predict chemotherapy response in patients with non-small-cell lung cancer. J Clin Oncol 7:1398–1406.
13. Skov BG, Sørensen JB, Hirsch FR, et al. 1991. Prognostic impact of histologic demonstra-

tion of chromogranin A and Neuron Specific Enolase in pulmonary adenocarcinoma. Ann Oncol 2:355–360.

14. Gazdar AF, Helman LJ, Israel MA, et al. 1988. Expression of neuroendocrine cell markers L-dopa decarboxylase, chromogranin A and dense core granules in human tumors of endocrine and nonendocrine origin. Cancer Res 48:4078–4082.

15. Bunn PA Jr, Linnoila RI, Minna JD, et al. 1985. Small cell lung cancer, endocrine cells of the fetal bronchus and other neuroendocrine cells express the Leu-7 antigenic determinant present on natural killer cells. Blood 65:764–768.

16. Hamid QA, Addis BJ, Springal DR, et al. 1987. Expression of the C-terminal peptide of human pro-bombesin in 361 lung endocrine tumours, a reliable marker and possible prognostic indicator for small cell carcinoma. Virchows Arch A 411:185–192.

17. Nybroe O, Linneman D, Bock E. 1988. NCAM biosynthesis in brain. Neurochem Int 12:251–262.

18. Souhami RI, Beverly PCL, Bobrow LG. 1987. Antigens of small-cell lung cancer. Lancet 2:325–326.

19. Carbone DP, Koros AC, Linnoila I, et al. 1991. Neural cell adhesion molecule expression and messenger RNA splicing pattern are correlated with neuroendocrine phenotype and growth morphology. Cancer Res 51:6142–6149.

20. Pujol JL, Simony J, Laurent JC, et al. 1989. Phenotypic heterogeneity studied by immunohistochemistry and aneuploidy in non-small cell lung cancers. Cancer Res 49: 2797–2802.

21. Broers JLV, Rot MK, Oostendorp T, et al. 1987. Immunocytochemical detection of human lung cancer heterogeneity using antibodies to epithelial, neuronal and neuroendocrine antigens. Cancer Res 47:3225–3234.

22. Mooi WJ, Wagenaar SS, Schol D, Hilgers J. 1988. Monoclonal antibody 123C3 in lung tumour classification-immunohistology of 358 resected lung tumours. Mol Cell Probes 2:31–37.

23. Berendsen HH, de Leij L, Poppema S, et al. 1989. Clinical characterization of non-small-cell lung cancer tumors showing neuroendocrine differentiation features. J Clin Oncol 7:1614–1620.

24. Komminoth P, Rothe J, Lackie PM, et al. 1991. Polisialic acid of the neural cell adhesion molecule distinguished small cell lung carcinoma from carcinoids. Am J Pathol 139: 297–304.

25. Gazdar AF, Kadoyama C, Venzon D, et al. 1992. The association between histological type and neuroendocrine differentiation on drug sensitivity of lung cancer cell lines. J Natl Monagr Natl Cancer Inst 13:191–196.

26. Kibbelaar RE, Moolenaar KEC, Michalides RJAM, et al. 1991. Neural cell adhesion molecule expression, neuroendocrine differentiation and prognosis in lung carcinoma. Eur J Cancer 27:431–435.

27. Moolenaar CEC, Muller EM, Schol DJ, et al. 1990. Expression of an N-CAM related sialoglycoprotein in small cell lung cancer and neuroblastoma. Cancer Res 50:1102–1106.

28. Sundarensan V, Reeve JG, Stenning S, et al. 1991. Neuroendocrine differentiation and clinical behaviour in non-small cell lung tumours. Br J Cancer 64:333–338.

29. Van Zandwijk N, Jassem E, Bonfrer JMG, et al. 1992. Serum neuron-specific enolase and lactate dehydrogenase as predictors of response to chemotherapy and survival in non-small cell lung cancer. Semin Oncol 19:37–43.

30. Carles J, Rosell R, Abad A, et al. 1992. Better outlook for patients with non-small cell lung cancer who expressed neuroendocrine differentiation markers (NSCLC-NE). Proc Ann Oncol 3(Suppl 5):27.

31. Ruckdeschel J, Linnoila RI, Mulchine JL, et al. 1991. The impact of neuroendocrine and epithelial differentiation on recurrence and survival in patients with lung cancer. Proc 6th World Conf Lung Cancer. Lung Cancer 7(Suppl):56.

32. Moody TW, Cuttitta F. 1993. Growth factor and peptide receptors in small cell lung cancer. Life Sci 52:1161–1173.

153

33. Moody TW, Pert CB, Gazdar AF, et al. 1981. High levels of intracellular bombesin characterize human small-cell lung carcinoma. Science 214:1246–1248.
34. Cuttitta F, Carney DN, Mulshine J, et al. 1985. Bombesin-like peptides can function as autocrine growth factors in human small-cell lung cancer. Nature 316:823–825.
35. Avis IL, Kovacs TOG, Kasprzyk PG, et al. 1991. Preclinical evaluation of an antiautocrine growth factor monoclonal antibody for treatment of patients with small-cell lung cancer. J Natl Cancer Inst 83:1470–1476.
36. Korman LY, Carney DN, Citron ML, Moody TW. 1986. Secretin/vasoactive intestinal peptide-stimulated secretion of bombesin/gastrin releasing peptide from human small cell carcinoma of the lung. Cancer Res 46:1214–1218.
37. Moody TW, Carney DN, Korman LY, et al. 1985. High affinity receptors for bombesin/GRP-like peptides on human small cell lung cancer. Life Sci 37:105–113.
38. Davis TP, Burgess HS, Crowell S, et al. 1989. Endorphin and neurotensin stimulate in vitro clonat growth of human SCLC cells. Eur J Pharmacol 161:283–285.
39. Mahmoud S, Staley J, Taylor J, et al. 1991. Bombesin analogues inhibit growth of small cell lung cancer in vitro and in vivo. Cancer Res 51:1798–1802.
40. Aguayo SM, Kine TE, Kane MA, et al. 1992. Urinary levels of bombesin-like peptides in asymptomatic cigarette smokers: A potential risk marker for smoking-related diseases. Cancer Res 52:2727–2731.
41. Miller YE, Aguayo SM. 1993. Bombesin-like peptides, neuroendocrine cells and pulmonary carcinogenesis. Proc 4th IASLC Lung Tumor Biology Workshop, VA, April.
42. Gazdar AF, Carney DN, Guccion JG, Baylin SB. 1981. Small cell carcinoma of the lung: Cellular origin and relationship to other pulmonary tumors. In Small Cell Lung Cancer, FA Greco, RK Oldham, and PA Bunn (eds.). Clinical Oncology Monographs. Grune & Straton, pp. 145–175.
43. Matthews MJ. 1973. Morphologic classification of bronchogenic carcinoma. Cancer Chemother Rep 4:299–301.
44. Hirsch FR, Matthews MJ, Aisner S, et al. 1988. Histopathologic classification of small cell lung cancer. Changing concepts and terminology. Cancer 62:973–977.

154

8. In vivo models for testing of cytostatic agents in non-small cell lung cancer

Henk B. Kal

Introduction

The limited progress in non-small cell lung cancer (NSCLC) in numerous clinical trials is rather disappointing. There is a need for more detailed information on the specific biological properties of the various forms of lung cancer before a more rational approach in the improvement of treatment can be made. In contrast to the situation in other forms of cancer, e.g., lymphoid and myeloid leukemia, mammary cancer, and colon cancer, there has been a noticeable scarcity of useful animal models for the study of the biological properties of lung tumors and their responsiveness to chemo-therapeutics and radiation. In general, a particular tumor model should be chosen based upon the specific question to be answered. One of the major areas of research is response to treatment. Human lung tumor xenografts have been used as tools to study responsiveness to treatment modalities, and rodent lung tumor models were developed that can be used for this purpose. In this chapter, the xenograft model and the rodent lung tumor models will be described with respect to their responsiveness to cytostatic agents.

Tumor xenografts

The use of human tumor xenografts in nude mice or immunosuppressed animals has received wide application for obvious reasons. Numerous large studies using subcutaneous transplantation have confirmed the human origin and described a close resemblance between xenografts and tumors of origin [1–4]. There is considerable evidence that this resemblance carries over into response rates and associated parameters [5–9].

For practical reasons, the most relevant way of validating the xenograft model for treatment responses is to compare directly xenograft response with the clinical response. A major study of this type was that of Shorthouse et al. [10]. The clinical response of small cell lung cancers was reflected in highly responsive xenografts, as was the lack of response of the non-small cell tumors.

Heine H. Hansen, (ed), Hansen: Lung Cancer.
© *1994 Kluwer Academic Publishers. ISBN 0-7923-2835-3. All rights reserved.*

Steel et al. [11] studied responses of a variety of human tumor xenografts and found good correlation between the response of xenografts and the clinical complete remission rates. Their overall impression is that chemo-responsive human cancers give rise to xenografts that also respond well to chemotherapy.

Ovejera [12] discussed the use of human tumor xenografts in large-scale drug screening. In the screening panel of the U.S. National Cancer Institute (NCI), three human xenografts were included, namely, the CX-1 colon carcinoma, the LX-1 undifferentiated small cell lung carcinoma, and the MX-1 mammary ductal carcinoma. Ovejera concluded that it appears that human tumor xenografts are unable to predict clinical activity of drugs based on tumor type. This lack of correlation may be attributed to the fact that panel testing is limited to one tumor xenograft of each type.

Bellet et al. [13] proposed the use of a disease-oriented approach employing a 14-tumor xenograft system of similar origin. Such a system is considered ideal in predicting the clinical efficacy of a drug against specific tumor types.

Responses were heterogeneous to a variety of chemotherapeutic drugs of four different experimental bronchial carcinomas that originated in the lungs of rats. A similar tumor-specific pattern of response was observed when these tumors were grown as xenotransplants in nude mice [14]. This observation strongly supports the notion that results of experiments performed with human xenografts in nude or immunosuppressed rodents are predictive for responses of tumors in human patients. This rat lung tumor model (to be discussed later) is a result of attempts to develop a multiple tumor system of similar origin with the aim, among others, of predicting of clinical efficacy of drugs.

Murine lung tumor models

Lewis lung carcinoma (3LL)

The Lewis lung carcinoma originated spontaneously in the lung of a C57BL/6 mouse in 1951 [15]. This tumor was maintained in vivo by subcutaneous (sc) passages. It is a weakly immunogenic, poorly differentiated epidermoid carcinoma. The 3LL has been used in many studies either for its claimed closeness to the human pattern [16] or for its metastasizing behavior, which allows the effect of chemotherapy against both primary and secondary outgrowth to be investigated. The Lewis lung carcinoma is one of the tumor systems that constitute the NCI anticancer screening panel [12].

NMU-1 adenocarcinoma

NMU-1 is a lung adenocarcinoma induced by N-nitroso-N-methyl-urea in a BALB/c Lac Dp mouse and maintained in vivo by subcutaneous passaging

156

of tumor fragments [17]. The tumor spontaneously metastasizes to the lung. It was found that mitomycin, cyclophosphamide, and cisplatin significantly modified tumor growth delay and increase of life span in treated mice. These three drugs show a certain degree of activity as single agents on human lung tumors.

CMT64

A spontaneous alveolar lung carcinoma originated in a female C57BL/ICRF a^t mouse. From this tumor, the lung tumor cell line CMT64 was developed [18]. Upon sc inoculation, local tumors can be produced that give rise to a small number of lung metastases within three weeks. It was concluded that the CMT64 system is a particularly useful model for experimental metastasis studies.

These are examples of tumors originating in the lungs of mice. Their resemblance to human lung cancers is poor, e.g., alveolar lung carcinomas are not frequently seen in humans, and the tumor doubling times are rather short. Due to passaging, an extensive selection has taken place, and therefore they are far removed from the tumor of origin and usually lack differentiation. Ideally, one would like to have several types of experimental small cell carcinomas, squamous cell carcinomas, large cell carcinomas, and adenocarcinomas, all with two characteristics: 1) rather long tumor doubling times, in order to allow treatments to be applied that last up to about one week, and 2) a resemblance to their human counterparts with respect to degree of differentiation and responsiveness to treatment. The TNO rat lung tumor model is an example of such a system.

TNO rat lung tumor model

During the past few years, a program was initiated for the development of realistic animal models for human bronchial cancer. Tumors were induced in the rat lung by ionizing radiation. Radiation was used because, in general with this agent, nonimmunogenic tumors could be expected. A method was developed to implant tumor fragments into the lung. These tumor implants grew to carcinomas resembling primary tumors in man. The development of the model, the growth characteristics of tumors growing intrapulmonarily or subcutaneously in the flank of the rat, and responses to chemotherapeutic drugs will be reported below.

Induction

Specific-pathogen-free derived WAG/Rij inbred rats 3 to 4 weeks old were used. Tumors were induced by means of iridium-192 wires or iodine-125 seeds implanted intrapulmonarily. Forty male rats received iridium-192 implants with an activity of 17.4 MBq. Twenty female rats received implants of iodine-125 seeds 4.5 mm long and 0.8 mm in diameter, with an activity of 14.8 MBq [19]. The operation procedure was as follows. The rats were anesthetized with ether. The skin of the thorax was shaved, and a lateral incision was made. A lobe of the right lung was brought outside the thoracic cavity while the animal was given artificial respiration. The radioactive source was implanted through the use of a trocar. After implantation, the lobe was returned into the thoracic cavity and the skin was closed with wound clips. The animals were housed in macrolon cages on an iron grid and were inspected regularly and monitored for the presence of the isotope.

In the 14-month observation period, 75% of the animals with implants of iridium-192 wires developed tumors, among which malignant hemangioendotheliomas occurred with the highest frequency (50%). Four transplantable squamous cell carcinoma lines were obtained. In 17 months of observation, three rats with implants of iodine-125 seeds developed tumors, among which one squamous cell carcinoma could be identified. The five squamous cell carcinomas were coded L17, L33, L37, L41, and L42.

In addition, an adenocarcinoma, L27, and an anaplastic tumor, L44, were obtained as by-products of other experiments. The L27 tumor originated in the lung of a BN rat after total body irradiation with a dose of 0.4 Gy; the L44 tumor originated in the lung of another BN rat after local irradiation of the thorax with a dose of 16 Gy 300 kV x-rays administered at a dose rate of 0.8 Gy per minute. Earlier passages of the L44 tumor were histologically characterized as adenosquamous carcinomas. After the tenth passage, on the basis of light and electron microscopy, the L44 tumor had to be classified as an anaplastic tumor (table 1). Tumor fragments were transplanted in syngeneic hosts for propagation.

The lung tumors are nonimmunogenic, as tested by irradiating subcutaneously growing tumors and by a subsequent challenge with cells. The

Table 1. Histological appearance and tumor volume doubling time of rat lung carcinomas growing subcutaneously (sc) and in the lung (tumor volumes of 200–400 mm³)

Tumor line	Rat strain	Sex	Histology (sc)	Induction method	$Td \pm SEM$ (d) sc tumor (n = 5)	$Td \pm SEM$ (d) lung tumor (n = 5)	Passage number
L17	WAG	M	md sq.c.c.	Ir-192	4.7 ± 0.7	9.6 ± 1.5	72
L33	WAG	M	wd sq.c.c.	Ir-192	5.6 ± 0.6	9.7 ± 0.5	75
L37	WAG	M	md sq.c.c.	Ir-192	5.9 ± 0.5	8.9 ± 1.9	54
L41	WAG	M	wd sq.c.c.	Ir-192	5.8 ± 0.9	10.9 ± 1.0	43
L42	WAG	F	wd sq.c.c.	I-125	4.1 ± 0.7	12.4 ± 1.6	27
L27	BN	F	md adeno ca	0.4 Gy	2.7 ± 0.3	5.4 ± 0.9	11
L44	BN	F	anaplastic	16 Gy	4.8 ± 1.0	4.7 ± 0.3	11

sq.c.c.: squamous cell carcinoma; wd: well differentiated; md: moderately differentiated; Td: tumor volume doubling time; SEM: standard error of the mean.

158

tumor take in the untreated and pretreated rats was similar. Only the L42 tumor is an exception. When small tumor fragments (about $2\,mm^3$) are implanted, the take rate is indeed 100%, but about a quarter of the tumors will regress spontaneously after reaching volumes up to $100\,mm^3$. When large tumor fragments of the L42 line (about $20\,mm^3$) are implanted, such regression was not observed. It is an advantage that one of the tumors in the panel is slightly immunogenic. Especially in studies in which the relative value of immunotherapy, e.g., cytokine gene therapy, is investigated, the L42 tumor line can be used to screen various regimens.

Cell lines were derived from the L17, L33, L37, L41, and L42 tumors either by using a specific feeder cell method described earlier by Klein et al. [20] or without feeder cells, as described by Barendsen et al. [21]. When needed, cells obtained from these in vitro cultures can be used to grow tumors.

Tumor volume and growth delay

Volume changes of tumors growing subcutaneously in the flanks of WAG/Rij or BN rats were derived from vernier caliper measurements of three tumor dimensions. Tumor volumes were calculated from the tumor diameters (a, b, and c) using the formula $V = \pi abc/6$. The tumor doubling times are shown in table 1.

Tumor volume growth delay (TGD) of treated tumors is defined as the time required to reach a volume equal to that at the time of treatment or the time required to reach a volume twice as great as that at the time of treatment, with subtraction of the value for the volume doubling time (Td) of the untreated tumor. The latter approach is applied when a volume reduction after treatment is not observed. For intercomparison of the responsiveness of tumors with different tumor doubling times, the method of specific growth delay (SGD) was used. The SGD is the tumor volume growth delay divided by the Td of the untreated control tumor (SGD = TGD/Td).

Intrapulmonary implantation of tumor fragments

It is not well known whether bronchial tumors growing at the unnatural subcutaneous site employed in most assays provide similar responses to orthotopically growing tumors. Studies concerned with this question have provided unequivocal answers [22,23], some showing that the intrapulmonary tumors were more sensitive than the subcutaneous tumors in the flank and others demonstrating the reverse relation or no difference [24,25]. To study the influence of the growth site, a technique was developed to grow and measure the progression of transplantable tumors in the lung of syngeneic rats [26]. The method of implantation of tumor fragments into the lung is comparable with the technique to implant the radioactive wired used for tumor induction. The (standardized) technique now is as follows: animals were anesthetized i.p. with 200 mg 2,2,2,-tribromoethanol/kg. A lateral incision of about 1.5 cm was made between the 7th and 8th ribs. The posterior lobe of the right lung was brought outside the thoracic cavity with forceps. In the meantime, a tumor fragment of about 2 mm^3 derived from a subcutaneous tumor was loaded in a trocar with an inner diameter of 1.3 mm and an outer diameter of 1.6 mm. Implantation was performed by piercing the lobe with the trocar and ejecting the tumor fragment. In several instances when breathing stopped, forced inhalation using a hand-operated pump was applied. After implantation, the wound in the lobe was coagulated and the lobe was placed back into the thoracic cavity. The incision was closed with a few stitches, and then the overlying skin was closed with several wound clips, after which the treated area was sprayed with Nobecutan. A more detailed description of the implantation technique has been published elsewhere [26].

Through this procedure, about six animals can be provided with intrapulmonary tumor implants in one hour by two skilled technicians. The mortality due to the surgical procedure is about 1%. With the standardized technique, 'take' rates varied between 90% and 100%. Starting 3 to 5 weeks after implantation, animals were inspected for the presence of tumors by chest radiographs in the ventrodorsal and lateral directions. Radiographs were made while the animals were kept in an upright position and immobilized with an i.m. injection of 1 ml Hypnorm/kg. Radiographs were taken once a week by technicians using a diagnostic Röntgen apparatus, CGR Senographe 1, operating at 30 kV.

Diameters of the lung implants were measured from the radiographs in two or three perpendicular directions, and the volume V was calculated using the formula $V = \pi abc/6$ or $V = \pi ab^2/6$, in which b is the smaller diameter. Doubling times for tumors growing intrapulmonarily are shown in table 1.

Histology and metastasizing capacity

For the determination of histological characteristics of the tumors, animals were killed with an overdose of pentobarbital at various times after implantation. A complete necropsy was performed. The lungs were fixed by intratracheal insufflation of 10% buffered formalin. Other tissues that showed abnormalities at necropsy were fixed by infusion in 10% buffered formalin. Tissue samples were routinely processed to 3-μm slides, stained with hematoxylin saffron, and examined histologically. The results of the histological examinations of subcutaneous and intrapulmonary tumors are shown in table 1.

All tumor lines showed a capacity to metastasize [27]. The intrapulmonary tumors disseminated to the mediastinum, lung, kidney, and subrenal area. Tumors of at least two lines, L17 and L37, growing subcutaneously, disseminated to the mediastinum, lungs, and kidneys. The majority of the metastases were observed when the primary tumors were relatively large ($>500\,mm^3$). Based on the distribution frequencies, the dissemination pattern of the subcutaneous tumors probably is to the lungs and from there to the mediastinum and kidneys. The dissemination pattern of intrapulmonary tumors is directly from the tumor to the kidneys, adrenals, and mediastinum.

Growth rate and histological characteristics

All tumors except the L44 grew faster at the subcutaneous location than in the lung (table 1). Since intrapulmonary tumors were derived from subcutaneous tumors, one might envisage that the lower growth rate might be due to adaptation to the other location. Therefore, we transplanted tumor fragments derived from intrapulmonary tumors to the lung for several passages. The change in tumor-volume doubling time was stable, as were differences in response to drugs.

Most of the subcutaneously growing squamous cell carcinoma lines developed cysts. These consist of large central areas of necrosis with keratinaceous debris surrounded by a rim of viable squamous cell carcinoma cells infiltrating into the surrounding connective tissue. Ulceration of overlying skin was frequent in L41 tumors.

The squamous cell carcinomas in the lung were more differentiated than their subcutaneous counterparts. Cyst formation was not observed, but the tumors had a dry keratinaceous center. The adenocarcinoma growing in the lung developed acini and tubuli. These features were less apparent in subcutaneous implants. Another difference between subcutaneous and intrapulmonary growing tumors was that the former were surrounded by a capsula of fibrous tissue, while in the latter there was no apparent border between tumor and normal tissue. All implants in the lung resulted in highly malignant carcinomas invading the surrounding lung parenchyma, bronchi, and vessels. All implants except those of the L37 tumor line caused compression of the surrounding lung tissue. Those of the L37 caused compression in only a quarter of the rats. L37 was further characterized by less necrosis and more frequent pleural metastasis.

Response of flank tumors to chemotherapeutic agents

Tumors were treated with a variety of chemotherapeutic drugs. The drugs used were mitomycin C (1.5 mg/kg, i.v.), methotrexate (3 × 10 mg/kg, every 3.5 h, i.p.), cisplatin (6 mg/kg, i.v.), adriamycin (doxorubicin) (7.5 mg/kg, i.v.), CCNU (30 mg/kg, p.o.), TCNU (20 mg/kg, p.o.), ifosfamide (200 mg/kg, i.v.), VP16 (30 mg/kg, i.p.), and flavone acetic acid (FAA) (275–500 mg/kg, i.v.).

A tumor is considered to be sensitive to a particular treatment when the SGD is at least 2. This value often corresponds to a volume reduction of about 50%. The responses of subcutaneously growing tumors to nine

Table 2. Chemosensitivity of rat lung tumors (flank implants)

Drug	Dose (mg/kg)	Specific growth delay						
		L17	L33	L37	L41	L42	L27	L44
Mitomycin C	1.5	0.1	0.5	0.2	0.4	6.3	Cures	0.4
Methotrexate	3 × 10	3.7	0	0	0.4	0.9	1.7	3.0
Cisplatin	6	0.3	1	0.6	0.8	5.9	7.5	5.3
Adriamycin	7.5	>12[a]	1.2	0.8	1.7	1.4	2.6	0
CCNU	30	0.5	0.3	0	1.1	>12[a]	Cures	13.9
TCNU	20	6.2	0.7	1.8	>5[a]	Cures	Cures	13;5c[b]
Ifosfamide	200	9.0	1.3	4	1.2	Cures	5.6;1c[b]	2.5
VP16	30	2.0		4.2	0.6	0.4		
FAA	275–300	0.4	0	0.9				
	500						0.7	0.3

[a] Specific growth delay is larger than the indicated figure; the exact value could not be determined because of the death of the experimental animals.
[b] 5c: 5 cures out of 5 treated animals; 1c: 1 cure out of 5 treated animals.
CCNU: N-(2-chloroethyl)-N-cyclohexyl-N-nitrosuourea; TCNU: 1-(2-Chloroethyl)-3-[2-(dimethylaminosulphonyl)ethyl]-1-nitrosourea (a new water-soluble nitrosourea, kindly provided by Leo Laboratories, Helsingborg, Sweden).

chemotherapeutic agents are presented in table 2. The responses are very heterogeneous, e.g., the L17 and L27 lines are sensitive to adriamycin, but the others are not. The L33 line is not responsive to any of eight drugs used. The L41 line is responsive to only one drug, and the L37 to only two drugs; the L42 and L44 lines are responsive to five drugs, and the L27 to six. TCNU and ifosfamide are effective in five of the seven tumor lines, and the other drugs in none or only two or three tumor lines. Responses of five rat lung tumors to the new drug FAA were almost absent. The SGD values were less than 1, in contrast to mouse colon 38, which resulted in 50% to 100% cures depending on the dose of FAA [28]. These results with the rat lung tumors are in line with clinical studies showing that for tumor FAA levels in patients similar to those achieved in mice, a lack of activity in human tumors was observed [29].

Response of intrapulmonary tumors to chemotherapeutic agents

The SGDs of tumors growing in the lung in response to selected drugs are listed in table 3. The combinations of tumors and drugs were selected on the basis of relatively low responses (SGD <2) and of a relatively large response (SGD >6) of tumors growing in the flank.

   In one experiment, we determined the response to ifosfamide of L17 tumors, growing at either location, as a function of tumor volume. No volume dependency was observed for the tumors growing subcutaneously, in

Table 3. Chemosensitivity of rat lung tumors (intrapulmonary implants)

Drug	Dose (mg/kg)	Specific growth delay				
		L17	L33	L37	L42	L44
Cisplatin	6		0.5			3.8
Adriamycin	5	6.3		0.3		
TCNU	20				9.5	
Ifosfamide	200	2.6^a;5.1^b	0.5		7.1	

^{a} Tumor volume 280–500 mm^3.
^{b} Tumor volume about 200 mm^3.

Table 4. Tumor volume doubling times of rat lung carcinomas growing subcutaneously in different hosts

Tumor line	Td ± SEM (d) syngeneic	n	Td ± SEM (d) nude mice	n
L17	4.5 ± 1.4	22	5.2 ± 1.7	13
L37	5.9 ± 1.5	14	8.8 ± 3.7	10
L42	5.8 ± 1.6	15	9.3 ± 4.2	18
L44	2.9 ± 0.8	17	5.0 ± 1.4	10

contrast to those growing in the lung. Small lung tumors were more sensitive to ifosfamide than large ones [30].

From tables 2 and 3, one may conclude that a drug ineffective in subcutaneous tumors is also ineffective in tumors growing in the lung; drugs that are effective on subcutaneous tumors are also effective in intrapulmonary tumors, although to a much lesser extent.

Responses of rat tumor xenografts in nude rodents

The same tests were performed on tumors growing in nude rodents to investigate whether the host stroma influences tumor response [14]. For the studies with athymic rodents, female C57BL/KaLwRy/nu/nu mice (18–25 g) and female WAG/Rij/rnu rats (135–170 g) were used. The volume-doubling times of tumors growing in the nude mice are, in general, larger than those of tumors growing in syngeneic hosts (table 4). The results of the experiments on drug sensitivity are shown in table 5. In this table, drug doses employed are also indicated. Tumor growth in nude mice after treatment with TCNU and ifosfamide could be monitored only up to about one month after treatment. Mice were then lost due to deteriorated health conditions with tumors still in regression. The SGD values in table 5 that are indicated

163

Table 5. Chemosensitivity of rat lung tumors growing subcutaneously in the flank of syngeneic hosts or in nude mice

| | Dose (mg/kg) | | Specific growth delay | | | | | | | |
| | | | L17 | | L37 | | L42 | | L44 | |
Drug	Rat	Mouse	Rat	Mouse	Rat	Mouse	Rat	Mouse	Rat	Mouse
Mitomycin	1.5	1	0.1	0.5	0.2	0.2	6.3	0.2	0.4	0.5
Methotrexate	3 × 10	10	3.7	1.0			0.9	0.6		
Cisplatin	6	8	0.3	0.1	0.6	0.2	5.9	4.9	11	6.1
Adriamycin	7.5	6	>12	8.2	0.4	0.5	1.4	0.4	0	0
CCNU	30	75					>12	4.3		
TCNU	20	20					Cures	>3.8		
Ifosfamide	200	400					Cures	>4.2		

by the '>' sign are therefore minimum values. In general, one can conclude from the data presented in table 5 that a tumor responsive in syngeneic hosts is also responsive as a xenograft in nude mice.

As shown in table 5, the L17 tumor line is very sensitive to adriamycin, while the L44 tumor line is not. As a matter of interest, a comparison was made between the response to this drug of the L44 tumor, which originated in the BN strain, and the L17 tumor that originated in a WAG/Rij rat, while both were grown in opposite flanks of the same WAG/Rij/rnu rat. A dose of adriamycin (6 mg/kg, i.v.) was given, and growth of the tumors was determined as a function of time after treatment. The growth curves obtained indicate that the L17 tumor is still very responsive, but the L44 tumor is not [14]. From these data, it is not likely that the host environment did influence significantly the response of the tumors. This observation strongly supports the notion that results of experiments performed with human xenografts in nude rodents or immunosuppressed animals are predictive for responses of tumors in human patients.

Cytokeratin expression

Cytokeratin expression in rat lung tumors was studied using polypeptide-specific monoclonal antibodies to human cytokeratins 4, 5, 7, 8, 10, 13, 14, 18, and 19. Experiments were performed on tumor fragments derived from the five squamous cell lung tumors and the L27 adenocarcinoma, as well as on cell lines obtained from the squamous cell carcinomas [31].

The panel of antibodies was tested in an earlier study on human epithelial tissues including lung tissue and human carcinomas [32]. It was shown that this panel of immunoreagents offers the possibility of differentiating between pulmonary squamous cell carcinoma, adenocarcinoma, and small cell carcinoma. Furthermore, it provides an indication of the degree of differentiation of the carcinomas.

Our results with the panel of antibodies and material obtained from rat tumors indicate that most monoclonal and polyclonal antibodies against human cytokeratins do cross-react with rat cytokeratins. The reactivity of all rat lung tumors as well as all rat lung carcinoma cell lines to the polyclonal antibody pKer confirms the epithelial nature of these tumors. In addition, the reaction patterns found with the chain-specific cytokeratin antibodies indicate that these antibodies can be used to differentiate between the two main subtypes of lung cancer examined, i.e., between squamous cell carcinomas and adenocarcinomas of the rat [31].

The results of the immunoperoxidase technique assay indicate that the rat cytokeratin homologues to human CKs 10, 13, and 14 were expressed in squamous cell carcinomas and not in the adenocarcinoma, while the rat counterparts of the human CKs 7, 18, and 19 were immunohistochemically only detectable in the adenocarcinoma. These findings indicate that the rat lung tumors examined show a more homogeneous type of differentiation as compared to human lung cancer, in which poorly differentiated squamous cell carcinomas generally show the expression of cytokeratins characteristic of simple epithelia or adenomateous tissue [32,33].

Within squamous cell carcinomas, the cytokeratin expression patterns confirmed the degree of differentiation as diagnosed by light and electron microscopy.

Gene transfer and therapy

Due to the availability of in vitro cell lines, a novel method to evoke host-derived antitumor immune response can be tested. L44 tumor cells were infected with the ecotropic retroviral vector pLJ-IL-2, encoding mouse IL-2, and the neomycin resistance gene (Neo^R).

Tumor take of parental L44 cells in BN rats that have been pretreated with a nontumorigenic dose of cells from this IL-2-producing L44 cell line was tested [34]. The preliminary data obtained indicate that IL-2 production of L44 lung tumor cells reduces their capacity to take in vivo. Furthermore, IL-2-producing cells are immunogenic. These observations implicate that it is possible to direct the immune system towards a nonantigenic tumor.

In another series of experiments, the intratumoral injection of IL-1β in an L42 tumor resulted in complete resolution of both injected and distant L42 deposits. This treatment induced long-lasting specific immunity toward the L42 tumor, but not to the other lines. The L42 cell line will be genetically modified with genes encoding for cytokines that are most promising. These modified L42 cell lines will be used for screening. Subsequently, the other lung tumor cell lines will be transduced with genes encoding the most effective cytokines. In vivo experiments will show the value of this approach in nonimmunogenic lung tumors.

165

9. In vitro models for testing of cytostatic agents in small cell lung cancer

Peter Buhl Jensen and Maxwell Sehested

Introduction

Small cell lung cancer (SCLC) is one of the solid tumors most responsive to chemotherapy. Despite the apparent initial sensitivity of SCLC, acquired drug resistance is the major problem; only a small proportion of patients will remain in remission beyond two years [1]. The overall treatment results have not changed markedly in the last decade, despite the application of numerous combination regimens, late intensification regimens, high-dose chemotherapy with autologous bone-marrow rescue, and various types of adjuvant radiotherapy. Resistance in SCLC may be associated with the concomitant occurrence of a less chemosensitive histological tumor type, such as adenocarcinoma or squamous cell carcinoma, but only in a minority of cases. The large majority (over 85%) of SCLC patients who after treatment die with disease still have SCLC histology at autopsy [2]. Although drug resistance in SCLC may have a pharmacological basis or be due to changes in cell kinetics during therapy, the resistance appears to be due primarily to cellular factors.

There is substantial experimental evidence that drug resistance in malignant cells arises as a result of specific biochemical alterations ensuing from specific mutations in the genome [3,4]. Accordingly, resistance is not a pan-resistance towards all types of drugs but is restricted to a single drug or to drug types with certain similarities, e.g., mechanism of action or drug transport. Therefore, progress in drug treatment of SCLC still appears to be possible by identifying active, non-cross-resistant agents that can be used in combination with the most effective agents available today. The clinical application of new agents in patients with SCLC is encumbered with difficulties [5], and, accordingly, only a small fraction of new drugs will be tested in patients. It was recently documented that only 23 agents have been tested thoroughly in patients with SCLC within the last two decades [6]. This figure is in contrast to the more than 20,000 agents submitted every year to the National Cancer Institute, U.S.A. (NCI) for evaluation of antitumor activity [7]. Thus, the number of new drugs or drug combinations for clinical trials is very large. It is therefore highly relevant to determine the

Heine H. Hansen, (ed), Hansen: Lung Cancer.

171

extent to which preclinical parameters can be used in the selection of new drugs or drug combinations for clinical trials. Several research groups have therefore aimed at developing preclinical therapeutic models of SCLC.

In vitro models of SCLC

A number of in vitro models are available for drug screening and for testing of new drugs. This reflects the fact that no single drug screening system is perfect, and, since there is no consensus as to what should be required from a new drug, different investigators examine for different drug characteristics.

It is debated whether drug selection for evaluation and screening ideally should be specific or random. It is a matter of opinion whether the optimal drug-discovery strategy should be based on our increasing knowledge of the molecular and biochemical mechanism of action of anticancer agents together with our knowledge of growth regulation to specifically design or seek new compounds, or whether the fact that many major discoveries in medicine were serendipitous should lead to a broad drug-discovery program including nondesigned 'random' drugs.

The new drug-discovery program at the NCI is directed at drugs with activity in a given type of tumor. This program investigates panels of human cell lines derived from histologically defined tumors, e.g., colon adenocarcinoma, small cell lung cancer, etc. It is hoped that this investigation will lead to the discovery of new drugs with activity in highly refractory tumors, e.g., colon cancer [7]. In contrast to this approach, the pharmaceutical industry often aims to find a new drug with broad activity, while the academic world is interested in a novel drug with a new mechanism of action that will also elucidate biological mechanisms.

A number of investigators have used specific models in drug screening. An example is the nuclear enzyme topoisomerase II (topo II), which is the cellular target of clinically active anticancer agents such as VP-16 and doxorubicin (adriamycin). Much effort has been devoted to screening for drugs with activity on this enzyme. Recently, Nitiss et al. [8–10] have selected a mutant yeast cell with a temperature-dependent topo II activity, where the enzyme activity decreases 5- to10-fold when the cells are grown at 30° as compared to 25°. Thus, if a drug is much more toxic at 25° than at 30°, it presumably has topo II as its target enzyme. Nitiss et al. suggest that this finding can be used in the screening for topo II active drugs. A similar approach to drug screening has recently been taken by Yamashita and Kawada et al. [11,12], who used functional assays with the purified enzymes to successfully test a number of drugs directly on the target enzymes topo I and II. They have thereby identified several new biologically interesting compounds with alternative mechanisms of action on the target enzymes.

Within the last decade, a large number of tumor cell lines have been established from patients with SCLC. This resource has inspired many

172

researchers to use SCLC cell lines to investigate mechanisms of drug resistance and to screen for new active compounds [13]. However, in our opinion, it has still not been convincingly demonstrated that tumor cell lines reflect the sensitivity patterns of the tumor type from which they were derived. For instance, although SCLC clinically is much more drug sensitive than non-SCLC, some non-SCLC cell lines exhibit higher in vitro sensitivities to different conventional anticancer agents than an array of SCLC cell lines [14]. Thus, it is reasonable to expect that new drugs for phase II trials in SCLC could be selected more rationally in a panel of yeast cell lines with relevant well-defined resistance mechanisms than in an arbitrary panel of SCLC cell lines.

The screening of 'random' drugs in a large panel of cell lines at the NCI drug-discovery program is still at its beginning, but appears to give fruitful information. It is very encouraging that the data from the testing of more than 60 cell lines demonstrate that drugs with a specific mechanism of action have specific sensitivity patterns in the panel, e.g., a tubulin-targeting drug exhibits a specific 'tubulin targeting' pattern in sensitivity [15,16]. This finding supports the notion that drug resistance is specific and therefore also that resistance may be overcome.

There are more than 10 established anticancer agents with activity in SCLC. With such a high number of active drugs, it appears that the main problem is no longer the identification of new drugs effective in reducing a bulky tumor in the initial phase of SCLC, but rather identification of agents with activity in resistant SCLC phenotypes. Our approach to drug evaluation has therefore been aimed at identifying drugs with activity in SCLC cells that are resistant to the most active agent used today, VP-16 (etoposide). VP-16 is highly active as a single agent [17,18], and combinations containing VP-16 are superior to those without [19]. Recent results have suggested that VP-16, or its analogue, VM-26 (teniposide), either as a single agent or in a two-drug combination with cisplatin, is as effective as multidrug combinations in producing initial responses [18]. VP-16 will undoubtedly be widely used in the future, and the mechanisms of resistance to VP-16 are therefore of special interest. Accordingly, the main theme in our preclinical drug screening setup has been to establish a panel of SCLC cell lines that would enable us to identify new drugs of potential value when used in combination with VP-16. However, as always when investigating biological systems, complementary assays are neccessary to secure specificity and to broaden our perception. With the clonogenic assay as the mainstay in our laboratory, a number of other assays, as described below, have proved to be of value in the preclinical evaluation of new drugs.

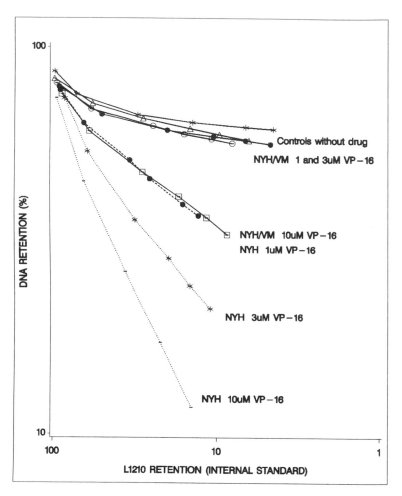

Figure 1. Alkaline elution assay demonstrating VP-16-mediated DNA cleavage in NYH/VM cells compared to the wild-type cell line NYH.

including VP-16, VM-26, adriamycin, daunorubicin, mitoxantrone, and amsacrine (m-AMSA) are all considered to exert their cytotoxic effect via topo II [34]. Also, topo I may be targeted with anticancer agents [35]. The first drug demonstrated to act on topo I was camptothecin, and at present a number of camptothecin analogues are being studied clinically. The catalytical process of topo II has been studied thoroughly and can be divided into distinct steps [36]. These steps involve noncovalent binding of topo II to DNA followed by the introduction of a double-stranded DNA cleavage. The cleaved topo II–DNA complex consists of four base-pair staggered nicks where the enzyme becomes covalently attached to the protruding 5'-ends. Following DNA cleavage, topo II passes a second DNA

176

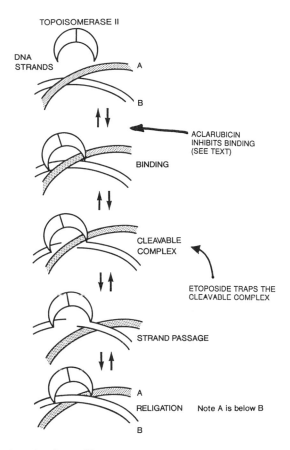

TOPOISOMERASE II

DNA
STRANDS

A

B

ACLARUBICIN
INHIBITS BINDING
(SEE TEXT)

BINDING

CLEAVABLE
COMPLEX

ETOPOSIDE TRAPS THE
CLEAVABLE COMPLEX

STRAND PASSAGE

A

RELIGATION   Note A is below B

B

Figure 2. The catalytic cycle of topo II.

helix through the break and finally religates the broken DNA [37] (figure 2).
Drugs such as VP-16 (etoposide) convert topo II into a toxic DNA cleaver
by trapping the enzyme in a nonfunctional state, the so-called *cleavable
complex*, in which neither the rejoining of the cleaved DNA strands nor the
passage of DNA through the broken DNA can occur [34]. Cells with a
decreased topo II content have fewer targets for VP-16, as illustrated with
NYH/VM in figure 1, and are therefore less susceptible to VP-16-mediated
toxicity [4].

Drug interactions with topoisomerases can be studied in vitro. Radiolabeled DNA is incubated with purified topoisomerase enzyme, and the
cleaved DNA fragments generated by the enzyme can be separated by gel
electrophoresis [38]. In this system, it is possible to investigate whether a
drug induces topoisomerase-mediated DNA breaks; also, the effect of drug
combinations can be tested in such an assay [28,29]. Only topo II can unlink
two intertwined DNA circles via its strand-passing activity [34]. The strand-

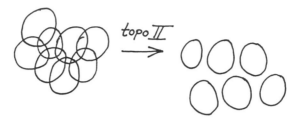

Figure 3. Topo II can mediate decatanation of intertwined DNA circles.

passing activity of topo II can be measured in a decatenation assay. The enzyme is incubated with catenated kinetoplast DNA (intertwined circular DNA) in the presence or absence of drug. Topo II allows the separation of the catenated DNA to free minicircles (figure 3). The free minicircles migrate with a higher mobility in a gel than do the intertwined circles; accordingly, gel electrophoresis can separate the two forms. The DNA is subsequently stained with ethidium-bromide and visualized under UV illumination, and possible drug inhibition of DNA decatenation can thereby be visualized. Also, the assay can be used to quantitate topo II activity in nuclear extracts from different cell lines. When the assay is used together with a Western blot for immunological quantization of topo II, it is possible to distinguish between drug resistance caused by a reduced amount of topo II or by an altered topo II activity, i.e., a mutated enzyme [4,39,40].

Drug transport assays

A common mechanism of drug resistance in both bacteria and cells is a change in membrane transport [41]. The most well known in cancer cells is the classical, or P-glycoprotein-associated, multidrug resistance (MDR) phenotype characterized by a decrease in drug accumulation due to an energy-dependent increase in drug efflux [42,43]. A 170-kDa plasma membrane glycoprotein called the P-glycoprotein (Pgp) appears to act as a molecular pump capable of extruding a wide variety of drugs [44]. The result is a lowered intracellular drug concentration leading eventually to drug resistance. Most anthracyclines, actinomycin D, and all vinca alkaloids are efficiently transported by the Pgp-mediated efflux system [45], while VP-16 is a poorer substrate [46]. It appears that Pgp-mediated efflux of very lipophillic drugs is ineffective. Although such drugs may be substrates for an efflux mechanism, their high membrane permeability makes pumping futile. Thus, the anthracyclines aclarubicin and iododoxorubicin are more lipophilic than doxorubicin and accumulate to the same degree in wild-type and classical MDR cells. The efflux mechanism is a basic problem that also has to be taken into account in the development of new drug types. Recent

178

Table 1. Daunorubicin accumulation in SCLC cells (pmol/10^6 cells)

Cell line	Glucose	Azid	Glucose + verapamil
NCI-H69	544	699	514
H69/DAU	170	488	333
H69/VP	324	719	588
OC-NYH	1156	1303	1125
NYH/VM	969	1066	868

Note: Cells were incubated with 3 µM daunorubicin for one hour. Glucose: medium with glucose; Azid: medium without glucose and with azide; Glucose + verapamil: medium with glucose and verapamil (5 µM). For description of cell lines, see table 2.

examples demonstrate this. It appears that two important new drugs in clinical trials, namely, the topo I targeting agent topothecan and taxol, are transported by Pgp. The topo I targeting agent camptothecin is very lipophilic and overcomes MDR, whereas Pgp MDR cells exhibit cross-resistance to more hydrophilic camptothecin analogues such as topothecan [47]. Also, the anthracycline iododoxorubicin (4'-deoxy-4'-iododoxorubicin) is quickly metabolized to the more hydrophilic 9-OH-iododoxorubicin in human erythrocytes. There is a lower intracellular accumulation of this metabolite in Pgp MDR cells and although it is active in many different cell lines, the metabolite is much less active than iododoxorubicin in Pgp MDR cells [48]. Thus, in order to establish whether a new drug should be included in the Pgp MDR family, accumulation studies in a Pgp-containing cell line, such as NCI-H69/DAU, are indicated. Intracellular drug concentrations are assessed either by use of radiolabeled drugs or by spectrofluoroscopy when possible (e.g., anthracyclines). The wild-type and MDR cell lines are typically incubated for one hour at 37°C in the presence of the drug to be investigated at 1–5 µM. Since the efflux is energy dependent, the experiments are performed both in medium with glucose and in medium where cellular energy is depleted by adding sodium azide and omitting glucose [45]. So-called MDR modulators — drugs such as verapamil and cyclosporine A — which increase the intracellular concentration of cytostatic drug by inhibiting its efflux can be tested in the same system. A typical experiment on SCLC MDR cells is shown in table 1.

The altered topoisomerase II or at-MDR phenotype (for a definition, see below) is characterized by equal drug accumulation in wild-type and resistant cells, and transport studies are therefore not relevant in this case (cell line NYH/VM). However, a third, still poorly defined MDR phenotype without Pgp expression but with cross-resistance to vincristine (so-called non-Pgp, non-at MDR) often shows a decrease in drug accumulation, indicating the usefulness of accumulation studies. An example is shown in table 1, in the cell line NCI-H69/VP. Several MDR drugs, e.g., vincristine and daunorubicin, are weak bases, and an increased exocytosis of basic drugs sequestered in acidic vesicles has been suggested to play a role in MDR [49,50]. Cole et al. [51] suggested that such an altered drug distribution within the cells may be responsible for the vincristine resistance in their cell line, H69AR, and, interestingly, Cole et al. [52] recently described an overexpression of a non-Pgp transporter gene in this cell line. The identification of such alternative transporters appears particularly promising since a reduced drug accumulation without the presence of Pgp has also been demonstrated by other groups [53,54] and in our investigations on *H69/VP* [24].

It is a controversial question whether experimentally developed resistant cell lines are at all clinically relevant. An argument against the experimental lines is that the high level of resistance often seen in these lines is far above what seems clinically relevant. Since maximum tolerated doses of cytostatics are most often used, a 2- to 3-fold decrease in cellular sensitivity is sufficient to explain clinical resistance. However, recent clinical investigations demonstrate that MDR is not only a laboratory phenomenon [55]. In several studies on patients with acute myelocytic leukemia, there is a significantly reduced survival of patients with overexpression of *mdr*1 mRNA or Pgp in the leukemia cells [56,57]. Because of the difficulty of obtaining biopsies in SCLC, it is still unsettled whether the classical Pgp MDR phenotype is involved in drug resistance in SCLC. Some overexpression has been described [58,59], and Pgp-positive SCLC cell lines have been generated in the laboratory by us and by others [60–62]. Thus, experimentally developed resistance mechanisms can be expected to be of relevance in SCLC.

Results from in vitro drug evaluation in SCLC

Our approach has primarily been to concentrate on the most active drug, VP-16. It is a curious fact that experimental resistance to VP-16 always confers cross-resistance to structurally unrelated drugs, and a VP-16-resistant cell line will therefore always have an MDR phenotype. There are at present at least three different MDR phenotypes, all of which are VP-16 resistant. In our panel of cell lines, we have included three sublines, each with a different VP-16-resistant MDR phenotype. In this way, evaluation of new drugs will be tested against the entire (known) VP-16 resistance spectrum.

H69/DAU4, primarily resistant to daunorubicin, is a classical MDR cell line with P-glycoprotein (Pgp) overexpression, decreased drug accumulation, and cross-resistance to vincristine [60].

NYH/VM, primarily resistant to VM-26, is an at-MDR (altered topoisomerase-MDR) [39] cell line with reduced topo II content as measured by Western blot and with reduced catalytic activity as measured by a decatanation assay. The cell line is without reduced drug accumulation and is

Table 2. DNA content, plating efficiency, relation to chemotherapy, and growth behavior in vitro of the cell lines used

Cell line	DNA index	%PE	Prior therapy	Growth	MDR type
NCI-H69	0.90	12	CTX MTX CCNU VCR ADR PRO	S	
H69/DAU4	0.87	12		S	Pgp
H69/VP	0.82	13		S	non-Pgp-non-at
OC-NYH	1.39	27	None	Mon	
NYH/VM	1.29	30		Mon	at
NCI-N592	1.48	30	MTX*	S	
OC-TOL	1.40	22	None	S	
GLC-16	1.80	17	CTX VP-16 ADR	S	
SCCL 86M1	1.45	15	None	S	

CTX: cyclofosfamide; MTX: methotrexate; VCR: vincristine; ADR: adriamycin; PRO: procarbazine; DNA index: DNA content of the cells in G1 relative to human diploid cells; PE: plating efficiency at approximately 3000 colonies; S: growth in suspension; Mon: growth as monolayer; MDR type: see text.

not cross-resistant to vincristine. The resistance mechanism is thus a change in drug target, i.e., topo II enzyme [33].

H69/VP, primarily resistant to VP-16, is a non-Pgp, non-at-MDR cell line with cross-resistance to vincristine and with reduced drug accumulation [24,63]. This resistance mechanism is the least defined.

In addition to these MDR cell lines, our panel has so far included six wild-type lines (see table 2).

The major benefit of using the panel of SCLC lines has been the information gained on patterns of differential sensitivity. Figure 4 shows the sensitivity patterns as determined by clonogenic assay to 19 drugs in the six wild-type and three MDR SCLC cell lines.

The data demonstrate that the variation in sensitivity to most drugs in the wild-type lines is within a factor of 2 to 10. As seen in figure 4, sensitivity patterns to VP-16 and BCNU are very different, whereas patterns to VP-16 and VM-26 are identical and similar to the pattern obtained with doxorubicin. Similarity in sensitivity patterns is also obtained between vincristine and vindesine as well as to BCNU and cisplatin. However, a more detailed visual comparison of patterns of all possible drug pairings is obviously not feasible. We therefore performed a correlation analysis using rank orders of sensitivity with all possible pairings of the 19 agents. From such an analysis, a high correlation coefficient for a given pair of compounds is indicative of a similar pattern of response in the set of cell lines. A numerically low coefficient indicates that the two compounds are acting in

181

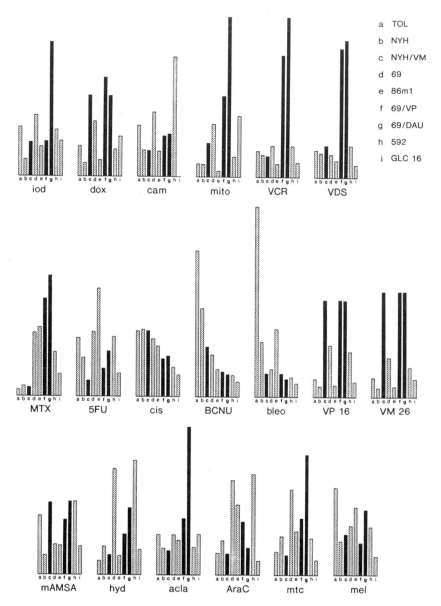

Figure 4. Sensitivity patterns to 19 anticancer agents on nine SCLC cell lines. The cell lines are sorted by increasing sensitivity to BCNU. The results are depicted as the mean LD50 values from at least two experiments. The three MDR lines are demarcated with solid bars. iod: iododoxorubicin; dox: doxorubicin; cam: camptothecin; mito: mitoxantrone; VCR: vincristine; VDS: vindesine; MTX: methotrexate; cis: cisplatin; BCNU: carmustine; bleo: bleomycin; hyd: hydroxyurea; acla: aclarubicin; AraC: cytarabin; mtc: mitomycin C; mel: melphalan. From [24]. Reproduced with permission.

182

Table 3. Correlation analysis on rank order of sensitivity with all possible pairings of 19 anticancer agents. Correlation coefficients (%) were obtained in six wild-type and three MDR lines

	BCNU	5FU	acla	dox	mel	AraC	bleo	cam	cis	hyd	iod	mAMSA	MTX	mito	mtc	VCR	VDS	VM26	VP16
BCNU	*																		
5FU	-26	*																	
acla	-37	22	*																
dox	-13	-47	59	*															
mel	-6	76	37	-12	*														
AraC	2	43	-8	-18	-1	*													
bleo	40	29	7	-32	36	0	*												
cam	-35	24	45	18	34	31	-2	*											
cis	89	24	-21	-2	12	-12	34	-12	*										
hyd	-47	6	14	20	-20	54	-61	47	-47	*									
iod	-31	28	76	43	52	0	-19	73	-9	42	*								
mAMSA	-44	-7	27	55	29	-23	-14	44	-22	15	47	*							
MTX	-66	44	56	22	13	30	-22	-2	-59	44	27	18	*						
mito	-45	-33	60	84	-17	-23	-55	23	-34	50	56	50	49	*					
mtc	-25	24	48	30	13	50	-22	13	-23	66	43	0	73	48	*				
VCR	-19	-4	67	67	15	1	-22	44	-18	52	63	56	41	76	55	*			
VDS	-10	-4	60	69	16	-2	-6	34	-13	30	54	59	41	62	41	89	*		
VM26	-19	-38	50	94	0	-13	-42	16	-7	32	48	71	29	83	36	72	71	*	
VP16	-21	-34	47	92	5	-15	-43	14	-6	31	48	72	29	81	37	73	71	99	*

acla, aclarubicin; dox, doxorubicin; mel, melphalan; bleo, bleomycin: cam, camptothecin; hyd, hydroxyurea; iod, iododoxorubicin; MTX, methotrexate; mito, mitoxantrone; mtc, mitomycin C; VCR, vincristine; VDS, vindesine. Data from [24].

different ways, and a negative correlation coefficient suggests that two drugs exhibit collateral sensitivity. Two separate experiments from each of the nine SCLC cell lines (i.e., 18 LD50 values for each drug) were used in the correlation analysis. Table 3 presents the correlation coefficients to all the possible pairings. In accordance with the visual interpretation of the data (figure 4), BCNU and cisplatin, VP-16 and VM-26, and vincristine and vindesine have very high correlation coefficients (89%, 99%, and 89%, respectively). Also, the sensitivity pattern to VP-16 is highly correlated with the pattern of doxorubicin (92%). Similar results from a large panel of 62 human tumor cell lines have recently been described from the NCI drug-discovery program by Wu et al. [64], with a correlation coefficient of 88% between VP-16 and DOX.

In our panel of cell lines, VP-16 also exhibits high correlation coefficients to the other topo II targeting agents mitoxantrone (81%) and m-AMSA (72%). Table 3 depicts a remarkable inverse correlation between BCNU and MTX (−66%) as well as between bleomycin and hydroxyurea (−61%). In addition, numerically smaller inverse correlation coefficients are observed a number of times. Thus, the alkylating agents (BCNU and cisplatin), the antimetabolites, and bleomycin are all inversely correlated to the MDR drugs; e.g., BCNU and bleomycin correlation to mitoxantrone is −45% and −55%, respectively.

The data demonstrate that 1) cells resistant to VP-16 are often but not always cross-resistant to vinca alkaloids, 2) cells resistant to vinca alkaloids are cross-resistant to VP-16, 3) cells resistant to VP-16 are not resistant to alkylating agents or cisplatin (in contrast, VP-16-resistant cells often exhibit collateral sensitivity to cisplatin and other alkylating agents), 4) cells resistant to alkylating agents are not resistant to topo II targeting agents and may exhibit collateral sensitivity to topo II targeting agents, and 5) cells resistant to one alkylating agent are not always cross-resistant to other alkylating agents.

The appearance of collateral sensitivity between MDR drugs and akylating agents suggests that an altered scheduling of the administration of these drugs may be advantageous, i.e., MDR drugs used before alkylating agents. However, it cannot be expected that an altered schedule of alkylating agents and topo II targeting drugs is 'sufficient' to improve substantially the therapeutic results in SCLC. Obviously, new drugs are needed with activity in the doubly resistant cells. From figure 4 and table 3, it is possible to get hints as to the identification of drugs with other cellular targets pontentially useful in combinations with alkylating agents and topo II drugs. Thus, sensitivity patterns to drugs, such as camptothecin and the antimetabolite ara-C, differ both from topo II targeting drugs and from alkylating agents.

We have recently been able to demonstrate that sensitivity patterns in an appropriate panel of cell lines may in fact reflect differences in the drugs' mechanisms of action.

In contrast to the uniform sensitivity pattern obtained with the epipodophllotoxins VP-16 and VM-26, different sensitivity patterns were found when various intercalating agents were compared [23,60]. Doxorubicin, daunorubicin, and mitoxantrone exhibited very similar sensitivity patterns on six SCLC wild-type cell lines, while the sensitivity pattern to aclarubicin was different. Specific interactions of doxorubicin, daunorubicin, and mitoxantrone with the nuclear enzyme topo II were known to play a role in the cytotoxic activity of these drugs as they stimulate DNA cleavage in the presence of purified topo II [65,66], presumably due to a stimulation in the formation of cleavage complexes between DNA and topo II as described with VP-16 [34] (figure 2). The discrepancy between aclarubicin and the other topo II active drugs guided us to investigate whether aclarubicin had a mode of action that was different than that of the other 'classical' anthracyclines. The drugs were tested together with the purified topo II enzyme and labeled DNA. Indeed, in contrast to what was observed with VP-16 and amsacrine (m-AMSA) [28] and daunorubicin [29], aclarubicin did not stimulate a topo-II-mediated DNA cleavage. In fact, aclarubicin inhibited the DNA cleavage obtained with amsacrine, VP-16, and daunorubicin in vitro. In accordance with this finding, we were able to demonstrate that aclarubicin also inhibited VP-16 and daunorubicin cytotoxicity in SCLC cells in the clonogenic assay and that aclarubicin inhibited DNA strand breaks in the alkaline elution assay. Our recent data suggest that aclarubicin is able to inhibit the binding of topo II to DNA [36]. By preventing the initial non-covalent binding of topo II to DNA, aclarubicin antagonizes all drugs that act by stimulating topo-II-mediated DNA cleavage (figure 2). Also, we now have data from both healthy and tumor-bearing mice demonstrating an inhibitory effect of aclarubicin on VP-16 in vivo [67]. These results convincingly show that sensitivity patterns in a relevant panel of cell lines can help pinpoint a drug's mode of action. In a similar fashion, Bai et al. [15] demonstrated by sensitivity testing on a panel of 60 cell lines that two new drugs, halichondrin B and homohalichondrin B, are tubulin inhibitors.

The described altered mechanism of action of aclarubicin in contrast to typical topo II inhibitors has the potentially clinically interesting consequence that at-MDR cells, such as NYH/VM, exhibiting resistance to doxorubicin, daunorubicin, and mitoxantrone, are *not* cross-resistant to aclarubicin [33] (figure 5).

We have studied which structures in the anthracycline molecule were critical of determining cross-resistance to VP-16 in at-MDR cells. Using six anthracycline derivatives on wild-type and at-MDR SCLC cells, as well as the alkaline elution and the DNA cleavage assays described above, we were able to show that one domain in the anthracycline molecule is of particular importance for interaction with topo II, namely, the positions C-10 and C-11 in the chromophore. We have further demonstrated that the at-MDR phenotype was circumvented by a $COOCH_3$ substitution at position C-10 in aclarubicin [33]. Our data show that the anthracyclines can be separated into two different types. One type has its cytotoxicity linked to topo II activity,

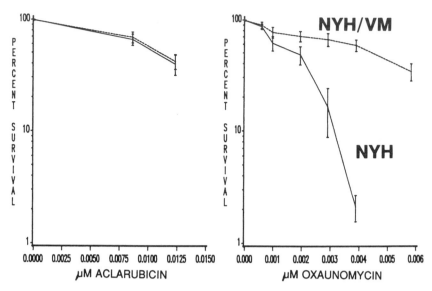

Figure 5. Dose–response curves obtained in a clonogenic assay with (A) aclarubicin on cell lines NYH (——) (N = 8) and NYH/VM (----) (N = 6), and (B) oxaunomycin on cell lines NYH (——) (N = 7) and NYH/VM (----) (N = 7). *Points*, mean; *bars*, SEM from N experiments. From [33]. Reproduced with permission.

while the other is independent of topo II activity. These findings may provide guidance for the synthesis and development of new analogues with activity in at-MDR cells.

In the above-mentioned structure–activity studies, the aclarubicin analogue oxaunomycin was found to be 50-fold more potent than doxorubicin and daunorubicin on the wild-type OC-NYH cell line. Such an increased potency detected in vitro is, however, of no practical significance if followed by a similar increase in toxicity. For example, a number of in vitro experiments have shown that VM-26 is 10-fold more potent than VP-16 [25], but when the two drugs are tested in equitoxic doses in vivo, there is no difference in their efficacy [68]. Our studies with oxaunomycin demonstrated that it was a potent stimulator of topo II cleavage; in accordance with this, we found that aclarubicin was able to inhibit its cytotoxicity and that the drug exhibited clear cross-resistance in NYH/VM (figure 5). This demonstrates that our system has identified oxaunomycin as a topo II cleavage-stimulating drug, but we cannot determine whether this topo II targeting agent has any advantages over other topo II stimulators, such as, e.g., VP-16. To clarify whether therapeutic differences exist between such analogues, comparative analysis in vivo should be performed of maximal tolerated doses, toxicological profiles, therapeutic activity in equitoxic doses, and the antineoplastic spectrum. Accordingly, our in vitro system is not suited to distinguish between analogues with the same mechanism of action, but is instead able to detect lack of cross-resistance between different drug leads.

Conclusions

The described in vitro methods are not sufficient for a thorough evaluation of new drugs. Such analysis requires a number of additional in vivo studies. However, by using a panel of wild-type and VP-16- (MDR-) resistant SCLC cell lines in a clonogenic assay together with other in vitro assays, we are able to detect modes of action of new as well as established drugs, leading to patterns of collateral sensitivity and cross-resistance. These patterns should facilitate the selection of a combination of non-cross-resistant agents. In addition to determining sensitivity patterns, the clonogenic assay is suitable for determining the effect of combining different drugs. In future, the panel of SCLC lines will be extended with sublines resistant to non-MDR drugs, such as cisplatin and topo I active drugs, in order to give a broader picture of sensitivity patterns. The panel will also be of potential use in evaluating other modes of therapy such as antisense inhibition, growth factor regulation, and drug targeting in conjunction with conventional chemotherapy in SCLC.

References

1. Hansen HH. 1992. Management of small-cell cancer of the lung. Lancet 339:846–849.
2. Sehested M, Hirsch FR, Østerlind K, Olsen JE. 1986. Morphologic variations of small cell lung cancer. A histopathologic study of pretreatment and posttreatment specimens in 104 patients. Cancer 57:804–807.
3. Goldie JH, Coldman AJ. 1984. The genetic origin of drug resistance in neoplasms: Implications for systemic therapy. Cancer Res 44:3643–3653.
4. Borst P. 1991. Genetic mechanisms of drug resistance. A review. Rev Oncol 4:87–105.
5. Cullen M. 1990. The design of phase II trials. Lung Cancer 5:214–220.
6. Grant SC, Gralla RJ, Kris MG, Orazem J, Kitsis EA. 1992. Single-agent chemotherapy trials in small-cell lung cancer, 1970 to 1990: The case for studies in previously treated patients. J Clin Oncol 10:484–498.
7. Monks A, Scudiero D, Skehan P, Shoemaker R, Paull K, Vistica D, Hose C, Langley J, Cronise P, Vaigro-Wolff A, Gray-Goodrich M, Campbell H, Mayo J, Boyd M. 1991. Feasibility of a high-flux anticancer drug screen using a diverse panel of cultured human tumor cell lines. J Natl Cancer Inst 83:757–766.
8. Nitiss J, Wang JC. 1988. DNA-topoisomerase-targeting antitumor drugs can be studied in yeast. Proc Natl Acad Sci USA 85:7501–7505.
9. Elsea SH, Osheroff N, Nitiss JL. 1992. Cytotoxicity of quinolones toward eukaryotic cells. Identification of topoisomerase II as the primary cellular target for the quinolone CP-15, 953 in yeast. J Biol Chem 267:13150–13153.
10. Nitiss JL, Liu Y-X, Harbury P, Jannatipour M, Wasserman R, Wang JC. 1992. Amsacrine and etoposide hypersensitivity of yeast cells overexpressing DNA topoisomerase II. Cancer Res 52:4467–4472.
11. Kawada S, Yamashita Y, Fujii N, Nakano H. 1991. Induction of a heat-stable topoisomerase

II-DNA cleavable complex by nonintercalative terpenoides, terpentecin and clerocidin. Cancer Res 51:2922–2925.

12. Yamashita Y, Kawada S, Fujii N, Nakano H. 1991. Induction of mammalian DNA topoisomerase I and II mediated DNA cleavage by saintopin, a new antitumor agent from fungus. Biochemistry 30:5838–5845.

13. Cole SPC. 1992. Multidrug resistance in small cell lung cancer. Cancer J Physiol Pharmacol 70:313–329.

14. Giaccone G, Gazdar AF, Beck H, Zunino F, Capranico G. 1992. Multidrug sensitivity phenotype of human lung cancer cells associated with topoisomerase II expression. Cancer Res 52:1666–1674.

15. Bai R, Paull KD, Herald CL, Malspeis L, Pettit GR, Hamel E. 1991. Halichondrin B and homohalichondrin B, marine natural products binding in the vinca domain of tubulin. Discovery of tubulin-based mechanism of action by analysis of differential cytotoxicity data. J Biol Chem 266:15882–15889.

16. Paull KD, Lin CM, Malspeis L, Hamel E. 1992. Identification of novel antimitotic agents acting at the tubulin level by computer-assisted evaluation of differential cytotoxicity data. Cancer Res 52:3892–3900.

17. Kristjansen PEG, Hirsch FR. 1989. A review of the 5th World Congress on Lung Cancer held by the International Association for the Study of Lung Cancer. Eur Respir J 2:275–279.

18. Bork E, Ersbøll J, Dombernowsky P, Bergman B, Hansen M, Hansen HH. 1991. Teniposide and etoposide in previously untreated small-cell lung cancer: A randomized study. J Clin Oncol 9:1627–1631.

19. Hirsch FR, Hansen HH, Hansen M, Østerlind K, Vindeløv LL, Dombernowsky P, Sørensson S. 1987. The superiority of combination chemotherapy including etoposide based on in vivo cell cycle analysis in the treatment of extensive small cell lung cancer: A randomized trial of 288 consecutive patients. J Clin Oncol 5:585–591.

20. Roper PR, Drewinko B. 1976. Comparison of in vitro methods to determine drug-induced cell lethality. Cancer Res 36:2182–2188.

21. Freshney RI. 1987. Culture of Animal Cells: A Manual of Basic Technique (2nd ed.). Wiley-Liss: New York, pp. 245–256.

22. Roed H, Christensen IJ, Vindeløv LL, Spang-Thomsen M, Hansen HH. 1987. Inter-experiment variation and dependence on culture conditions in assaying the chemosensitivity of human small cell lung cancer cell lines. Eur J Cancer Clin Oncol 23:177–186.

23. Jensen PB, Roed H, Vindeløv L, Christensen IJ, Hansen HH. 1989. Reduced variation in the clonogenic assay obtained by standardization of the cell culture conditions prior to drug testing on small cell lung cancer cell lines. Invest New Drugs 7:307–315.

24. Jensen PB, Christensen IJ, Sehested M, Hansen HH, Vindeløv L. 1993. Differential cytotoxicity of 19 anticancer agents in wild type and etoposide resistant small cell lung cancer cell lines. Br J Cancer 67:311–320.

25. Roed H, Vindeløv LL, Christensen IJ, Spang-Thomsen M, Hansen HH. 1987. The effect of the two epipodophyllotoxin derivatives etoposide (VP-16) and teniposide (VM-26) on cell lines established from patients with small cell carcinoma of the lung. Cancer Chemother Pharmacol 19:16–20.

26. Sehested M, Skovsgaard T, Jensen PB, Demant EJF, Friche E, Bindslev N. 1990. Transport of the multidrug resistance modulators verapmil and azidopine in wild type and daunorubicin resistant Ehrlich ascites tumor cells. Br J Cancer 62:37–41.

27. Friche E, Jensen PB, Nissen NI. 1992. Comparison of cyclosporin A and SDZ PSC 833 as multidrug resistance modulators in a daunorubicin resistant Ehrlich ascites tumor. Cancer Chemother Pharmacol 30:235–237.

28. Jensen PB, Sørensen BS, Demant EJF, Sehested M, Jensen PS, Vindeløv L, Hansen HH. 1990. Antagonistic effect of aclarubicin on the cytotoxicity of etoposide and 4'-(9-acridinylamino) methanesulfon-m-anisidide in human small cell lung cancer cell lines and on topoisomerase II mediated DNA cleavage. Cancer Res 50:3311–3316.

29. Jensen PB, Jensen PS, Demant EJF, Friche E, Sørensen BS, Sehested M, Wasserman K, Vindeløv L, Westergaard O, Hansen HH. 1991. Antagonistic effect of aclarubicin on daunorubicin-induced cytotoxicity in human small cell lung cancer cells: relationship to DNA integrity and topoisomerase II. Cancer Res 51:5093–5099.

30. Roed H, Vindeløv LL, Christensen IJ, Spang-Thomsen M, Hansen HH. 1988. The cytotoxic activity of cisplatin, carboplatin and teniposide alone and combined determined on four human small cell lung cancer cell lines by the clonogenic assay. Eur J Clin Oncol 24:247–253.

31. Carmichael J, Mitchell JB, Degraff WG, Gamson J, Gazdar AF, Johnson BE, Glatstein E, Minna JD. 1988. Chemosensitivity testing of human lung cancer cell lines using the MTT assay. Br J Cancer 57:540–547.

32. Kohn KW. 1991. Principles and practice of DNA filter elution. Pharmac Ther 49:55–77.

33. Jensen PB, Sørensen BS, Sehested M, Demant EJF, Kjeldsen E, Friche E, Hansen HH. 1993. Different modes of anthracycline interaction with topoisomerase II: separate structures critical for DNA-cleavage, and for overcoming topoisomerase II related drug resistance. Biochem Pharmacol 45:2025–2035.

34. Liu LF. 1989. DNA topoisomerase poisons as antitumor drugs. Annu Rev Biochem 58:351–371.

35. Hsiang Y, Herzberg R, Hect S, Liu LF. 1985. Camptothecin induces protein-linked DNA breaks via mammalian DNA topoisomerase I. J Biol Chem 260:14873–14878.

36. Sørensen BS, Sinding J, Andersen AH, Alsner J, Jensen PB, Westergaard O. 1992. Mode of action of topoisomerase II targeting agents at a specific DNA sequence: uncoupling the DNA binding, cleavage, and religation events. J Mod Biol 228:778–786.

37. Osheroff N. 1989. Biochemical basis for the interactions of type I and type II topoisomerases with DNA. Pharmacol Ther 41:223–241.

38. Andersen HA, Christiansen K, Zechiedrich EL, Jensen PS, Osheroff N, Westergaard O. 1989. Strand specificity of the topoisomerase II mediated double-stranded DNA cleavage reaction. Biochemistry 28:6237–6244.

39. Danks MK, Schmidt CA, Cirtain MC, Suttle DP, Beck WT. 1988. Altered catalytic activity of and DNA cleavage by DNA topoisomerase II from human leukemic cells selected for resistance to VM-26. Biochemistry 27:8861–8869.

40. Bugg BY, Danks MK, Beck WT, Suttle DP. 1991. Expression of a mutant DNA topoisomerase II CCRF-CEM human leukemic cells selected for resistance to teniposide. Proc Natl Acad Sci (USA) 88:7654–7658.

41. Hayes JD, Wolf CR. 1990. Molecular mechanisms of drug resistance. Biochem J 272: 281–295.

42. Danø K. 1973. Active outward transport of daunomycin in resistant Ehrlich ascites tumor cells. Biochim Biophys Acta 323:466–483.

43. Juliano RL, Ling V. 1976. A surface glycoprotein modulating drug permeability in Chinese hamster ovary cell mutants. Biochim Biophys Acta 455:152–162.

44. Endicott JA, Ling V. 1989. The biochemistry of p-glycoprotein mediated multidrug resistance. Annu Rev Biochem 58:137–171.

45. Skovsgaard T. 1978. Mechanism of cross-resistance between vincristine and daunorubicin in Ehrlich ascites tumor cells. Cancer Res 38:4722–4727.

46. Sehested M, Friche E, Jensen PB, Demant EJF. 1992. Relationship of VP-16 to the classical multidrug resistance phenotype. Cancer Res 52:2874–2879.

47. Chen AY, Yu C, Potmesil M, Wall ME, Wani MC, Liu LF. 1991. Camptothecin overcomes MDR1-mediated resistance in human KB carcinoma cells. Cancer Res 51:6039–6044.

48. Ballinari D, Pezzoni G, Giuliani FC, Grandi M. 1989. Biological profile of 13-OH-iododoxorubicin: preclinical data. Proc Am Assoc Cancer Res 30:482.

49. Sehested M, Skovsgaard T, van Deurs B, Winther-Nielsen H. 1987. Increased plasma membrane traffic in daunorubicin resistant P388 leukaemic cells. Effect of daunorubicin and verapamil. Br J Cancer 56:747–751.

189

50. Demant EJF, Sehested M, Jensen PB. 1990. A model for computer simulation of P-glycoprotein and transmembrane delta pH mediated anthracycline transport in multidrug resistant tumor cells. Biochim Biophys Acta 1055:117–125.

51. Cole SPC, Chanda ER, Dicke FP, Gerlach JH, Mirski SEL. 1991. Non-P-glycoprotein-mediated multidrug resistance in a small cell lung cancer cell line: evidence for decreased susceptibility to drug-induced DNA damage and reduced levels of topoisomerase II. Cancer Res 51:3345–3352.

52. Cole SPC, Bhardwaj G, Gerlach JH, Mackie JE, Grant CE, Almquist KC, Stewart AJ, Kurz EU, Duncan AMV, Deeley RG. 1992. Overexpression of a transporter gene in a multi-drug-resistant human lung cancer cell line. Science 258:1650–1654.

53. Versantvoort CHM, Broxterman HJ, Pinedo HM, de Vries EGE, Feller N, Kuiper CM, Lankelma J. 1992. Energy-dependent processes involved in reduced drug accumulation in multidrug-resistant lung cancer cell lines without P-glycoprotein expression. Cancer Res 52:17–23.

54. Scheper RJ, Broxterman HJ, Scheffer GL, Kaaijk P, Dalton WS, van Heijningen THM, van Kalken CK, Slovak ML, de Vries EGE, van der Valk P, Meijer CJLM, Pinedo HM. 1993. Overexpression of a Mr 110,000 vesicular protein in non-P-glycoprotein-mediated multidrug resistance. Cancer Res 53:1475–1479.

55. Nooter K, Herweijer H. 1991. Multidrug resistance (mdr) genes in human cancer. Br J Cancer 63:663–669.

56. Pirker R, Walner RJ, Geissler K, Linkesch W, Haas OA, Bettelheim P, Hopfner M, Scherrer R, Valent P, Havelec L, Ludwig H, Lechner K. 1991. MDR1 gene expression and treatment outcome in acute myeloid leukemia. J Natl Cancer Inst 83:708–712.

57. Sehested M, Ersbøl J, Friche E, Jensen PB, Demant EJF. 1993. Detection of P-glycoprotein in adult AML. In The Clinical Value of Drug Resistance Assays in Leukemia and Lymphoma, P Twentyman and G Kaspars (eds.). Harwood Academic Publishers, pp. 49–54.

58. Lai SL, Goldstein LJ, Gottesman MM, Pastan I, Tsai CM, Johnson BE, Mulshine JL, Ihde DC, Kayser K, Gazar AF. 1989. MDR1 gene expression in lung cancer. J Natl Cancer Inst 81:1144–1145.

59. Holzmayer TA, Hilsenbeck S, Vonhoff DD, Roninson IB. 1992. Clinical correlates of mdrl (P-glycoprotein) gene expression in ovarian and small-cell lung carcinomas. J Natl Cancer Inst 84:1486–1491.

60. Jensen PB, Vindeløv L, Roed H, Demant EJF, Sehested M, Skovsgaard T, Hansen HH. 1989. In vitro evaluation of the potential of aclarubicin in the treatment of small cell carcinoma of the lung (SCCL). Br J Cancer 60:838–844.

61. Reeve JG, Rabbitts PH, Twentyman PR. 1989. Amplification and expression of mdr1 gene in a multidrug resistant variant of small cell lung cancer cell line NCI-H69. Br J Cancer 60:339–342.

62. Minato K, Kanzawa F, Nishio K, Nakagawa K, Fujiwara Y, Saijo N. 1990. Characterization of an etoposide-resistant human small-cell lung cancer cell line. Cancer Chemother Pharmacol 26:313–317.

63. Jensen PB, Roed H, Sehested M, Demant EJF, Vindeløv L, Christensen IJ, Hansen HH. 1992. Doxorubicin sensitivity pattern in a panel of small cell lung cancer cell lines: Correlation to etoposide and vincristine and inverse correlation to carmustine sensitivity. Cancer Chemother Pharmacol 31:46–52.

64. Wu L, Smythe AM, Stinson SF, Mullendore LA, Monks A, Scudiero DA, Paull KD, Koutsoukos AD, Rubinstein LV, Boyd MR, Shoemaker RH. 1992. Multidrug-resistant phenotype of disease-oriented panels of human tumor cell lines used for anticancer drug screening. Cancer Res 52:3029–3034.

65. Tewey KM, Rowe TC, Yang L, Halligan BD, Liu LF. 1984. Adriamycin-induced DNA damage mediated by mammalian DNA topoisomerase II. Science 226:466–468.

66. Bodley A, Liu LF, Israel M, Seshadri R, Koseki Y, Giuliani FC, Kirschenbaum R, Silber R, Potmesil M. 1989. DNA topoisomerase II-mediated interaction of doxorubicin and daunorubicin congeners with DNA. Cancer Res 49:5969–5978.

67. Holm B, Jensen PB, Sehested M, Hansen HH. In vivo inhibition of etoposide (VP-16) mediated apoptosis, toxicity, and antitumor effect by the topoisomerase II uncoupling anthracycline aclarubicin. Cancer Chemother Pharmacol (in press).
68. Jensen PB, Roed H, Skovsgaard T, Friche E, Vindeløv L, Hansen HH, Spang-Thomsen M. 1990. Antitumor activity of the two epipodophyllotoxin derivatives VP-16 and VM-26 in preclinical systems: a comparison of in vitro and in vivo drug evaluation. Cancer Chemother Pharmacol 27:194–198.

10. Multidrug resistance in lung cancer

Henk J. Broxterman, Carolien H.M. Versantvoort, and Sabine C. Linn

Introduction

Lung cancer is divided into four major histological types: squamous cell carcinomas, adenocarcinomas, and large cell carcinomas, which are collectively referred to as non-small cell lung cancers (NSCLC), and a distinct type of lung cancer, small cell lung cancer (SCLC) [1]. Surgery, radiotherapy, and chemotherapy are used for the treatment of lung cancer, but long-term survival is obtained in only 5% to 10% of the patients. Thus, improvements in lung cancer therapy are urgently required [2,3].

SCLC has a high initial response rate (about 90%) to chemotherapy, with the most active single agents being doxorubicin (DOX), etoposide (VP-16), and cisplatin. However, despite this high sensitivity, patients with SCLC will relapse, and resistance to subsequent chemotherapy develops in almost all patients who initially demonstrated a clinical complete response to combination chemotherapy. Therefore, these patients will die, because no active chemotherapeutic agent is available after relapse. This type of resistance seems to pre-exist or to emerge in the population of tumor cells, regrowing after relapse, and could therefore be regarded as a clinically acquired form of multidrug resistance (MDR).

The treatment history of SCLC is in contrast with NSCLC, the most common form of lung cancer, for which no single chemotherapy treatment has emerged as a standard for patients with advanced disease. In general, 20% to 25% of these patients have a partial response, and single or multidrug therapy has no significant impact on survival. Thus, NSCLC is for the great part a primary (intrinsic) multidrug-resistant disease [1].

Primary and acquired cellular drug resistance may be based in part on the same biochemical mechanisms, since both originate as a consequence of the genetic instability of malignant cells leading to (spontaneous) generation of variants that may result in cellular drug resistance [4].

Definition

Clinically speaking, when a tumor does not respond to any chemotherapeutic treatment modality available, the tumor is said to be resistant to multiple drugs. In the experimental cancer literature, forms of (multiple) drug resistance are mostly defined based on the pharmacological, cellular, or biochemical mechanism that is thought to underlie each one. Such a subdivision allows the investigator to isolate a certain resistance mechanism in his or her mind and experiments. The advantage is clear: individual resistance mechanisms can be identified and described in terms of a single gene (mutation), and ways to circumvent a particular form of resistance can be developed in a rational way. The disadvantage is clear also: the elimination of just one mechanism used by tumor cells to defend themselves against toxic cytostatic drugs is not likely to create a situation that will cure the patient. Therefore, information derived from such experimental studies must be translated into clinical studies in order to identify the clinically relevant resistance mechanisms.

In this chapter, we will discuss one such form of MDR, defined by in vitro resistance to antitumor agents that are derived from natural sources and that are thought to kill cancer cells by acting at different primary targets. In practice, this definition means that this form of resistance will almost certainly be caused by mechanisms leading to a lower accumulation of the drugs at their cellular target sites via decreased drug influx, increased drug efflux, or increased detoxification of the drug before it reaches its target. By far the best studied mechanism is the P-glycoprotein- (Pgp-) mediated form of MDR, which is caused by an increase of energy-dependent drug transport from the cell (see figure 1A). Pgp is a plasma-membrane efflux pump for lipophilic drugs with a wide variety of chemical structures and mechanisms of action [5]. The Pgp encoding gene, called MDR1, is the only human gene cloned so far that has been proven by transfection experiments to confer MDR to otherwise drug-sensitive tumor cells [6] or to murine bone marrow cells [7].

Pgp/MDR1 overexpression causes resistance to some of the most active anticancer agents, such as the anthracyclines, DOX and daunorubicin (DNR), the vinca alkaloids, VP-16 and mitoxantrone, and also to the newer agent taxol. However, recently it has been recognized that other drug transporter molecules may exist in MDR lung cancer cell lines [8–10]. An important consequence of the identification of drug transporter molecules in cancer cells is that this form of MDR offers an obvious possibility for developing pharmacological means of modulating the resistance by intervening with (i.e., blocking) the drug transport (figure 1B). Indeed, numerous compounds have been tested in vitro for their potential to block Pgp, such as verapamil, cyclosporin A, and nontoxic analogues of vinca alkaloids and anthracyclines [11]. These approaches are now in the stage of clinical testing [12,13] (see below).

194

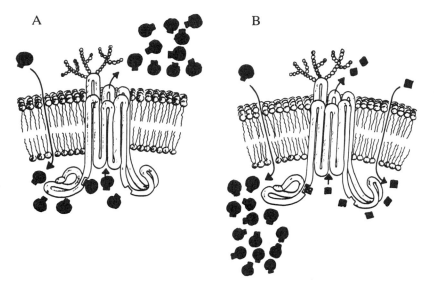

Figure 1. Proposed model for P-glycoprotein. (A) Antitumor drug diffuses through the plasma membrane lipid bilayer into the cells, binds to Pgp, and is translocated by this protein to the outer side of the plasma membrane in an ATP hydrolysis-dependent mechanism. (B) Resistance modifiers such as verapamil or cyclosporin A may bind to the Pgp and competitively or noncompetitively inhibit binding and/or transport of antitumor drugs. (Drawing by Kees Smid.)

In addition to this form of MDR, we will also discuss some data on altered target-related, mainly topoisomerase II-related, drug resistance. This resistance is not MDR in the real sense, since only one target is involved, but it often occurs in conjunction with MDR and implicates some of the MDR drugs most important in the treatment of lung cancer, namely, doxorubicin and VP-16. Of importance is that resistance to cisplatin is thought not to be involved in the forms of MDR we will discuss here.

In vitro chemosensitivity tests in lung cancer

Ideally, the response of a cancer patient to chemotherapy should be predicted from a short-term laboratory test measuring the effect of cytostatic drugs on the patient's tumor cells obtained from a biopsy. In theory, if we were able to select an effective therapy in this way [14], we would not have to know what the particular resistance mechanisms to certain drugs are.

As for many other tumor types and also for lung cancer, in vitro drug sensitivity assays using fresh human tumor specimens have been used in order to try to predict the clinical response of a tumor to chemotherapy from in vitro data [15]. Despite some limited success in chemosensitivity testing in some studies, especially those using non-cell-growth-dependent

195

but cytolysis endpoint assays such as the dye exclusion assay [16,17], these types of assays are still too difficult to perform in a routine clinical setting [18–20]. One study using the incorporation of ^{3}H-uridine in freshly isolated stage III lung adenocarcinoma cells showed a statistically significant positive correlation between in vitro resistance or sensitivity to doxorubicin and survival [21]. It cannot be inferred from those data, however, whether a form of MDR was responsible for the phenomenon. Of particular relevance for the present discussion, there are no published studies available that by using a cell culture or cytotoxicity assay of fresh lung cancer specimens have been able to assess the presence of the MDR phenotype in those lung cancer cells.

Therefore, to analyze the potential importance of the MDR phenotype in lung cancer, we have three types of data available:

1. Determination of the expression level of specific MDR-related mRNA or proteins in lung *tumor tissue*.
2. Determination of MDR-related parameters, including mRNA or protein (over) expression and chemosensitivity tests, in *cell lines* established from tumor specimens.
3. Identification of specific resistance mechanisms in *in vitro selected drug resistant* lung cancer cell lines.

These types of data will be discussed below.

Gene-specific MDR analysis in lung cancer

MDR1 RNA analysis

Specific mechanism-based screening for MDR has only been performed until now for the MDR1 gene product Pgp.

The highest levels of Pgp/*MDR1* expression are generally found in tumors originating from Pgp-expressing normal human tissues such as liver, kidney, adrenal, colon, and pancreas, where Pgp is thought to function as an extrusion mechanism for naturally occurring toxins [22] (see figure 2).

The most extensive study into the expression levels of the *MDR1* gene in nontumorous lung tissue and lung tumors has been performed by Lai et al. [23]. They found a generally low, but detectable level of *MDR1* mRNA by a slot blot analysis (see table 1) in lung tumors as well as normal lung tissue; this finding was confirmed by Shin et al. [24]. Furthermore, equally low levels of *MDR1* RNA were found in lung cancer cell lines originating from treated as well as untreated patients [23]. However, no correlation was found between *MDR1* mRNA expression level and in vitro chemosensitivity of these cell lines. Only in one type of lung cancer cell line, NSCLC with neuroendocrine properties (NSCLC-NE), studied in a limited number, was the level of *MDR1* mRNA significantly higher. Although the results from this study suggest that *MDR1* mRNA overexpression cannot solely explain

196

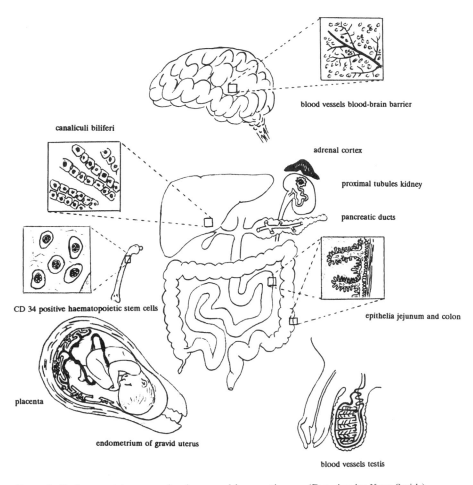

Figure 2. P-glycoprotein expression in normal human tissues. (Drawing by Kees Smid.)

the clinical multidrug resistance of many lung cancers, and certainly not the acquired drug resistance after relapse in SCLC, some role for Pgp cannot be excluded. A recent study using a sensitive polymerase-chain-reaction-based assay for *MDR1* RNA found that three of three SCLC patients with MDR1-negative tumors responded to chemotherapy (including at least one MDR drug), while four out of four patients with MDR1 positive tumors did not [25]. Since this very sensitive analysis could mean that only a few MDR1-positive (tumor or nontumor) cells in the sample were detected, it cannot be easily seen what the implications of such low-level expression for the treatment of a patient would be, especially since Pgp-positive macrophages in the tumor might obscure the interpretation of these data [26]. Prospective studies are needed to confirm the hypothesis that the presence of (even a

197

Table 1. Summary of MDR1 expression in nontumorous lung tissue, lung cancer tissue, and lung cancer cell lines

	No. of samples with >2 units of MDR1 RNA[a]	Mean MDR1 RNA level (range)[a]
Nontumorous lung	7/10 (70%)	2.5 (1–4)
Lung cancer		
SCLC	3/6 (50%)	3.0 (1–6)
NSCLC	8/13 (61%)	2.6 (<1–6)
NSCLC-NE	1/2 (50%)	15.5 (<1–30)
Carcinoid	2/3 (67%)	3.7 (<1–8)
Total	14/24 (58%)	3.9 (<1–30)
Lung cancer cell lines		
SCLC[b]	4/14 (28%)	1.6 (1–6)
SCLC[c]	0/9 (0%)	1.0 (<1–1)
Extra pulmonary	0/4 (0%)	1.0 (1)
SC	11/29 (38%)	1.8 (<1–10)
NSCLC	5/6 (83%)	12.3 (<1–30)
NSCLC-NE	2/5 (40%)	1.0 (1)
Carcinoid	22/67 (33%)	2.9 (<1–30)
Total		

[a] One unit MDR1 RNA is the level of the drug-sensitive KB3-1 cell line; about 6 units is the level of KB8 cells, which have a resistance factor of 1–2, according to Noonan et al. [32].
[b] Cell lines established from untreated patients.
[c] Cell lines established from treated patients.
Adapted from [23].

few) *MDR1* expressing cells in SCLC may be useful as a predictive marker for clinical resistance to combination chemotherapy.

Immunohistochemical studies

The previous section discussed the detection of *MDR1* by bulk methods, which do not allow appreciation of the level of gene expression in the individual cells. Since the above-mentioned considerations reveal that cellular heterogeneity might affect the interpretation of the results, immunohistochemical techniques to detect Pgp or in situ hybridization studies are indicated. A number of monoclonal antibodies suited for different immunohistochemical methods are available now, including C219, C494, JSB-1, MRK16, and 4E3. All these antibodies have their own technical problems with reference to specificity, cross-reactions, stability problems of the epitope recognized, etc. [27]. Therefore, insufficient quality control, together with the inherent lower sensitivity of immunohistochemical techniques as compared to sensitive RNA detection, is likely to be responsible for the highly inconsistent picture emerging from many immunohistochemical studies of Pgp expression in tumor types (including lung tumors) that have a low expression of this protein. If anything can be said from the few published studies, it is that in general the expression of Pgp in lung tumor cells as assessed by immunohistochemistry is below the limit of detection [26,28,29]. However, one paper reporting a high percentage of Pgp-positive tumor cells has appeared [30]. This finding is not consistent with the very low *MDR1* RNA levels found in lung cancer (vide supra). One observation that suggests that Pgp/*MDR1* might be related to resistance of lung cancer in certain cases was that out of seven xenografted human (epidermoid) lung tumors, one, which was resistant in vivo (in the mouse) to vincristine, dactinomycin, and DOX, also expressed Pgp as measured with a monoclonal antibody (Mab 265/F4) [31].

In conclusion, no evidence is available from immunohistochemical studies to suggest a major role of Pgp in the overall MDR of lung tumors. However, from another point of view, it must be said that a very low level of *MDR1* expression (as in KB8 cells [32]) may confer a very low degree of resistance to drugs such as vincristine or DOX in these cells. Thus, if a low level of *MDR1* expression is present in a lung tumor (see table 1) it might contribute to clinical resistance, especially if an MDR drug elicits some (partial) response, indicating that at least some drug is reaching the tumor cells and the intracellular targets. Even a very low Pgp density may then lower the effective dose of the drugs at their target sites at the maximum tolerated dose.

Chemosensitivity and MDR1 analysis in lung cancer cell lines

Comparison of SCLC cell lines established pre- and posttreatment

The obvious way to study the relevance of *MDR1* (or other gene) expression and its possible causal relationship to the clinical response of lung tumors to chemotherapy would be to perform prospective clinical studies correlating both parameters (see below). A second approach, namely, the correlation between *MDR1* expression and the in vitro measured response to cytotoxic drugs by freshly obtained tumor cells from effusions or tumor biopsies had very limited success due to poor in vitro growth of tumor cells, as discussed above. Therefore, as another approach, the resistance phenotype of lung cancer cell lines is often studied. Such studies might give clues to the cellular mechanisms involved in intrinsic resistance to lung cancer. Great caution must of course be exercised regarding the interpretation of such studies, since selection of discrete tumor-cell populations upon in vitro growth may occur. This possibility was suggested, e.g., by a recent study of Smit et al. [33]. These authors established three SCLC cell lines from patients with a complete response to chemotherapy and three SCLC cell lines from patients with no response, but they found no correlation at all between the clinical behavior of the tumor and the in vitro chemosensitivity of the cell lines, which therefore in this case cannot be considered representative of the clinical situation. From a different point of view, the establishment of a cell line may be indicative of a more aggressive type of SCLC [34], and it may therefore still be worthwile to study the chemosensitivity phenotype of such cell lines. Moreover, in contrast to the above-mentioned study, Campling et al. [20] have reported that SCLC cell lines established from untreated patients were more sensitive to 15 out of 16 cytotoxic drugs (the one exception was vincristine) than cell lines from treated patients, but the differences were small and only statistically significant for two drugs. A remarkable correlation between in vitro chemosensitivity and pretreatment status in SCLC and NSCLC was also found by Carmichael et al. [35] and Carney et al. [36]. It is unclear at present why the data of Smit et al. [33] differ from these latter studies, but selection of tumor cell populations in vitro remains one plausible possibility.

An interesting study design was followed by Berendsen et al. [37], who established three human SCLC cell lines from one patient during longitudinal follow-up. During the course of the study, the tumor changed from sensitive (complete response to cyclophosphamide, DOX, and VP-16) to completely resistant to chemotherapy. The chemosensitivity of the three cell lines was measured and showed at most a twofold increase in resistance to VP-16, DOX, melphalan, and vinblastine, but not to the MDR drugs VCR and actinomycin D. An investigation into the putative resistance mechanisms of these cell lines [38] showed no evidence for the involvement of Pgp/ MDR1 overexpression or increased detoxification mechanisms for DOX or cisplatinum as major mechanisms to explain the clinical resistance of the patient. Another study that followed the same approach was from Hida et al. [39]. They established three cell lines from one patient with SCLC, the first before treatment (SK1) and the second after the tumor relapsed following a partial response to cyclophosphamide, DOX, VCR, and VP-16 with radiotherapy (SK2). Then a second round of chemotherapy was given (cisplatin and VP-16) that was effective for two months, after which the third cell line (SK3) was established. The in vitro chemosensitivity of SK1 and SK2 was remarkably similar, but SK3 was more resistant to cisplatin, VP-16, VCR, and cyclophosphamide. No attempts were made in this study to pinpoint a particular resistance mechanism. Finally, Milroy et al. [40] describe seven SCLC cell lines that do not express Pgp as measured by immunohistochemistry.

Comparison of SCLC and NSCLC cell lines

Only two studies have appeared that have analyzed cell lines in any detail in order to investigate putative mechanism(s) explaining the remarkable difference in chemosensitivity between SCLC and NSCLC. The rationale for such studies is that if the difference in clinical behavior between SCLC and NSCLC tumors has an underlying cellular, biochemical mechanism that also occurs in cell lines, their analysis would be greatly facilitated. Lai et al. [23] have reported on the chemosensitivity and *MDR1* RNA analysis of SCLC and NSCLC cell lines. They concluded that there was no correlation between *MDR1* RNA (over)expression and chemosensitivity to DOX, VP-16, cisplatin, melphalan, and carmustine. However, the NSCLC lines were 4- to 20-fold more chemoresistant to these drugs than the SCLC lines. A study by Kasahara et al. [41] tried to dissect the contribution of two types of resistance mechanisms to VP-16 and DOX in SCLC and NSCLC cell lines, namely, alterations in (one of) the target(s) of these drugs, topoisomerase II, and altered drug uptake, e.g., by Pgp. These authors found a statistically significant greater chemosensitivity of four SCLC cell lines to VP-16 and DOX than three NSCLC cell lines. The uptake of VP-16 was only marginally lower in the NSCLC cell lines, while the content and activity of the primary target for DOX and VP-16, namely, topoisomerase II, were twofold higher in the SCLC cell lines. Any (combination) of the following conclusions could be drawn from these studies:

1. The cell lines do not represent the clinical situation (in vitro selection of just one clonal line in each case)
2. The single most important resistance mechanism has not been identified yet
3. A number of resistance mechanisms all contribute in part to the MDR phenotype, even at apparently low levels of resistance (see also next section)
4. The tumor was not resistant because of cellular resistance (see below)
5. Some evidence for a cellular basis for the different chemosensitivity of SCLC compared to NSCLC exists, but again, this difference may be multifactorial.

To obtain more definite data about the cellular resistance mechanisms that might play a role in lung cancer, systematic studies into in vitro selected (low-level) resistant cell lines are now being pursued in a number of laboratories. These studies will be described below.

In vitro selection of MDR lung cancer cell lines

Non-P-glycoprotein-mediated MDR

A classical way to study possible causes for the resistance of cancer cells to chemotherapy is to expose in vitro growing cell lines to gradually increasing doses of a particular drug, after which stably resistant mutants usually will emerge. In this way, many MDR cell lines originating from various tumor types (including lung cancer) have been established, many of them overexpressing Pgp [42]. The first MDR cell lines established were the SCLC cell lines GLC4/ADR [43] and H69AR [44]. Remarkably, although these cell lines had an MDR phenotype that included drugs directed at different targets such as vincristine and etoposide, they did not have Pgp/*MDR1* overexpression. Later MDR cell lines were developed from NSCLC cell lines that did not overexpress Pgp/*MDR1*, namely, SW-1573/1R50, 2R50, and 2R120 [45] and COR-L23/R [46]. This form of MDR has been named non-P-glycoprotein-mediated MDR (non-Pgp MDR).

Characteristics of non-Pgp MDR

Some important characteristics of experimental MDR in lung cancer are summarized below and in table 2.
1. In lung cancer cell lines, there was a relatively frequent selection for non-Pgp MDR. It has to be noted, however, that all these selections were done with DOX.
2. Non-Pgp MDR may develop at lower drug (DOX) concentrations than Pgp MDR (e.g., SW-1573/1R50 and 2R50 selected at 50 nM DOX have non-Pgp MDR, while 1R500 and 2R160 selected at 500 and 160 nM DOX, respectively, have Pgp MDR [45]). The inverse situation, namely, Pgp-MDR followed by non-Pgp MDR at a higher selecting DOX concentration, has not been reported so far.

   Somatic cell fusion experiments have shown the non-Pgp MDR phenotype expressed in SW-1573/1R50 cells to be due to a dominant mutation [47]. Interestingly, in these cell lines the emergence of the non-Pgp MDR phenotype was accompanied by downregulation of the MDR1 gene expression.

Table 2. Multidrug resistant lung cancer cell lines

Cell line	Lung cancer type	Selecting drug	Type of MDR	P190/MRP RNA[a]	Reference
GLC4/ADR	SCLC	Doxorubicin	Non-Pgp	+	[9,43]
H69/AR	SCLC	Doxorubicin	Non-Pgp	+	[8]
H69/LX4	SCLC	Doxorubicin	Pgp	−	[92]
H69/VP	SCLC	VP-16	Pgp	?	[93]
COR-L23/R	NSCLC	Doxorubicin	Non-Pgp	+	[10,50]
MOR/0.4R	Adenocarc.	Doxorubicin	Non-Pgp	+	[51]
SW-1573/1R50 2R50, 2R120	NSCLC[b]	Doxorubicin	Non-Pgp	+?	[45,48,94]
SW-1573/1R500 2R160, 4R50	NSCLC[b]	Doxorubicin	Pgp	−	[45,48,61,94]
SW-1573/mitox	NSCLC[b]	Mitoxantrone	Pgp	?	Unpubl.
U1285-100/250	SCLC	Doxorubicin	Non-Pgp	?	[66]
U1690-40/150	SCLC	Doxorubicin	Non-Pgp	?	[66]
N592/DOX	SCLC	Doxorubicin	Non-Pgp	?	[95]

[a] See text for P190 and MRP RNA.
[b] SW-1573 is a cell line established by Dr. A. Leibovitz (see [94]) from a papillary/alveolar cell bronchial cell carcinoma, obtained at passage 10 (two populations; one was lost). The cell line could not be clearly identified as squamous or adenocarcinoma (unpublished).

3. Non-Pgp MDR mostly, if not always, accompanies reduced intracellular drug accumulation, and may be (partly) reversible by resistance modifiers, such as verapamil [48,49] or more lipophilic anthracyclines [50], which were first used to circumvent Pgp function.

4. Upon selection with DOX (even at low concentrations), non-Pgp MDR or Pgp MDR is usually accompanied by selection for cells with alterations in topoisomerase II and possibly still other mutations. This situation probably contributes to the resistance phenotype and makes the analysis of the genotype more difficult [43,45,47].

5. The accumulation defects for anthracyclines and VP-16 in non-Pgp MDR lung cancer cell lines GLC4/ADR and SW-1573/2R120 [9] and for daunorubicin in COR-L23/R [50] were shown to be dependent on cellular energy, which indicates the presence of an active drug transport process in these cells.

6. The efflux of daunorubicin and VP-16 was more rapid in GLC4/ADR cells as compared to GLC4 cells, but was energy dependent in the GLC4/ADR cells only (see figures 3 and 4B). In SW1573-2R120 cells, no such rapid efflux was measured. On the basis of this kinetic evidence, we postulated the existence of at least two mechanistically different types of non-Pgp MDR [9], the SW-1573 type and the GL4/ADR type.

7. In the GLC4/ADR type of non-Pgp MDR cell lines, a protein with an apparent M_r of 190 kDa (P190) has been found to be overexpressed, as

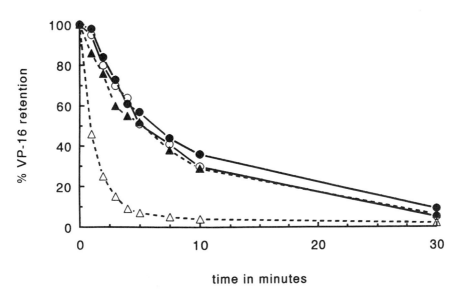

time in minutes

Figure 3. VP-16 efflux from GLC4 and GLC4/ADR SCLC cells. Cells were loaded with VP-16 (5 µM) for 60 minutes, the GLC4/ADR cells in the presence of sodium azide and deoxyglucose to deplete cellular ATP to obtain equal levels of intracellular VP-16 in GLC4 and GLC4/ADR. Then VP-16 retention in the cells was measured in GLC4 (circles) and GLC4/ADR (triangles) in energy-rich (open symbols) or energy-poor conditions (closed symbols).

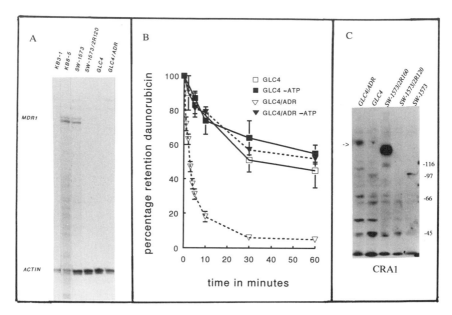

Figure 4. (A) MDR1/Pgp expression in SW-1573/2R120, GLC4, and GLC4/ADR cells is undetectable by RNAse protection assay (see [45]), but was detectable in parental SW-1573 cells. For comparison, the Pgp MDR cell line KB8-5 and its parental KB3-1 cell line are shown. (B) Daunorubicin efflux from GLC4 and GLC4/ADR cells. Cells were loaded with daunorubicin (0.5 μM) for 60 minutes, the GLC4/ADR cells in the presence of sodium azide and deoxyglucose to deplete cellular ATP to obtain equal levels of intracellular daunorubicin in GLC4 and GLC4/ADR cells. Then daunorubicin retention in the cells was measured in GLC4 (squares) and GLC4/ADR (inverted triangles) in energy-rich (open symbols) or energy-poor conditions (solid symbols). (C) Overexpression of a 190-kDa protein in GLC4/ADR cells, as detected with antiserum CRA-1 on a Western blot (courtesy of Dr. Peter Twentyman, Cambridge). CRA-1 was raised against an epitope present in Pgp (see the 170-kDa band in Pgp-expressing SW-1573/2R160 cells) as well as in the MRP protein [8].

    detected by an antibody against an epitope near the ATP binding site of Pgp [10,51,52] (figure 4C). This protein has been described earlier in a non-Pgp MDR variant of the human leukemia cell line HL-60 (HL-60/Adr) [53].

8. Preliminary data have also shown an ATP-binding protein of 190 kDa in GLC4/ADR as detected with azido-ATP photoaffinity labelling (Versantvoort et al., unpublished data).

9. Recently, a novel gene (*MRP*, or multidrug resistance associated protein) has been identified, which was overexpressed in H69AR non-Pgp MDR cells and which, based upon alignment of its nucleotide sequence, could be classified as a putative transporter gene [8]. It is, however, remarkable that this cell line has been reported not to have an enhanced drug efflux [54]. Other cell lines that have been found to overexpress the MRP gene are GLC4/ADR [55], COR-L23/R and MOR/R (P.

Twentyman, personal communication), all non-Pgp MDR lung cancer cell lines, and HL-60/ADR, a non-Pgp MDR leukemia cell line (M. Center, personal communication). In addition, these cell lines all have overexpressed P190 as well as reduced drug accumulation or enhanced drug efflux. Indeed, antibodies raised against peptide sequences of *MRP* recognized a 190-kDa protein in the H69AR [56] cells. Thus, for the GLC4/ADR type of non-Pgp MDR, it can be hypothesized that the P190 protein is coded for by the *MRP* gene and is a drug transporter molecule like Pgp. Alternatively, the *MRP* gene could be coamplified in all these cell lines with an as yet unknown transporter gene in the same amplicon [55]. The mechanism of overexpression of MRP in these human cell lines seems for the most part to occur by an increase in gene copy number [8,55], while Pgp overexpression in human cells usually takes place mainly by transcriptional activation.

10. The overexpression of a number of antigens has been described in non-Pgp MDR cell lines, for which the functional significance with respect to drug resistance is not known. A 110-kDa protein, as detected with monoclonal antibody LRP56 raised against SW-1573/2R120 cells, was found to be overexpressed in a number of non-Pgp MDR cell lines [57]. This protein is, like Pgp, also highly expressed in epithelial tissues chronically exposed to xenobiotic agents, such as the kidney tubules and bronchial cells [57]. Consistent with this expression pattern, this protein is also highly expressed in several non-in-vitro-selected renal cancer and lung cancer cell lines (Versantvoort et al., unpublished observations). Cole et al. [58] described an antibody Mab 3.186, raised against the H69/AR cell line and overexpressed in it, which was found to recognize a 36-kDa phosphorylated protein identical to lipocortin II, a calcium- and phospholipid-binding protein. The functional significance of this protein with respect to MDR is not known.

Gene-specific analysis of non-Pgp MDR

As discussed above, the usual options to analyze the occurrence of the MDR phenotype in human cancer are in vitro cell growth or cell survival inhibition assays, or gene-product-specific probes or antibodies. The analysis of *MDR1* has been discussed above. For the non-Pgp MDR phenotype, no studies have been reported so far. The first putative new transporter gene since the discovery of Pgp, namely, the Multidrug Resistance-associated Protein (*MRP*) gene, has only recently been cloned [8]. Therefore, whether or not *MRP* expression or the detection of P190 or P110 protein may have clinical application remains to be seen. Both the P110 (LRP56) protein and *MRP* mRNA are widely expressed in human tissues [55] and human cancers (e.g., MRP expression in leukemias, Broxterman et al., unpublished; or LRP56 staining, e.g., in adenocarcinomas of the gastro-intestinal tract and lung, Izquierdo et al., unpublished). So far, translation of the expression of these gene products into levels of clinical resistance does not seem straight-forward. However, it remains a possibility that these or any future probes might have more value for clinical applications in lung cancer than the detection of Pgp/*MDR1*.

Detection of drug transporter function

An entirely different way of screening for MDR is possible because it is related to energy-dependent drug transport leading to reduced steady-state cellular drug accumulation. We have developed a number of tests based on the principle that reduced drug accumulation in a cell, when caused by an active drug transport mechanism, is characterized by a lower cytoplasmic drug concentration than in a sensitive cell and therefore to a lower binding of drug to intracellular binding sites.

1. Decreased drug accumulation can be determined by measurement of the uptake of (fluorescent or radioactively labeled) drug in the cells, with and without the addition of a transport blocker. The difference will be the active transport-related drug accumulation defect, which causes (part of) the resistance. For Pgp, many transport blockers are known [59]. These compounds may or may not be active on other drug transporters. Recently we obtained some evidence that certain (iso)flavonoids such as genistein might be inhibitors of other daunorubicin transporters, but not of Pgp [60]. If viable cells can be recovered from human tumors, such tests can be done in principle to detect MDR in the clinic.
2. Another method developed by us to detect the presence of *any* active drug transport mechanism (Pgp or other) uses digitonin. Digitonin at low concentration makes the cellular plasma membrane permeable to a drug such as daunorubicin, which subsequently binds to DNA target sites if these are not yet saturated at the particular extracellular daunorubicin concentration by the action of drug transporters [65]. This method requires either equal intracellular and extracellular pH or a correction for the pH difference [65].
3. For the anthracyclines, DOX and daunorubicin, a lower binding to the nuclear DNA leads to a decrease in nuclear drug concentration. In Pgp and non-Pgp MDR cell lines, this has been shown as a relative decrease of the nuclear DOX fluorescence (or a decrease of the nuclear to cyto-plasic fluorescence ratio (N/C ratio) [61]. An example is shown in figure 5 for SW-1573 and SW-1573/2R160 Pgp-expressing cells. An advantage of this technique is the detection of a functional drug transporter on single-cell level, which can be quantified by laser scan microscopy. Therefore, a small number of viable cells would be sufficient, and heterogeneity can be studied [61].

Significantly, this method has been shown to be applicable to Pgp as well as non-Pgp MDR cell lines with a low resistance factor [49,62]. Again,

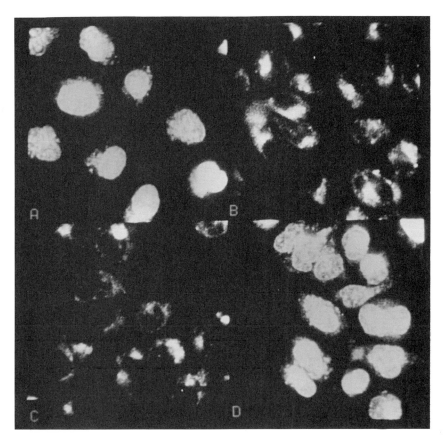

Figure 5. Intracellular doxorubicin fluorescence distribution in SW-1573 non-small cell lung cancer cells (A) and in SW-1573/2R160 Pgp-expressing cells (B). Cells were incubated in 8 μM (SW-1573) or 32 μM (SW-1573/2R160) doxorubicin for 1.5 hours. Doxorubicin fluorescence was visualized and quantified by laser scan microscopy in the nucleus and cytoplasmic compartment. It can be clearly seen that doxorubicin is mainly in the nucleus in SW-1573, but not in 2R160 cells. DOX fluorescence in 2R160 is reversed by 32 μM verapamil (D), but not 200 μM genistein (C), from the 'resistant' to the 'sensitive' pattern.

transport blockers are a powerful tool in this assay, since in the same cell population a comparison with and without addition of transport blocker might indicate the type of MDR, or even given opportunities to predict the effectiveness of clinical application of such compounds (see, e.g., figures 5C and 5D, where an effect of verapamil but not of genistein on nuclear DOX fluorescence in SW-1573/2R160 cells indicates that Pgp is involved in this effect).

This method has been applied to acute myeloid leukemias, in which a lowered nuclear DOX fluorescence appeared to correlate with pretreatment status [63]. Some progress has also been made in nuclear localization of fluorescent drug in cells prepared from solid tumors [64]. Therefore, this method may have future potential to detect the function of drug transporters in human malignancies.

Modulation of non-Pgp MDR in vitro

The modulation of MDR by administration of blockers of putative drug transporters present in lung cancer cells is an appealing approach in attempts to circumvent resistance.

In vitro experiments have shown that, in general, Pgp drug transport modulators such as verapamil and cyclosporin A also have some capacity to reverse resistance in non-Pgp-expressing cell lines, although a somewhat higher concentration seems to be needed for optimal modulatory effects [48,66].

Moreover, verapamil has been shown to increase the daunorubicin and VCR accumulation in several non-Pgp MDR cell lines [48,60].

The latter data might suggest that verapamil is able to interfere in some way with drug transporter action in these non-Pgp MDR cells. Interestingly, we recently found that the (iso)flavonoid-type compounds such as genistein decrease the enhanced daunorubicin and etoposide efflux in the non-Pgp MDR cell line GLC4/ADR, but not in a number of Pgp-MDR cell lines, indicating a preferential interaction of genistein with the transporter (MRP) present in GLC4/ADR cells as compared to its affinity for Pgp [60].

Another study suggests that a combination of cyclosporin A (another Pgp resistance modulator) and the glutathione-depleting agent buthionine sulfoximine (BSO) modified resistance in the non-Pgp MDR SCLC cells U-1690 [67] (see also table 2).

Another approach that has been suggested to circumvent Pgp-mediated MDR is the use of cytotoxic agents that either are not substrates for the drug pump or are so lipophilic that their passive transport into the cells is too rapid to be influenced to a significant extent by the limited pumping capacity. An example of the latter compounds, the lipophilic anthracyclines such as 4'-deoxy-4'-iododoxorubicin and aclarubicin, have also been shown to display very limited cross-resistance in the non-Pgp MDR large cell lung cancer cell line COR-L23/R [50] (see also table 2).

Although these data indicate that non-Pgp in principle might be modulated by following the same approach as for Pgp, it is clear that these hypotheses can be investigated in more detail only after identification of drug transporter(s) and proof of their involvement in non-Pgp MDR in lung cancer cell lines and finally in clinical resistance in lung cancer patients. Moreover, in analogy to Pgp, it can be anticipated that these transporters will have (a) role(s) in normal physiology. Future attempts to block these proteins will have to take these functions into account.

Topoisomerase II and multidrug resistance in lung cancer

In addition to Pgp- and non-Pgp-mediated MDR, other mechanisms for resistance to multiple cytostatic agents of different chemical classes have been described. Foremost among these is target-related resistance such as that caused by alterations in topoisomerase II activity, which of course is only of importance for drugs that act on topoisomerase II, such as the anthracyclines and VP-16, but not the vinca alkaloids. A decreased drug accumulation is not involved in this type of resistance.

In this section, we will not discuss topoisomerase-II-related resistance (sometimes referred to as 'atypical' MDR) in detail, but rather show some examples that may serve to illustrate that Pgp or non-Pgp MDR is frequently accompanied by topoisomerase-II-mediated resistance. For a recent review on the role of topoisomerase II (and topoisomerase I) in drug resistance, we refer to Pommier [68].

Topoisomerase II is a nuclear enzyme that regulates the topological configuration of DNA, which is essential for DNA replication, recombination, transcription, and repair, through a concerted breaking and rejoining of both DNA strands. Anthracyclines and epipodophyllotoxins stimulate DNA strand breaks by stabilizing the transient cleavable enzyme–DNA complexes. Therefore, a decrease in the topoisomerase II concentration decreases the number of potential drug targets (cleavable complexes), thus rendering cells resistant [68]. Another type of topoisomerase-II-mediated resistance may be due to alterations in topoisomerase II activity [69]. Topoisomerase II also may become less sensitive to inhibition by drugs, presumably by point mutations.

In most if not all lung cancer cell lines selected in vitro for resistance to DOX, non-Pgp MDR is accompanied by a decreased topoisomerase II gene expression and reductions of drug-induced DNA breaks, which may contribute to the reduced cytotoxic effects [47,54,70]. By somatic cell fusions of sensitive SW-1573 and low-resistance non-Pgp MDR SW-1573/1R50 cells with lowered topoisomerase II levels, Eijdems et al. [47] reported that the SW-1573 non-Pgp MDR phenotype is a dominant genetic alteration. Furthermore, they showed that the decreased topoisomerase II expression was not cotransferred to the acceptor cells. From these data, it appeared that already in the low-resistance SW-1573/1R50 cells more than one mutation occurred during the selection for resistance to low concentrations of DOX.

A correlation between topoisomerase II expression levels and drug sensitivity for DOX and VP-16 was found in lung tumor cell lines not selected for resistance in vitro. Kasahara et al. [41] found a twofold higher topoisomerase II gene expression in four SCLC as compared to three NSCLC cell lines, while the SCLC cell lines were significantly more sensitive ($\approx$10-fold) to doxorubicin and VP-16 than the NSCLC cell lines. In another study by Giaccone et al. [71] in seven lung cancer cell lines, a correlation of topoisomerase II gene expression and activity was found with sensitivity to the epipodophyllotoxins and doxorubicin. In one NSCLC cell line with neuro-endocrine properties, the topoisomerase II gene expression was very low despite a high sensitivity to drugs. Remarkably, in that study, the correlation of topoisomerase II activity was not restrained to drug sensitivity of topoiso-merase II inhibitors but included cisplatin. Such a cross-resistance spectrum is not commonly observed in drug-selected cell lines with an altered topoiso-merase II phenotype, and might indicate that several defense mechanisms against chemically induced stress are already operative concomitantly at a low level in untreated lung cancer.

Little is known about the mechanisms that could cause lowered topoiso-merase II gene expression, since the genetic changes determining the decreased expression are recessive. Therefore, it is not possible to select for such genes by gene transfer. Two studies [72,73] reported that in P388 murine leukemia-resistant cell lines, the lowered topoisomerase II expres-sion was probably due to rearrangements and hypermethylation of the topoisomerase II gene. A novel approach was followed by Roninson's group [74]. Their strategy was to select for changes in genetic elements that might suppress the function of recessive drug-resistance genes. They showed that genetic suppressor elements (GSEs) could induce topoisomerase-II-mediated resistance in HeLa cells.

From the above studies, it was suggested that topoisomerase II expression could become a useful tool in predicting the response of a patient to therapy involving topoisomerase II inhibitors. GSEs might be very useful to elucidate the mechanisms of altered topoisomerase II activities.

Clinical implications of multidrug resistance in lung cancer

Drug resistance in the clinical setting

During the last 20 years, research on drug resistance has focussed more and more on biochemical strategies of the tumor cell to survive the attack of cytotoxic drugs. Other factors, however, may make a tumor appear resistant in the clinical setting, e.g., an inadequate treatment schedule. 'Apparent' drug resistance, for instance due to poor drug absorption, poor tumor vascularization, or an unfavorable tumor pH, may be overcome by another route of administration, a higher drug dosage, a longer treatment duration, or a more suitable drug (or combination of drugs). Furthermore, intrinsic resistance may be due to a low growth fraction of the tumor or to a localiza-tion at a pharmacological sanctuary (brain, testis, etc.); also, though rarely, drug interactions may be the cause of a lack of response to chemotherapy.

The development of cellular drug resistance in tumor cell lines in most cases results from mutations, which are thought to occur with a frequency of 10^{-6}–10^{-8} per DNA base pair per cell division [75]. This rate can be increased by mutagenic agents, including many cytotoxic drugs. The occurrence of cellular drug resistance in a patients' tumor might develop in a similar way. When a tumor becomes clinically detectable, it consists of at least 10^9 cells and will contain heterogeneous subpopulations of tumor cells. The eradication of this mixture of tumor cells is usually more successfully achieved by a combination of different anticancer drugs, since monotherapy will more easily select for a resistant subpopulation.

However, even multiagent chemotherapy together with radiotherapy, which is currently considered to be the treatment modality that gives the best results in SCLC [76], does not cure SCLC. At present, only some hematological malignancies, several childhood tumors, and most testicular cancers can be cured by chemo(radio)therapy. These malignancies make up only a few percent of the total number of cancers treated with chemotherapy or radiotherapy. Therefore, new strategies are being developed, based on in vitro experiments, to overcome clinical drug resistance. One of these is the use of resistance-modifying agents (RMAs), such as verapamil [77], that have been shown to reverse Pgp-mediated multidrug resistance in vitro [59].

Resistance modifiers as a strategy to overcome MDR

Since the discovery of verapamil as an RMA, numerous compounds have been identified with MDR-reversing potential in vitro [59]. Among these are calcium channel blockers, calmodulin inhibitors, steroids and hormonal analogues, antiarrhythmic agents, cyclosporin-A and derivatives, and non-cytotoxic analogs of vinca alkaloids and anthracyclines. Reversing capacity in vivo in mice has been shown for (R-)verapamil, quinine, quinidine, cyclosporin-A, and some investigational RMAs.

Various clinical trials have been reported using RMAs in combination with MDR-related anticancer drugs. Most investigators have used verapamil in combination with doxorubicin, a vinca alkaloid, and/or etoposide. While results are promising in several hematological malignancies [78,79], few responses have been reported in solid tumors thus far. A major problem encountered with most RMAs is their prohibitive toxicity occurring at plasma concentrations that can modulate MDR in vitro. Severe cardiotoxicity was observed with verapamil at plasma levels of 2–3 μmol/l [80], the concentration needed in vitro to give effective MDR reversal. Therefore, other RMAs that have appeared to be more potent resistance modifiers with less toxicity than verapamil in animal experiments [82] are currently under investigation in clinical trials [79,81].

The only phase I/II study in SCLC using resistance-modulating agents has been performed by Figueredo et al. [83]. They studied the addition of verapamil and tamoxifen to an induction therapy of doxorubicin, vincristine, and etoposide in previously untreated patients with extensive SCLC. The most prominent toxicity encountered was febrile neutropenia in 24% of patients, which resulted in 9% toxic deaths. This percentage was higher than expected when compared with similar studies using the same anticancer drugs without RMAs. Nevertheless, these reported results compared favorably with those obtained in another study of doxorubicin, vincristine, and etoposide in extensive SCLC patients without concomitant use of RMAs [84]: 24% versus 21% response rate and a 46-week versus 24-week median survival time [83]. Although these results are encouraging, they are difficult to interpret. For instance, none of the patients had received prior chemotherapy; therefore, it was not known whether these patients were in fact resistant to the administered chemotherapy. Furthermore, Pgp expression in the tumors was not studied, while a generally low MDR1/Pgp expression in lung tumors has been reported [23], implicating a minor role for Pgp in drug resistance of lung cancer. Another matter of concern is the increasing evidence for a pharmacokinetic interaction between some RMAs and anticancer drugs, leading to an increase in the area under the curve (AUC) of the anticancer drug(s) used [85,86]. It is known that temporary drug resistance can be overcome by dose intensification of anticancer drugs. Therefore, pharmacokinetic monitoring of the anticancer drugs both before and after addition of RMAs in the same patient is warranted to exclude a response obtained by a dose-intensification effect. At present, such pharmacokinetic data have been reported in only one study [86].

The only study on resistance modulation in NSCLC was recently reported by Millward et al. [87], who used a randomized design. Both arms ($n = 68$) received chemotherapy consisting of intravenous vindesine 7 mg bolus followed by ifosfamide $5.0 \, g \, m^{-2}$ continuous infusion over 24 hours. One arm ($n = 34$) received verapamil 480 mg/day in addition for three days starting 24 hours prior to chemotherapy. Results were in favor of the chemotherapy + verapamil group; the overall response rate was 41% in this group versus 18% in the no verapamil group. Furthermore, median overall survival was 41 weeks in the verapamil arm versus 22 weeks in the no verapamil arm. Major toxicity encountered from the combination of verapamil with vindesine/ifosfamide was neurological, e.g., constipation and peripheral neuropathy. Again, the lack of information on pharmacokinetic interaction and Pgp expression in tumor tissue makes interpretation of the results difficult.

Trial design to study the relevance of MDR in lung cancer

Figure 6 shows a proposed schedule to investigate the relevance of Pgp-mediated MDR in clinical practice. The key points are as follows:
1. Assessment of Pgp expression (and activity) in the patients' tumor before entering the first part of the trial, e.g., treatment with a regimen consisting of MDR drugs solely. Subsequent treatment outcome will provide an answer to the question of whether Pgp expression may serve as a predictor of response to therapy.
2. Pharmacokinetic studies of the MDR drugs administered during the first

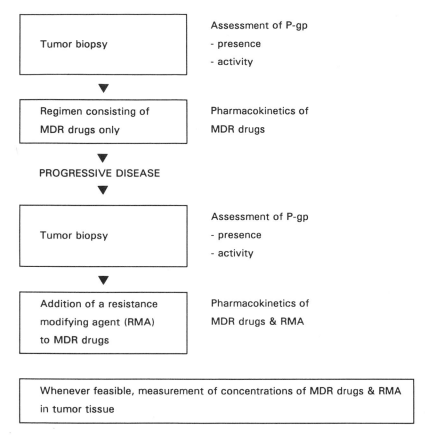

Tumor biopsy	Assessment of P-gp - presence - activity
Regimen consisting of MDR drugs only	Pharmacokinetics of MDR drugs

PROGRESSIVE DISEASE

Tumor biopsy	Assessment of P-gp - presence - activity
Addition of a resistance modifying agent (RMA) to MDR drugs	Pharmacokinetics of MDR drugs & RMA

Whenever feasible, measurement of concentrations of MDR drugs & RMA
in tumor tissue

Figure 6. Proposed trial design of MDR drugs with RMA.

part of the trial, providing the possibility to compare the AUCs of MDR drugs without a modifier with the AUCs of MDR drugs when combined with a modifier in the same patient.

3. Reassessment of Pgp expression when the patient has shown progression on the MDR regimen. An increased Pgp expression would support the hypothesis that Pgp plays a role in the development of clinical MDR.

4. Second part of the trial: Addition of an RMA to the MDR regimen. Pharmacokinetic studies of both RMA and MDR drugs. Comparison with AUCs determined before addition of the RMA.

5. In the case of pharmacokinetic interaction: Randomization in the second part of the trial. One arm continues the MDR regimen/RMA combination. The other arm receives an intensified MDR regimen without the RMA, with AUCs of the MDR drugs comparable to those obtained in the arm receiving the combination. If a dose-intensification effect is the sole cause of responses observed after addition of the modifier, then no

differences in response should be noted between the two treatment arms of this randomized design.

6. Whenever possible, assessment of adequate tumor tissue levels of both RMA and MDR drugs.

7. Monitoring of toxicities that might be related to effective blocking of the physiological functions of Pgp in several organs (figure 2).

The above proposed study design may give insight into the role of Pgp expression for the development of clinical MDR. The use of MDR drugs solely will provide a clean model of clinical MDR and thus will facilitate the evaluation of Pgp as a marker for response. Progression on an MDR drug-containing regimen is required before addition of an RMA in order to assess its resistance-modifying potential. Furthermore, information on pharmacokinetic interaction will be available with this design and an MDR modulation effect will be distinguished from a dose-intensification effect caused by addition of the modifier to therapy.

Another, perhaps more challenging approach is to give an MDR regimen in combination with an RMA in first line, since this approach might eradicate tumor cells with a low Pgp expression before repeated cycles of conventional chemotherapy may induce the outgrowth of highly resistant mutants. A proper study design in this setting would be a randomized trial with pharmacokinetics of anticancer drugs in both arms. Response rate and overall survival would be the endpoints of the study, provided that patients and AUCs of anticancer drugs in both arms are comparable.

Assessment of Pgp activity and effect of RMAs

One of the key questions in clinical trials using RMAs is whether the RMA reaches its target, e.g., the Pgp molecule present in the plasma membrane of multidrug-resistant tumor cells. Pgp supposedly causes a decreased intracellular concentration of certain anticancer drugs, and an effective RMA would increase this intracellular concentration.

One possible way to determine the effect of Pgp expression on cytostatic drug uptake in a patient's tumor is to isolate viable tumor cells and expose these in vitro to radioactively labeled or fluorescent drugs with and without an RMA. For solid tumors, this approach is still technically difficult, and improvements in purification of tumor cells from solid tumors are needed [14,64].

Measurement of the levels of an RMA in tumor tissue (biopsies) obtained after administration of the RMA could at least give some useful information about the approximate levels of the RMA reaching the target cells. Tumor tissue levels capable of modulating MDR in vitro have been measured in humans only for cyclosporin-A, quinidine, and bepridil [22].

An imaging technique would be more elegant than taking tumor biopsies in order to detect adequate target concentrations of an RMA. Moreover, a suitable imaging technique would help us to detect the presence of the MDR phenotype in a given tumor and would allow us to measure the MDR-reversing capacity of any RMA administered. Recently, promising results have been reported for a commonly used radioisotope in planar and single photon emission computed tomography, [^{99m}Tc]SESTAMIBI, which appears to be a Pgp substrate [88]. After inoculation of a Pgp-expressing xenograft and its sensitive counterpart in the flanks of a nude mouse, the radioisotope showed a reduced uptake on scintigraphic imaging in the Pgp-expressing xenograft as compared with the sensitive parent xenograft, while tumor vascularization was equal in both xenografts [88]. Information on the expected increase in [^{99m}Tc]SESTAMIBI uptake in the Pgp-expressing xenograft after systemic administration of a potent RMA to the mouse was not available. Results of pilot studies in patients are awaited.

Another, more indirect way to obtain information on effective blocking of Pgp in patients is to monitor toxicities that are expected to occur in organs that normally express Pgp, such as the liver, kidney, adrenals, CD34 positive hematopoietic stem cells, and intestine (see figure 2). However, as long as the physiological function of Pgp remains a matter of speculation, it is difficult to anticipate the kind of toxicities to be closely monitored.

Radiotherapy and MDR

There is increasing evidence that the combination of multiagent chemotherapy with radiotherapy for the treatment of advanced lung cancer is superior to chemotherapy or radiotherapy alone [76]. Critical in the design of combined chemotherapy/radiotherapy schedules is optimal timing together with the optimal drug and radiation doses to be administered [76]. Important with regard to timing is the question whether application of radiotherapy might be related to the development of chemoresistance and vice versa. A small number of studies have addressed this question and have found an increased Pgp expression in tumor cells after fractionated X-irradiation [89,90]. At least five fractions were needed before increased expression was observed. However, increased Pgp expression was not accompanied by an increase in MDR1 mRNA or gene amplification [89,90]. Moreover, resistance to vincristine, colchicine, and etoposide, but not to doxorubicin, was observed [89]. Further experiments are needed to elucidate the mechanism regulating the expression of this distinctive MDR phenotype [91]. Interestingly, X-irradiated cell lines remained sensitive to radiation [89,90]. These data suggest that radiation may play a role in the development of drug resistance but not radiation resistance of tumor cells. Additional studies are warranted to provide a biological basis for the design of rational treatment schedules combining chemotherapy- and radiotherapy.

MDR1/Pgp expression as a prognostic factor

While a relationship between MDR1/Pgp expression and poor prognosis has been demonstrated for de novo acute myeloid leukemia, neuroblastoma, sarcoma, and breast cancer [22], little is known about the prognostic significance of MDR1 expression in lung cancer.

MDR1/Pgp expression as a predictor for response to therapy

Few investigators have attempted to correlate MDR1/Pgp expression in lung cancer with response to chemotherapy. Lai et al. [23] studied MDR1 expression in 21 cell lines using RNA slot blot analysis and compared the results with response to chemotherapy (usually etoposide and cisplatin) of the corresponding patients. No significant difference in increased MDR1 expression was found between responders (2/12) and nonresponders (2/9). This result is in contrast with those reported by Holzmayer et al. [25], who determined MDR1 expression in SCLC tumor biopsies with a sensitive assay based on the polymerase chain reaction (PCR). They found a significant difference in subsequent response to chemotherapy (containing at least one MDR drug): responses were observed in 3 of 3 MDR1-negative cases, while none of the four MDR1-positive cases responded to chemotherapy. Studies including larger numbers of patients are awaited in order to give a more definite answer to the question of whether Pgp expression may serve as a predictor of therapy outcome.

Conclusions

Given the data currently available, the role of Pgp-mediated MDR in drug resistance of lung cancer remains speculative. This might be one of the reasons that only a few investigators have conducted a clinical trial combining MDR drugs with an RMA in lung cancer. The study design of these trials made interpretation of the results difficult. Therefore, if we want to know the clinical relevance of Pgp-mediated MDR in lung cancer, a trial design as described (vide supra) is warranted. If the interest is mainly to assess the therapeutic advantage of the addition of an RMA to therapy, regardless of the underlying mechanism(s), a randomized trial in first line with an RMA with proper pharmacokinetic studies might be a challenging alternative.

General conclusions

The study of the chemotherapeutic resistance of lung cancer has not identified one single, specific mechanism as a major cause for the multiple drug resistance (MDR) in the clinic. In vitro, several mechanisms, including overexpression of cytostatic drug transporters (MDR1, MRP) and alterations in topoisomerase II activity, have been identified as determinants for MDR. Typically, in the GLC4/ADR SCLC cell line, the resistance to DOX and VP-16 is caused by a rapid energy-dependent efflux of these drugs, as well as alterations in levels of their target enzyme topoisomerase II.

Since it is readily conceivable that tumors in the lung, like those in the digestive tract, might originate from cells chronically exposed to environmental carcinogens, it is a reasonable hypothesis that inherent MDR in human lung cancer represents general mechanisms to protect the organism against naturally occurring toxins [31]. Therefore, it is the hope that the further unraveling of those mechanisms that prevail in conferring MDR to lung tumor cells will lead to possibilities of interfering with them by pharmacological means and thereby will improve chemotherapeutic treatment.

References

1. Minna JD, Pass H, Glatstein E, Ihde DC. 1989. Cancer of the lung. In Cancer Principles and Practice of Oncology, vol. 1, VT DeVita, S Hellman, and SA Rosenberg (eds.). J.B. Lippincott: Philadelphia, pp. 591–705.
2. Blechen NM. 1990. Lung cancer — still a long road ahead. Br J Cancer 61:493–494.
3. Kristjansen PEG, Hansen HH. 1990. Management of small cell lung cancer: a summary of the Third International Association for the Study of Lung Cancer Workshop on small cell lung cancer. J Natl Cancer Inst 82:263–266.
4. Goldie JH, Coldman AJ. 1985. Genetic instability in the development of drug resistance. Semin Oncol 12:222–230
5. Juranka PF, Zastawny RL, Ling V. 1989. P-glycoprotein: multidrug-resistance and a superfamily of membrane-associated transport proteins. FASEB J 3:2583–2592.
6. Choi K, Frommel TO, Kaplan Stern R, Perez CF, Kriegler M, Tsuruo T, Roninson IR. 1991. Multidrug resistance after retroviral transfer of the human MDR1 gene correlates with P-glycoprotein density in the plasma membrane and is not affected by cytotoxic selection. Proc Natl Acad Sci USA 88:7386–7390.
7. Mickisch GH, Pastan I, Gottesman MM. 1991. Multidrug resistant transgenic mice as a novel pharmacologic tool. BioEssays 13:381–387.
8. Cole SPC, Bhardwaj G, Gerlach JH, et al. 1992. Overexpression of a transporter gene in a multidrug-resistant human lung cancer line. Science 258:1650–1654.
9. Versantvoort CHM, Broxterman HJ, Pinedo HM, De Vries EGE, Feller N, Kuiper CM, Lankelma J. 1992. Energy-dependent processes involved in reduced drug accumulation in multidrug-resistant human lung cancer cell lines without P-glycoprotein expression. Cancer Res 52:17–23.
10. Barrand MA, Rhodes T, Center MS, Twentyman PR. 1993. Chemosensitisation and drug accumulation of cyclosporin A, PSC 833 and verapamil in human MDR large cell lung cancer cells expressing a 190 kD membrane protein distinct from P-glycoprotein. Eur J Cancer 29A:408–415.
11. Beck WT. 1990. Multidrug resistance and its circumvention. Eur J Cancer 26:513–515.
12. Dalton WS. 1993. Drug resistance modulation in the laboratory and the clinic. Semin Oncol 20:64–69.
13. Kaye SB. 1993. P-glycoprotein (P-gp) and drug resistance — time for reappraisal? Br J Cancer 67:641–643.
14. Dietel M, Bals U, Schaefer B, Herzig I, Arps H, Zabel M. 1993. In vitro prediction of cytostatic drug resistance in primary cell cultures of solid malignant tumours. Eur J Cancer 29A:416–420.
15. Miller TP, Young LA, Perrot L, Salmon SE. 1984. Feasibility of a prospective randomized

correlative trial of advanced non-small cell lung cancer using the human tumor clonogenic assay. In Human Tumor Cloning, SE Salmon and JM Trent (eds.). Grune and Stratton: Orlando, FL, pp. 535–542.

16. Weisenthal LM. 1992. Antineoplastic drug screening belongs in the laboratory, not in the clinic. J Natl Cancer Inst 84:466–469.

17. Wilbur DW, Camacho ES, Hilliard DA, Dill PL, Weisenthal LM. 1992. Chemotherapy of non-small cell lung carcinoma guided by an in vitro drug resistance assay measuring total tumour cell kill. Br J Cancer 65:27–32.

18. Gazdar AF, Steinberg SM, Russell EK, et al. 1990. Correlation of in vitro drug-sensitivity testing with respons to chemotherapy and survival in extensive-stage small cell lung cancer: a prospective clinical trial. J Natl Cancer Inst 82:117–124.

19. De Vries EGE, Meijer C, Mulder NH, Postmus PE. 1987. In vitro chemosensitivity of human lung cancer for vindesine. Eur J Cancer Clin Oncol 23:55–60.

20. Campling BG, Pym J, Baker HM, Cole SC, Lam Y-M. 1991. Chemosensitivity testing of small cell lung cancer using the MTT assay. Br J Cancer 63:75–83.

21. Volm M, Drings P, Hahn EW, Mattern J. 1988. Prediction of the clinical chemotherapeutic response of stage III lung adenocarcinoma patients by an in vitro short-term test. Br J Cancer 57:198–200.

22. Linn SC, Giaccone G, Van Kalken CK, Pinedo HM. 1992. P-glycoprotein mediated multidrug resistance and its clinical relevance in cancer treatment. FORUM Trends Exp Clin Med 2:642–657.

23. Lai S-L, Goldstein LJ, Gottesman MM, et al. 1989. MDR1 gene expression in lung cancer. J Natl Cancer Inst 81:1144–1150.

24. Shin HJC, Lee JS, Hong WK, Shin DM. 1992. Study of multidrug resistance (MDR1) gene in non-small-cell lung cancer. Anticancer Res 12:367–370.

25. Holzmayer TA, Hilsenbeck S, Von Hoff DD, Roninson IB. 1992. Clinical correlates of MDR1 (P-glycoprotein) gene expression in ovarian and small-cell lung carcinomas. J Natl Cancer Inst 84:1486–1491.

26. Schlaifer D, Laurent G, Chittal S, et al. 1990. Immunohistochemical detection of multidrug resistance associated P-glycoprotein in tumour and stromal cells of human cancers. Br J Cancer 62:177–182.

27. Finstad CL, Yin BWT, Gordon CM, Federici MG, Welt S, Lloyd KO. 1991. Some monoclonal antibody reagents (C219 and JSB-1) to P-glycoprotein contain antibodies to blood group A carbohydrate determinants: a problem of quality control for immunohistochemical analysis. J Histochem Cytochem 39:1603–1610.

28. Van der Valk P, Van Kalken CK, Ketelaars H, et al. 1990. Distribution of multidrug-resistance associated P-glycoprotein in normal and neoplastic human tissues. Ann Oncol 1:56–64.

29. Brambilla E, Moro D, Gazzeri S, et al. 1991. Cytotoxic chemotherapy induces cell differentiation in small-cell lung carcinoma. J Clin Oncol 9:50–61.

30. Radosevich JA, Robinson PG, Rittman-Grauer LS, et al. 1989. Immunohistochemical analysis of pulmonary and pleural tumors with the monoclonal antibody HYB-612 directed against the multidrug resistance (MDR1) gene product, P-glycoprotein. Tumor Biol 10: 252–257.

31. Volm M, Bak M, Mattern J. 1988. Intrinsic drug resistance in a human lung carcinoma xenograft is associated with overexpression of multidrug-resistance DNA-sequences and of plasma membrane glycoproteins. Arzneim Forsch Drug Res 38(II):1189–1193.

32. Noonan KE, Beck C, Holzmayer TA, et al. 1990. Quantitative analysis of MDR1 (multidrug resistance) gene expression in human tumors by polymerase chain reaction. Proc Natl Acad Sci USA 87:7160–7164.

33. Smit EF, De Vries EGE, Timmer-Bosscha H, et al. 1992. In vitro response of human small-cell lung cancer cell lines to chemotherapeutic drugs; no correlation with clinical data. Int J Cancer 51:72–78.

34. Masuda N, Fukuoka M, Matsui K, et al. 1991. Establishment of tumor cell lines as an

218

independent prognostic factor for survival time in patients with small-cell lung cancer. J Natl Cancer Inst 83:1743–1748.

35. Carmichael J, Mitchell JB, DeGraff WG, et al. 1985. Chemosensitivity testing of human lung cancer cell lines using the MTT assay. Br J Cancer 57:540–547.

36. Carney DM, Mitchell JB, Kinsella TJ. 1983. In vitro radiation and chemosensitivity of established cell lines of human small cell lung cancer and its large cell morphological variants. Cancer Res 43:2806–2811.

37. Berendsen HH, De Leij L, De Vries EGE, et al. 1988. Characterization of three small cell lung cancer cell lines established from one patient during longitudinal follow-up. Cancer Res 48:6891–6899.

38. De Vries EGE, Meijer C, Timmer-Bosscha H, Berendsen HH, De Leij L, Scheper RJ, Mulder NH. 1989. Resistance mechanisms in three human small cell lung cancer cell lines established from one patient during clinical follow-up. Cancer Res 49:4175–4178.

39. Hida T, Ueda R, Takahashi T, et al. 1989. Chemosensitivity and radiosenstivity of small cell lung cancer cell lines studied by a newly developed 3-(4,5-dimethylthiazol-2-yl)-2,5-diphenyltetrazolium bromide (MTT) hybrid assay. Cancer Res 49:4785–4790.

40. Milroy R, Plumb JA, Batstone P, et al. 1992. Lack of expression of P-glycoprotein in 7 small cell lung cancer cell lines established both from untreated and from treated patients. Anticancer Res 12:193–200.

41. Kasahara K, Yasuhiro F, Sugimoto Y, et al. 1992. Determinants of response to the DNA topoisomerase II inhibitors doxorubicin and etoposide in human lung cancer cell lines. J Natl Cancer Inst 84:113–118.

42. Nielsen D, Skovsgaard T. 1992. P-glycoprotein as multidrug transporter: a critical review of current multidrug resistant cell lines. Biochim Biophys Acta 1139:169–183.

43. Zijlstra JG, De Vries EGE, Mulder NH. 1987. Multifactorial drug resistance in an adriamycin-resistant human small cell lung cancer cell line. Cancer Res 47:1780–1784.

44. Mirski SEL, Gerlach JH, Cole SPC. 1987. Multidrug resistance in a human small cell lung cancer cell line selected in adriamycin. Cancer Res 47:2594–2598.

45. Baas F, Jongsma APM, Broxterman HJ, et al. 1990. Non-P-glycoprotein mediated mechanism for multidrug resistance precedes P-glycoprotein expression during in vitro selection for doxorubicin resistance in a human lung cancer cell line. Cancer Res 50:5392–5398.

46. Reeve JG, Rabbitts PH, Twentyman PR. 1990. Non-P-glycoprotein mediated multidrug resistance with reduced EGF receptor expresssion in a human large cell lung cancer cell line. Br J Cancer 61:851–855.

47. Eijdems EWHM, Borst P, Jongsma APM, et al. 1992. Genetic transfer of non-P-glyco-protein-mediated multidrug resistance (MDR) in somatic cell fusion: Dissection of a compound MDR phenotype. Proc Natl Acad Sci USA 89:3498–3502.

48. Kuiper CM, Broxterman HJ, Baas F, et al. 1990. Drug transport variants without P-glycoprotein overexpression from a human squamous lung cancer cell line after selection with doxorubicin. J Cell Pharmacol 1:35–41.

49. Broxterman HJ, Schuurhuis GJ, Lankelma J, Baak JPA, Pinedo HM. 1990. Towards functional screening for multidrug resistant cells in human malignancies. In Drug Resistance: Mechanisms and Reversal, E. Mihich (ed.). John Libbey CIC: Rome, pp. 309–319.

50. Coley HM, Workman P, Twentyman PR. 1991. Retention of activity by selected anthra-cyclines in a multidrug resistant human large cell lung carcinoma cell line without P-glycoprotein hyperexpression. Br J Cancer 63:351–357.

51. Barrand MA, Broxterman HJ, Wright KA, Rhodes T, Twentyman PR. 1992. Immuno-detection of a 190 kD protein in atypical MDR cells derived from small cell and non-small cell lung tumours. Br J Cancer 65(Suppl XVI):21.

52. Versantvoort CHM, Twentyman PR, Barrand MA, Lankelma J, Pinedo HM, Broxterman HJ. 1992. Overexpression of 110 kD and 190 kD proteins in cancer cells may be involved in drug resistant phenotype. Proc Am Assoc Cancer Res 33:456.

53. Marquardt D, McCrone S, Center MS. 1990. Mechanism of multidrug resistance in HL60 cells: detection of resistance-associated proteins with antibodies against synthetic peptides

that correspond to the deduced sequence of P-glycoprotein. Cancer Res 50:1426–1430.

54. Cole SPC. 1992. The 1991 Merck Frost Award. Multidrug resistance in small cell lung cancer. Can J Physiol Pharmacol 70:313–329.

55. Zaman GJR, Versantvoort CHM, Smit JJM, et al. 1993. Analysis of the expression of MRP, the gene for a new putative transmembrane drug transporter, in human multidrug resistant lung cancer cell lines. Cancer Res 53:1747–1750.

56. Cole SPC. 1993. A novel ATP-binding cassette transporter gene overexpressed in multidrug-resistant human lung tumour cells. Proc Am Assoc Cancer Res 34:579.

57. Scheper RJ, Broxterman HJ, Scheffer GL, et al. 1993. Overexpression of a M_r 110,000 vesicular protein in non-P-glycoprotein -mediated multidrug resistance. Cancer Res 53: 1475–1479.

58. Cole SPC, Pinkoski MJ, Bhardwaj G, Deeley RG. 1992. Elevated expression of annexin (Lipocortin II, p36) in a multidrug resistant small cell lung cancer cell line. Br J Cancer 65:498–502.

59. Ford JM, Hait WN. 1990. Pharmacology of drugs that alter multidrug resistance in cancer. Pharmacol Rev 42:155–199.

60. Versantvoort CHM, Schuurhuis GJ, Pinedo HM, Eekman CA, Kuiper CM, Lankelma JA, Broxterman HJ. 1993. Genistein modulates the decreased drug accumulation in non-P-glycoprotein mediated multidrug resistant tumour cells. Br J Cancer 68:939–946.

61. Schuurhuis GJ, Broxterman HJ, Cervantes A, Van Heijningen THM, De Lange JHM, Baak JPA, Pinedo HM, Lankelma J. 1989. Quantitative determination of factors contributing to doxorubicin resistance in multidrug-resistant cells. J Natl Cancer Inst 81:1887–1892.

62. Schuurhuis GJ, Broxterman HJ, De Lange JHM, et al. 1991. Early multidrug resistance, defined by changes in intracellular doxorubicin distribution, independent of P-glycoprotein. Br J Cancer 64:857–861.

63. Schuurhuis GJ, Broxterman HJ, Pinedo HM, et al. 1992. Multidrug resistance phenotype in acute myeloid leukemia, characterized by altered subcellular drug distribution and decreased drug accumulation, independent of P-glycoprotein. Proc Am Assoc Cancer Res 33:454.

64. Seidel A, Pest S, Kaufmann O, Dietel M. 1993. Intracellular distribution of cytostatic drugs in low degree resistant tumor cell lines and primary tumor cell preparations. Proc Am Assoc Cancer Res 34:25.

65. Versantvoort CHM, Broxterman HJ, Feller N, Dekker H, Kuiper CM, Lankelma J. 1992. Probing daunorubicin accumulation defects in non-P-glycoprotein expressing multidrug-resistant cell lines using digitonin. Int J Cancer 50:906–911.

66. Nygren P, Larsson R, Gruber A, Peterson C, Bergh J. 1991. Doxorubicin selected multidrug-resistant small cell lung cancer cell lines characterised by elevated cytoplasmic Ca^{2+} and resistance modulation by verapamil in absence of P-glycoprotein overexpression. Br J Cancer 64:1011–1018.

67. Larsson R, Bergh J, Nygren P. 1991. Combination of cyclosporin A and buthionine sulfoximine (BSO) as a pharmacological strategy for circumvention of multidrug resistance in small cell lung cancer cell lines selected for resistance to doxorubicin. Anticancer Res 11:455–460.

68. Pommier Y. 1993. DNA topoisomerase I and II in cancer chemotherapy: update and perspectives. Cancer Chemother Pharmacol 32:103–108.

69. Danks MK, Schmidt CA, Cirtain MC, Suttle DP, Beck WT. 1988. Altered catalytic activity of DNA cleavage by DNA topoisomerase II from human leukemic cells selected for resistance to VM-26. Biochemistry 27:8861–8869.

70. De Jong S, Kooistra AJ, De Vries EGE, Mulder NH, Zijlstra JG. 1993. Topoisomerase II as a target of VM-26 and 4'-(9-acridinylamino)methanesulfon-m-aniside in atypical multidrug resistant human small cell lung carcinoma cells. Cancer Res 53:1064–1071.

71. Giaccone G, Gazdar AF, Beck H, Zunino F, Capranico G. 1992. Multidrug sensitivity

220

phenotype of lung cancer cells associated with topoisomerase II expression. Cancer Res 52:1666–1674.

72. Tan KB, Mattern MR, Eng W-K, McCabe FL, Johnson RK. 1989. Nonreproductive rearrangement of DNA topoisomerase I and II genes: correlation with resistance to topoisomerase inhibitors. J Natl Cancer Inst 81:1732–1735.

73. Deffie AM, Bosman DJ, Goldenberg GJ. 1989. Evidence for a mutant allele of the gene for DNA topoisomerase II in adriamycin-resistant P388 murine leukemia cells. Cancer Res 49:6879–6882.

74. Gudkov AV, Zelnick CR, Kazarov AR, Thimmapaya R, Suttle DP, Beck WT, Roninson IB. 1993. Isolation of genetic suppressor elements, inducing resistance to topoisomerase II — interactive cytotoxic drugs, from human topoisomerase-II cDNA. Proc Natl Acad Sci USA 90:3231–3235.

75. Borst P. 1991. Genetic mechanisms of drug resistance. Reviews in Oncology. Acta Oncologica 30:87–105.

76. Haraf DJ, Devine S, Ihde DC, Vokes EE. 1992. The evolving role of systemic therapy in carcinoma of the lung. Semin Oncol 19(S11):72–87.

77. Tsuruo T, Iida H, Tsukagoshi S, et al. 1981. Overcoming of vincristine resistance in P388 leukemia in vivo and in vitro through enhanced cytotoxicity of vincristine and vinblastine by verapamil. Cancer Res 41:1967–1972.

78. Miller TP, Grogan TM, Dalton WS, et al. 1991. P-glycoprotein expression in malignant lymphoma and reversal of clinical drug resistance with chemotherapy plus high dose verapamil. J Clin Oncol 9:17–24.

79. Sonneveld P, Durie BGM, Lokhorst HM, et al. 1992. Modulation of multidrug-resistant multiple myeloma by cyclosporin. Lancet 340:255–259.

80. Pennock GD, Dalton WS, Roeske WR, et al. 1991. Systemic toxic effects associated with high-dose verapamil infusion and chemotherapy administration. J Natl Cancer Inst 83:105–110.

81. Yahanda AM, Adler KM, Fisher GA, et al. 1992. Phase I trial of etoposide with cyclosporine as a modulator of multidrug resistance. J Clin Oncol 10:1624–1634.

82. Boesch D, Gavériaux C, Jachez B, et al. 1991. In vivo circumvention of P-glycoprotein-mediated multidrug resistance of tumor cells with SDZ PSC 833. Cancer Res 51:4226–4233.

83. Figueredo A, Arnold A, Goodyear M, Findlay B, Neville A, Normandeau R, Jones RN. 1990. Addition of verapamil and tamoxifen to the initial chemotherapy of small cell lung cancer. A phase I/II study. Cancer 65:1895–1902.

84. Abratt RP, Wilcox PA, Hewitson RH. 1987. Etoposide combination therapy for small cell carcinoma of the lung. Cancer Chemother Pharmacol 20:83–84.

85. Kerr DJ, Graham J, Cummings J, Morrison JG, Thompson GG, Brodie MJ, Kaye SB. 1986. The effect of verapamil on the pharmacokinetics of adriamycin. Cancer Chemother Pharmacol 18:239–242.

86. Lum BL, Kaubisch S, Yahanda AM, et al. 1992. Alteration of etoposide pharmacokinetics and pharmacodynamics by cyclosporine in a phase I trial to modulate multidrug resistance. J Clin Oncol 10:1635–1642.

87. Millward MJ, Cantwell BMJ, Munro NC, Robinson A, Corris PA, Harris AL. 1993. Oral verapamil with chemotherapy for advanced non-small cell lung cancer: a randomised study. Br J Cancer 67:1031–1035.

88. Piwnica-Worms D, Chiu ML, Budding M, Kronauge JF, Kramer RA, Croop JM. 1993. Functional imaging of multidrug-resistant P-glycoprotein with an organotechnetium complex. Cancer Res 53:977–984.

89. Hill BT, Deuchars K, Hosking LK, Ling V, Whelan RDH. 1990. Overexpression of P-glycoprotein in mammalian tumor cell lines after fractionated X irradiation in vitro. J Natl Cancer Inst 82:607–612.

90. Mattern J, Efferth T, Volm M. 1991. Overexpression of P-glycoprotein in human lung

carcinoma xenografts after fractionated irradiation in vivo. Radiat Res 127:335–338.

91. McClean S, Hosking LK, Hill BT. 1993. Dominant expression of multiple drug resistance after in vitro X-irradiation exposure in intraspecific Chinese hamster ovary hybrid cells. J Natl Cancer Inst 85:48–53.

92. Reeve JG, Rabbits PH, Twentyman PR. 1989. Amplification and expression of mdrl gene in a multidrug resistant variant of small cell lung cancer cell line NCI-H69. Br J Cancer 60:339–342.

93. Minato K, Kanzawa F, Nishio K, Nakagawa K, Fujiwara Y, Saijo N. 1990. Characterization of an etoposide-resistant human small-cell lung cancer line. Cancer Chemother Pharmacol 26:313–317.

94. Keizer HG, Schuurhuis GJ, Broxterman HJ, et al. 1989. Correlation of multidrug resistance with decreased drug accumulation, altered subcellular drug distribution, and increased P-glycoprotein expression in cultured SW-1573 human lung tumor cells. Cancer Res 49:2988–2993.

95. Supino R, Binaschi M, Capranico G, Gambetta RA, Prosperi E, Sala E, Zupino F. 1993. A study of cross-resistance pattern and expression of molecular markers of multidrug resistance in a human small-cell lung-cancer cell line selected with doxorubicin. Int J Cancer 54:309–314.

11. New techniques in the diagnosis and staging of lung cancer

David Kaplan and Peter Goldstraw

Introduction

In the treatment of a patient with lung cancer, the clinician must establish diagnosis and stage efficiently (without causing needless delay), practically (without performing unnecessary invasive procedures), and pragmatically (without incurring extra cost). The end result should not rest on inferences of interpretation, but must be established beyond doubt on the basis of pathological material. There is a close relationship between pathological TNM stage and patient prognosis. Dramatic improvements in modern imaging techniques have not resulted in equally impressive improvement in the accuracy of appraising clinical stage. Using present technologies, determination of stage is still based on balancing probabilities, and is very much dependent on the quality of the interpretation. An open diagnostic procedure remains the standard against which all other modalities must be compared.

Herein lies the dilemma: the surgeon must reconcile the conflict between two mutually exclusive imperatives. On the one hand, patients should only be exposed to the hazards and discomfort of surgery when the procedure is curative. On the other, all patients with potentially curative lesions should be offered the benefits of surgery.

Diagnosis

No new technology is ever likely to replace the diagnostic power of a complete history and physical examination. Most lung cancers are symptomatic and in an advanced stage at the time of presentation. Symptoms are usually respiratory and/or constitutional. Patients often have symptoms due to years of smoking; a change in the pattern of respiratory symptoms can be just as important as symptoms arising de novo. Hemoptysis occurs in less than 20% of sufferers, but since it frequently brings the patient to medical attention, it carries a disproportionate power of emphasis. Thorough systematic enquiry is obligatory to screen for symptoms of underlying occult metastatic disease. There are no physical signs specific to lung cancer, nor is

Heine H. Hansen, (ed), Hansen: Lung Cancer.

there a constellation of signs that constitute a syndrome. These facts do not obviate the need for a complete physical examination. On the contrary, a vigorous search for evidence of possible extrapulmonary disease is mandatory.

A persistently abnormal chest radiograph (four weeks) requires accurate diagnosis. Only a firm diagnosis based on the pathological examination of clinical material is acceptable. Imaging may help to direct the sequence or conduct of invasive investigation, but tissue is ultimately required to make a firm diagnosis.

There are six ways to obtain material for histological examination. Sputum collection is easily the least invasive, and if positive can save a patient with advanced disease the necessity of hospitalization and the discomfort of further investigation. A diagnostic bronchoscopy, usually under local anesthesia, is performed when sputum is either nondiagnostic or unobtainable. Central tumors are biopsied. Washings and brushings are obtained from appropriate segmental or subsegmental bronchi when the lesion is peripheral. Transbronchial biopsy of enlarged (subcarinal) lymph nodes is now a standard technique [1]. Percutaneous transthoracic biopsy is widely available. It is performed at different centers with markedly different levels of enthusiasm. False negatives are not uncommon, although a positive result after an initial negative has been reported with an incidence of 45% [2,3]. The difficulties in making a specific benign diagnosis make the procedure less attractive. If the patient will proceed to thoracotomy regardless of the result, there is little point in delaying formal exploration.

Tissue from mediastinal lymph nodes and from the primary tumor can be obtained at mediastinoscopy, particularly for central left upper lobe tumors. Thoracoscopy has been an important maneuver in the staging of lung cancers, particularly those associated with pleural effusions. As instrumentation improves, one expects thoracoscopy to make an increasingly important contribution to the diagnosis and staging of lung cancer, especially in those areas of the chest not accessible to mediastinoscopy.

The final arbiter is, of course, thoracotomy. It can be appropriate to proceed to thoracotomy without prior histological diagnosis, provided that frozen section facilities for immediate histological diagnosis are available. It is hugely speculative to perform pneumonectomy without the benefit of confirmation of the diagnosis.

Screening as it applies to early diagnosis

What role does screening have in the diagnosis and treatment of lung cancer? There is little doubt that resected stage I lung cancers have a very favorable prognosis. When early-stage disease is detected and treated as part of a screening program, improved survival must be shown not to be due to lag-time phenomena or errors due to length-biased sampling. Screening

STAGE 1 DISEASE

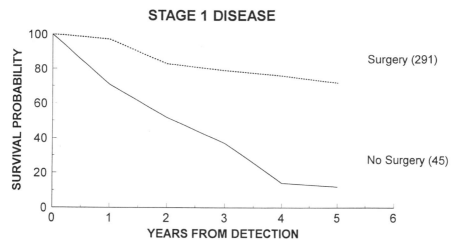

Figure 1. Kaplan–Meier estimates of survival from stage 1 (T1–T2, N0, M0) lung cancer. Deaths are due to lung cancer. Deaths from other causes are withdrawn.

by mass chest radiography in the general population has been shown to be of little value [4,5], and repeated studies in at-risk smoking populations have been equally disappointing [6,7].

To accept that mass chest radiography is not an effective screen does not mean that early diagnosis and treatment have no influence on the natural history of the disease. A joint study between the Mayo Clinic, Johns Hopkins, and Sloan-Kettering has compared surgical versus nonsurgical treatment in patients with clinical stage I lung cancer [8]. Patients were included in the nonsurgical group if they refused surgical intervention or had a noncancer-related contraindication to surgery. Deaths from causes other than lung cancer were withdrawn from the analysis. A clear survival advantage was gained by patients who underwent surgical excision (figure 1). This study reemphasizes that renewed efforts must be made to improve the yield of screening programs for lung cancer.

There is new evidence that screening might be more productive in identifying populations at increased risk by using biochemical and genetic markers of predisposition. Recent studies have identified genetic abnormalities including mutations [9–13], amplifications [14–16], deletions [17,18], and overexpression of proto-oncogenes [19–21]. These genetic lesions may be helpful as markers for at-risk populations and may serve in developing strategies to screen for lung cancer (table 1). A fuller comprehension of the genetic events occurring in patients with lung cancer is still outstanding. The chronological sequence of these events is yet to be determined. The presence of abnormal genes expressed in exfoliated cells in sputum samples, coupled with new techniques for identifying these abnormalities in ever decreasing samples of tissue, offer new possibilities for effective screening programs.

225

Table 1. Known genetic mutations in lung cancer

Oncogenes	Mechanism	Histology
Dominant		
ras (H-ras, K-ras, N-ras)	Point mutation	NSCLC
myc (c-myc, L-myc, N-myc)	Gene amplification	SCLC
erb B family	Gene amplification	NSCLC
Recessive		
Retinoblastoma	Delection	NS & SCLC
p53 gene	Point mutation	NS & SCLC
3p gene	Deleted	SCLC
Other genes		
raf genes	Expressed	NS & SCLC
jun family	Expressed	NS & SCLC
src family	Expressed	NS & SCLC
retinoic acid receptor gene	Deleted?	SCLC
phosphatases	Deleted?	SCLC

Plain chest radiograph

In an attempt to overcome the recognized inadequacies of the standard chest x-ray, several new approaches to routine chest radiography have been developed and are currently being evaluated. Scanning equalization radiography is a generic term for a family of new techniques improving the quality of image by using a smaller source beam with a detector behind the patient that modulates the x-ray tube output. At present, the only system that utilizes this technique and is commercially available is the Advanced Multiple Beam Equalization Radiography system (AMBER).

The technique relies on multiple beams, each with its own modulator in front of the x-ray tube in a feedback loop with a corresponding detector. When the image is obtained, the detector output signal is used to adjust the corresponding modulator to deliver the proper exposure to the part of the film covered by the detector (figure 2). This technique augments the dynamic range of the standard PA projection [22]. Demonstration of both mediastinal detail and pulmonary abnormalities is greatly enhanced (figure 3). Controlled studies have demonstrated that simulated nodules projected over the mediastinum and diaphragm were more readily seen using the AMBER technique [23,24].

Another approach, which is likely to have far-reaching effects, is Phosphor Plate Computed Radiography (PPCR, or digital radiography). This technology is ultimately expected to replace conventional film radiography. A phosphor plate is handled in a conventional cassette (which does not contain film) and is exposed in the normal fashion. The energy of the incident x-ray beam is stored on the plate as a latent image. The plate is, in turn, scanned with a laser beam, and the light emitted from the excited latent image is

AMBER ARCHITECTURE

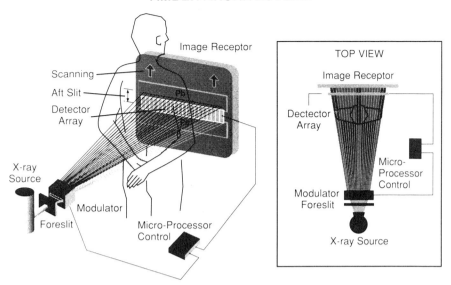

Figure 2. Advanced Multiple Beam Equalization Radiography (AMBER). The detector behind the patient modulates x-ray tube output.

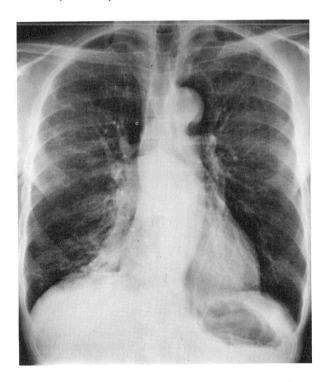

Figure 3. An AMBER radiograph. The contours of medistinal structures are outstanding. There is collapse of the right lower lobe. There is also a subcarinal lymph node mass. Note the obliteration of the azygo-esophageal line.

detected by a photomultiplier. Thereafter the signal is processed in digital form. The digital image may be viewed either on a television monitor or laser printed onto film.

PPCR holds a number of real advantages over conventional radiographic techniques. It has a wider dynamic range. Because the image can be manipulated and enhanced at the display station, patients on average receive a lower dose of radiation. The necessity of repeated examinations for technical reasons is reduced. The images can be stored on optical disks and/or laser printed onto film. Finally, the digital record can be transmitted by telephone to remote sites. It must be accepted that present technology limits the spatial resolution to that of present-day video display units. If hard copy is to be abandoned, secure and rapidly accessible computer archives will be mandatory. Clinical information cannot be subject to the whims of computer glitches, power surges, or computer vandalism. Digital storage and display currently does not compare favorably with a packet of films. It is expensive, retrieval is slow, and simultaneous comparison of multiple images is awkward.

Solitary pulmonary nodule (SPN)

Definition: SPN is a single pulmonary opacity, surrounded by normal lung, not associated with hilar enlargement or atelectasis. Size criteria vary from 1–4 cm in diameter.

The incidence of SPN is variable. In areas where granulomatous disease is endemic, the incidence of SPN can be as high as 0.2% of the adult population [25]. Risk factors for malignancy include age, history of smoking, size, and prior malignancy. A best-management strategy has been derived based on probability of malignancy [26].

Historical films, if existent, are essential for comparison. Tumor doubling times have been ascertained to lie within a range of 21 to 400 days [27]. A lesion that has doubled in size within a month or is unchanged over a two-year period is unlikely to be malignant.

Trans-Thoracic Needle Biopsy (TTNB) is clearly indicated in undiagnosed patients who are unsuitable for or unwilling to undergo surgical excision and in those who require a preoperative diagnosis. The procedure is not without attendant morbidity; pneumothorax occurs in 15% [28] and the incidence of false negatives is high [2,3].

The choice of continued observation of an indeterminate nodule or its excision is a matter of individual preference and never a comfortable decision. The patient may have strong feelings on the subject and should be invited to contribute to the discussion.

228

CT scanning

Computerized tomography of the thorax is a powerful imaging tool and is now widely accessible. It has been rapidly accepted because it overcomes many of the limitations of two-dimensional projection and produces images with a 10-fold improvement in resolution compared to standard tomography. Few patients with lung cancer experience the diagnostic or staging process without the benefit of axial imaging. Yet we are still unsure of the exact contribution this examination should make to the assessment of non-small cell lung cancer.

CT scanning times are continually falling. By reducing scanning time, resolution improves because motion artefacts due to breathing and cardiac action become less important. Generations of scanners refer to their scanning times. Modern fourth-generation scanners scan in less than two seconds. There is a limit to the speed at which the anode can be forced to spin around the patient; consequently, a fifth generation of scanners based on speed alone is unlikely. Electron beam technology is beginning to make a contribution. A hybrid of the two techniques is an attractive path of future investigation.

One of the limitations of current protocols for CT scanning is that non-contiguous slices may miss small lesions. Patient motion or inconsistent levels of inspiration from scan to scan may cause omission of some anatomic levels with repeated scanning of others. Continuous data acquisition over multiple rotations is now possible with many of the latest-generation scanners (figure 4). The patient table is advanced synchronous with continuous scanning, and the examination volume is scanned in a spiral path. Spiral volumetric CT with a single breath-hold has been shown to be a reliable

SPIRAL CT

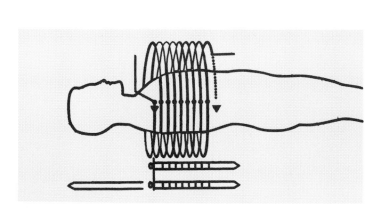

Figure 4. Continous data acquisition during a single breath-hold using spiral CT.

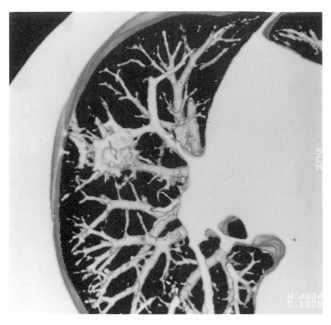

Figure 5. Spiral CT three-dimensional reconstruction of a peripheral carcinoma of the right upper lobe.

means of obtaining fully continuous data acquisition [29]. Complete organ volumes can be scanned in a single breath (12 seconds), or perhaps more importantly during vascular enhancement. Images can be reconstructed at observer-nominated table positions. Thus, the center of the lesion can be used to generate the level of interest, allowing a better basis for comparison between sequential scans.

In addition, spiral CT can produce very dramatic three-dimensional constructs (figure 5), elegantly exposing and displaying the relationship between the tumor and intrathoracic structures. Motion artifact (gantry rather than respiratory) has yet to be eliminated. Presently, spiral volumetric CT is limited primarily by available x-ray power (limited mAmpere settings). Truly continuous scanning, independent of breathing or other patient motion, demands continuous data acquisition and patient transport. The limitations encountered with the technique can be overcome by further improvements in x-ray and computer power.

The Imatron ultrafast CT scanner dispenses with a moving x-ray source. The electron beam is tightly focused and directed at a tungsten target ring, producing a useful array of radiaton. Static detectors mounted in an arc of 210° simultaneously accrue all the information at each level. This technique can produce images at up to 17 frames per second. A loop can be made of images obtained at a single level and projected as a real-time dynamic study.

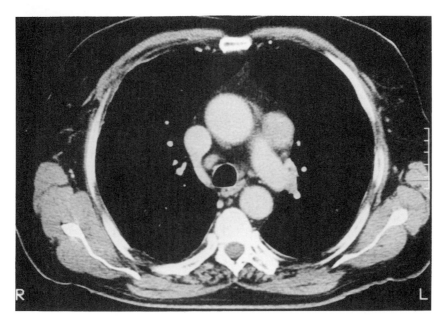

Figure 6. Imatron (ultra-fast CT scan): exquisite detail of mediastinal structures. Note the enlarged lymph node adjacent to the azygos vein as it joins the superior vena cava.

The structures of the mediastinum are demonstrated with uncommon detail and resolution (figure 6).

Tumor characteristics

Conventional radiology can only exclude malignancy in a pulmonary nodule if there is absence of growth with time or if specific patterns of calcification are present [30]. It is doubtful if CT scanning is any more helpful than conventional radiology in determining the malignant potential of a pulmonary nodule. CT densimetry has been used to discriminate between benign and malignant lesions. Masses with a density greater than 164 Hounsfield units are thought to be benign [31]. There are considerable technical problems associated with such an estimate, which are related to the volume of the opacity, the individual characteristics of the scanner, and even the time of day of the reading [32]. Some of these dynamic variables can be controlled for by using an 'anthropomorphic' reference phantom as a basis for comparison [33]. The mere demonstration that a nodule contains calcification is not proof positive of benign disease. Calcification has been demonstrated in up to 13% of lesions shown, at resection, to be malignant [34].

Nuclear imaging

A considerable amount of interest has been generated by positron emission tomography (PET) and single photon emission tomography (SPECT). There is significant uptake and retention of thallium-201 by lung cancers and metastases within mediastinal lymph nodes [35]. Resolution is, at present, limited to lesions of 1.5 cm. PET has been used as a detector of malignancy in patients with SPN. In a prospective study of 20 patients, PET (radio-labeled glucose: 2-fluoro-18-fluoro-2-deoxy-D-glucose) correctly demonstrated focal hypermetabolism in 13 of 13 malignant lesions; there were no areas of increased uptake in the remaining seven lesions, which proved to be benign [36]. In a single patient with positive sputum cytology and negative conventional imaging, [201]Ti SPECT was able to detect an otherwise radiologically occult carcinoma of the bronchus [37]. However attractive the concept becomes, cost considerations will seriously limit the availability of these techniques. The specialized scanners cost several millions of dollars, and an on-site cyclotron is necessary to produce the extremely short half-life radiotracers.

Finally, detection of lung cancer and mediastinal disease using radiolabeled monoclonal antibodies has largely been disappointing. Conceptually, the technique is very exciting, and has treatment as well as diagnostic implications. Expectations are high that radioimmunodetection should make an increasingly important contribution to the diagnosis and staging of lung cancers.

Thoracoscopy

With the advent of modern fiber-optic techniques and camera miniaturization, thoracoscopy has progressed from a century of diagnosing pleural disease to a much more effective tool for diagnosing staging of lung cancer. The surgical community is at present exploring the potential of this exciting technique. The ability to perform complex maneuvers will be facilitated by a new range of instruments developed specifically for thoracoscopic use. How large a role thorascopy is likely to play in the treatment of lung cancer has yet to be established.

Thoracoscopy can clearly make a contribution to the diagnosis of SPNs, particularly when the nodule is peripheral and in contact with a visceral pleural surface. A needle aspirate or true-cut biopsy can be obtained under direct visual control, if for some reason the excision of the lesion is contraindicated. However, with the advent of instruments suitable for minimally invasive techniques, a small peripheral lesion can be excised in its entirety. The ability to excise a peripheral nodule without the need for thoracotomy has served as a catalyst to an already heated debate regarding the suitability of local excision versus formal lung resection in peripheral tumors. The Lung Cancer Study Group has looked into this in meticulous detail. Survival in patients who had lesions that were excised as wedge resection is comparable to formal lung resection at two years. However, local recurrence is more common in patients having local excision alone. An absolutely essential aspect of the protocol was that these patients were fully staged at the time of operation, prior to randomization.

Diagnosis of small lesions that are not in direct contiguity with a pleural surface is more subtle. A number of centers have now reported CT-guided needle localization of small pulmonary nodules, which are transferred directly from the CT scanning suite to the operating theatre for excision. Pneumothorax following this procedure has not been clinically apparent. Dislodgement of the needles during transfer or at the time of controlled collapse of the lung at endoscopy have led most units to include an injection of a marker dye, such as methylene blue, at the time of needle localization. Although far from ideal, a number of ultrasound probes are suitable for use at thoracoscopy. When collapsed, the lung is a suitable organ for ultrasonic examination, and the detection of nodules deep within the parenchyma is straightforward.

The thoracoscope can be a useful adjunct in patients about to undergo thoracotomy for carcinoma of the bronchus. Units are now incorporating thoracoscopy as a preliminary staging investigation prior to thoracotomy in all patients with lung cancer. Previously undiagnosed malignant pleural disease has been exposed by this technique in a number of patients. Direct inspection of lesions abutting the chest wall can determine invasion and help to plan the incision accordingly. Central tumors are more difficult to assess because of the mechanical problems afforded by the relative immobility of the pulmonary hilum in such cases.

Staging

The first attempt to collate the disparate clinical material in patients with lung cancer was made by the Union Internationale Contre Cancer (UICC) in 1968 [38]. This attempt was followed in 1973 by the incorporation of the TNM system, as suggested by the American Joint Committee on Cancer (AJCC) [39]. If international staging systems are to have any value, they must be easy to apply and must be widely practiced for a long enough time for their inherent strengths and faults to become apparent. The AJCC system evolved through several manifestations. In order to take into account new trends in therapy and certain discrepancies in prognosis, an international task force was employed to create a meaningful and workable staging system. An international consensus was achieved in 1985 at the World Conference on Lung Cancer [40] (tables 2 and 3).

The goal of staging patients who have a diagnosis of lung cancer is to identify the extent of the disease process both locally and at distant sites

Table 2. New international staging system for lung cancer

Tx Tumor proven by the presence of malignant cells in bronchopulmonary secretions but not visualized roentgenographically or bronchoscopically, or any tumor that cannot be assessed, as in a retreatment staging.

T0 No evidence of primary tumor.

Tis Carcinoma in situ.

T1 A tumor that is 3.0 cm or less in its greatest dimension surrounded by lung or visceral pleura and without evidence of invasion proximal to a lobar bronchus at bronchoscopy.

T2 A tumor greater than 3.0 cm in any dimension, or a tumor of any size that either invades the visceral pleura or has associated atelectasis or obstructive pneumonitis extending to the hilar region. At bronchoscopy, the proximal extent of demonstrable tumor must be within a lobar bronchus or at least 2.0 cm distal to the main carina. Any associated atelectasis or obstructive pneumonitis must involve less than the entire lung.

T3 A tumor of any size with direct extension into the chest wall (including superior sulcus tumors), diaphragm, or the mediastinal pleura or pericardium without involving the heart, great vessels, trachea, esophagus, or vertebral body, or a tumor in the main bronchus within 2 cm of the carina without involving the carina, or associated pneumonitis or obstructive pneumonitis involving an entire lung.

T4 A tumor of any size with invasion of the mediastinum or involving the heart, great vessels, trachea, esophagus, vertebral body, or carina, or the presence of malignant pleural effusion.

Nodal involvement

N0 No demonstrable metastasis to regional lymph nodes.

N1 Metastasis to lymph nodes in the peribronchial or the ipsilateral hilar region, or both (including direct extension).

N2 Metastasis to the ipsilateral mediastinal lymph nodes and/or subcarinal lymph nodes.

N3 Metastasis to contralateral mediastinal lymph nodes, contralateral hilar lymph nodes, scalene lymph nodes, or supraclavicular lymph nodes.

Table 3. Using TNM to define stage subsets

Occult carcinoma		Tx	N0	M0
Stage 0	TIS			
Stage I	T1	N0	M0	
		T2	N0	M0
Stage II	T1	N1	M0	
		T2	N0	M0
Stage IIIa		T3	N0	M0
		T3	N1	M0
		T1–3	N2	M0
Stage IIIb		Any T	N3	M
		T4	Any N	M0
Stage IV		Any T	Any N	M1

throughout the body. Accurate staging is critical in the selection of treatment and in the estimation of patient prognosis. Pretreatment staging is a logical and progressive process whose purpose is to obtain sufficient information to arrive at a treatment decision. The minimal staging for an individual case must depend not only on the extent of the tumor but also on other aspects of patient care, such as availability of investigative techniques, access to treatment modalities, and patient fitness. The staging process should be structured so that as it continues there is a logical progression to more elaborate, expensive, and invasive investigations.

Under no circumstances should clinical staging be confused or equated with pathological staging. Surgery with complete removal of all tumor remains the only effective treatment for patients with lung cancer. Patients must be given every benefit of the doubt when clinical findings are equivocal. Clearly, the primary goal of staging is to ensure that all patients suitable for surgical resection receive prompt and expert surgical attention. Secondary goals are to minimize the rate of exploration for incurable or unresectable disease and to identify meaningful subpopulations of patients. These objectives allow direct comparison of results obtained at the same center over a period of time or comparisons of different treatments offered in separate centers. Endpoints other than cure can be identified and used as measures against which adjuvant treatments can be compared.

There is pressure today to include more than histological cell type and TNM status in the next incarnation of international staging classification. Factors that take into account the biological behavior and biochemical characteristics of tumors should be included if they predictably influence the natural history of the disease. There is now some very coherent evidence suggesting that measurable and reproducible markers of tumor biology profoundly effect the behavior of lung cancers.

One such parameter is the DNA ploidy status. In normal tissue, DNA is largely diploid, representing the G0/G1 phase of the cell cycle. There is a small amount of tetraploid DNA in preparation for normal cell division. Disturbances in the process of cell division due to chromosomal anomalies are characteristic of malignant cell kinetics. Regardless of pTNM stage and cell type, euploid tumors are associated with a better prognosis than aneuploid tumors [41]. The heterogeneity within tumors presents the most fundamental barrier to widespread acceptance of these data [42]. In addition, there is inconsistency between the ploidy status of the primary tumor and its lymph node metastases [7,43]. Given this degree of variability, it is difficult to accept the present evidence for inclusion as a staging criterion. A second observation worth considering when staging tumors is the presence or absence of peritumoral blood and lymphatic invasion. Ample experimental evidence shows that tumors with blood and lymphatic invasion have a higher metastatic potential [44,45]. When comparing survival in patients with T1/T2 N0 M0 non-small cell lung cancers treated by wedge resection, the presence of blood and lymphatic invasion was a highly discriminating factor [46].

Computed tomography

Tumors of any size extending beyond the boundaries of the lung, be it into parietal pleura, chest wall, diaphragm, or mediastinum, receive T3 or T4 status (vide supra). The pleurae present a natural, but not impenetrable, barrier to malignant invasion. Special attention should be given to patients complaining of chest pain suggestive of chest wall invasion. Bone erosion on conventional radiography is due to extensive malignant infiltration. CT scanning can disclose more subtle degrees of chest wall invasion with the loss of the extrapleural fat plane, tumor extension between ribs, or sometimes tumor extension into the extrathoracic muscles (table 4). The obliquity of successive ribs may make this assessment difficult (particularly in the upper hemi-thorax), and a slice may suggest tumor extension out with the arc of the rib above, an artefact created by the bulging of intercostal bundles displaced but not necessarily involved by tumor. A tumor with more than 3 cm contact with the mediastinum, or forming less than an angle of 90° contact with the mediastinum, is further supportive evidence of mediastinal invasion [47]. The most reliable indicator of chest wall invasion is rib destruction. Pleural thickening and extensive contact between mass and chest wall are sensitive signs, but show much less specificity.

A neat maneuver that can improve the diagnostic accuracy of CT is to induce a small pneumothorax by introducing 300 to 500 ml of air during the examination [48]. The authors use air in this study, but surely CO_2 must be a preferable contrast medium. Positive and negative predictive accuracy of the examination improves to 65% and 100%, respectively. Fortunately, the presence of chest wall invasion does not preclude successful resection, and excellent survival (50%–55% at five years) has been achieved for T3N0 tumors [49–51]. Nonetheless, it is helpful for the surgeon to be aware of chest wall invasion on CT scanning, since this knowledge aids tactical planning. Surgical resection of T3N1 and T3N2 tumors gives little chance of long-term survival [36,37,52]. The preoperative assessment of N1 disease in lower-stage tumors is a minor issue. Intraoperative assessment with frozen section will dictate appropriate action; lesser resections converted either to sleeve resection or pneumonectomy. In stage III tumors, node status pro-

---

Table 4. CT criteria for chest wall involvement

1. CT identifies tumors involving trachea and the main carina, although submucosal extension can lead to an underestimate of T status (T3)
2. Rib destruction (T3)
3. Irregular interdigitation of tumor within chest wall or mediastinal fat planes (T3)
4. Compression of the superior vena cava, the aorta, or pulmonary arteries outside the pleural reflection (T4)
5. Extension of tumor into cardiac chambers (T4)
6. Vertebral body destruction (T4)

---

foundly influences prognosis. The inability of CT to reliably judge the nature of intrapulmonary nodes is a major shortcoming when evaluating patients with advanced-stage disease. Recent studies employing preoperative induction chemotherapy and radiotherapy suggest that modern adjuvant treatment can improve poor resectability and survival rates in patients with stage III (A and B) non-small cell lung cancer [53,54]. These studies are compared against nonmatched historical controls and must be examined critically. The treatment group represents the best functional group of patients with stage III disease and would be expected to do well regardless of what treatment they received. As in every other aspect of treatment for lung cancer, there are no generalizations that can extend to every patient. Each case must be treated on its own merits. CT evidence alone should not contraindicate thoracotomy.

Nodal metastases

Mediastinal lymph nodes are identified on axial CT images as nonenhancing, oval soft-tissue densities surrounded by mediastinal fat. Nodal size can be estimated by measuring the long- or short-axis diameters. Short-axis diameter is less dependant on the spatial orientation of the node and is thus a more reliable and reproducible measurement. Computed tomography criteria for lymph node malignancy theoretically include morphological features such as nodal shape, density, and margination, as well as nodal size. In practice, however, most of these features are not helpful, and increased nodal size is the only useful criterion for malignancy.

CT can identify mediastinal lymph nodes in 88% of normal individuals [55]. The great majority of these nodes are less than 1 cm in diameter. However, over 5% of nodes are between 1 cm and 1.5 cm in diameter. While this study [55] evaluates the size of normal mediastinal nodes in one country, in the context of carcinoma of the bronchus enlarged nodes are not necessarily malignant. As node size increases, the probability of their being malignant becomes greater. However, there is no absolute size above which glands are certainly malignant, and glands greater than 2 cm in diameter are benign in at least 45% to 80% of case [56,57]. The corollary is also true; 8% to 36% [58] of lymph nodes with a diameter less than 1 cm excised as a part of routine mediastinal sampling at thoracotomy are malignant.

It therefore follows that in assessing the sensitivity with which CT scanning can detect nodal metastases, the surgeon must excise for analysis all detectable nodes, not merely those which appear macroscopically abnormal. Routine nodal sampling is now an established part of surgical staging procedure. The failure to be less than rigorous in lymph node sampling is a major source of bias in many of the studies assessing the accuracy of CT. In our practice, such sampling discloses unsuspected N2 disease in over 20% of our patients [59].

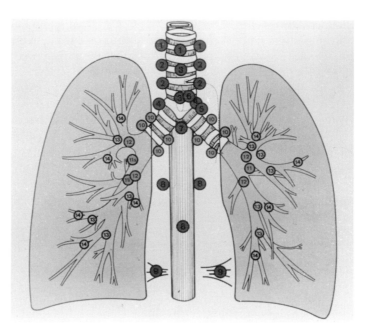

Figure 7. The Naruke map or a close equivalent is essential to the staging process.

Philosophically, it is unlikely that even the most exacting dissection will prove 100% sensitive in detecting nodal metastases, owing to sampling errors on the part of the surgeon and the pathologist processing the tissue. Whether N status reflects the natural history of the tumor or differences in tumor biology is one of the fundamental questions still awaiting clarification.

Recent studies demonstrating reasonable salvage in patients with N2 disease has only succeeded in clouding the issue further. In patients with resected N2 disease, the best long-term survival is obtained in patients with ipsilateral, single-station disease with squamous cell cancers [60].

The American Thoracic Society proposed a standard lymph node staging system [61] in 1983 largely based upon the Naruke map [62], which allows standard recognition and recording of lymph node status at anatomical stations within the mediastinum and lung parenchyma (figure 7).

Hilar nodes. The presence of ipsilateral hilar node metastases, N1 disease, does not contraindicate surgery, but does adversely affect prognosis and usually necessitates a more extensive resection. The preoperative determination of N1 disease is important in patients of great age or those with limited lung function in whom pneumonectomy would be hazardous. It can influence treatment decisions in situations such as chest wall invasion. N1 status is a

238

Table 5. CT assessment of mediastinal lymph node metastasis

Author	#Patients	Generation	Size	Sensitivity (%)	Specificity (%)	Accuracy (%)	Prevalence (%)
Moak	41	2nd	10	76	67	71	41
Underwood	18	2nd	NS	44	89	67	50
Lewis	75	2nd	10	91	94	92	NS
Modini	41	2nd	NS	50	96	83	29
Goldstraw	44	2nd	15	57	86	76	NS
Khan	50	2nd	<10	83	90	88	36
Hirleman	50	2nd	NS	96	73	84	60
Osbourne	42	3rd	5	94	62	76	43
Rea	22	3rd	All	80	76	77	23
McKenna	102	3rd	10	60	60	61	25
Glazer	49	3rd	10	95	64	78	43
Richey	48	3rd	10	95	68	79	42
Daly	146	3rd	15	80	91	88	28
Musset	44	3rd	10	91	82	84	25
Nakata	59	3rd	10	50	62	56	37
Heelan	20	3rd	15	100	70	85	50
Baron	94	4th	9	92	80	85	41
Patterson	84	4th	10	71	89	82	NS

critical determinant in patients with small cell lung cancer. CT is no more accurate in hilar assessment than conventional chest radiographs [63] or standard tomography [64,65]. There is some evidence that MRI is superior to CT in this respect (vide infra).

The CT interpretation of the normal [66] and abnormal [67] hilum is well understood, but the accuracy with which it can predict hilar node metastases varies greatly in reported series (table 5), with sensitivity varying from 38% to 90% and specificity from 64% to 100% [68,69]. This variation is not accounted for by differences in scan time or patient selection. Where the primary tumor or consolidated lung is adjacent to the hilum, difficulty is to be expected in distinguishing hilar node metastases, but studies including such patients [70] report results similar to studies that specifically excluded them [71]. The explanation may lie in the size of the gland found to contain deposits. The two studies reporting the highest sensitivity for CT scan detection of hilar node metastases report that such glands had a mean size of 2.2 cm [55] or that the majority of glands were greater than 2 cm in size [72]. One study [54] reporting a sensitivity far lower than these studies noted that the majority of hilar glands were 'only slightly enlarged.' The difference in size of involved glands between these studies may be chance or may reflect less critical node sampling at surgery. If small involved glands are escaping detection at thoracotomy, then the number of false-negative scans will be underestimated, leading to a falsely high sensitivity value. We are very aware that the figures given in our study [73] are unduly pessimistic, since we have come to appreciate the value of contrast enhancement with rapid sequence scanning through the hilum. Given the above, it seems reasonable to suggest that the CT scan assessment of the hilum has a sensitivity of 65%–70% with a specificity of 90%–95%. With this degree of accuracy, CT scanning of the hilum is unlikely to influence the decision regarding thoracotomy except in a small proportion of patients.

Mediastinal nodes. The earliest studies suggested CT scanning might prove useful in the staging of the mediastinum prior to surgery [74], and the subsequent literature on this topic has been prolific. Studies presenting the sensitivity and specificity of CT in predicting mediastinal node involvement have been made obsolete, almost before publication, by the introduction of later generations of scanners with improved resolution. The failure of later-generation scanners to provide presurgical assessment objectively superior to conventional imaging has been disappointing.

What then is our endpoint? It is tempting to say positive histology; but if, as we hope, most of our patients will be node negative, how far does one have to go to be sure that the histology is not falsely negative? It is not sufficient to say 'no abnormal nodes were detected at thoracotomy,' even if this assessment is made by an experienced thoracic surgeon. Meticulous routine sampling of mediastinal nodes is mandatory [75]. There are several studies documenting the accuracy of computed tomography of the mediastinum. The sensitivity of this assessment lies between 50% and 70% with a specificity of 90%–100%. The range is likely to reflect as much on the diligence of the surgeon concerned as on the technique and interpretation of the radiologists.

No firm pattern to the accuracy of these studies exists, but there is a trend, which seems eminently reasonable, that as the size criteria for abnormality increases, the sensitivity with which glands are discovered will fall while specificity will improve. There is an important source of bias in each of these studies: there is a variable degree of vigilance as to which mediastinal nodes are sought and subjected to microscopic analysis at thoracotomy.

A number of studies have examined the ability of CT to predict the status of lymph nodes on a station-by-station basis as determined by the ATS. The accuracy of CT falls dramatically when each station is assessed independently. CT sensitivity was only 33% when each node station was determined individually; when the mediastinal nodes were considered as a group, the sensitivity was more in keeping with previous studies at 73% [76]. These findings were supported by two carefully structured prospective studies in which sensitivity of CT on an individual node basis was 29%–44% [77,78]. The sensitivity on a per-patient basis was 64%, with a specificity of 62%.

There was a wide range of sensitivity at individual node stations. CT was most sensitive in assessing paratracheal nodes (79%). It was least sensitive for subcarinal glands (25%) and the left hilum (17%). At least 30% of nodes greater than 2 cm in diameter were found to have reactive changes. It was noted that, once again, adenocarcinoma had metastasized to a relatively large proportion of normal-sized lymph nodes. This work demands that the previous litany on this subject be reexamined and underscores the need to be even more circumspect in the CT evaluation of lymph node status. The relative insensitivity of CT makes formal lymph node sampling at the time of mediastinoscopy or thoracotomy essential to detect lymph node metastasis.

Magnetic resonance imaging

Magnetic resonance imaging (MRI) is now an established diagnostic procedure in patients with bronchogenic carcinoma. When comparing MRI with CT, it is important to keep in mind that CT is cheaper, more easily obtained, usually takes less time, is easier for sick patients to tolerate, and usually provides more ancillary information. If MRI provides diagnostic information equivalent to that provided by CT, CT is the more appropriate mode of study. However, it is a mistake to think of CT and MRI as mutually exclusive examinations; in certain instances, CT and MRI complement each other.

Several techniques are common to all MRI protocols. Gating images to the ECG reduces artifacts related to cardiac action and blood flow, which greatly improves the spatial resolution of MRI. Respiratory motion artifacts are problematic in thoracic MRI. Rapid scanning techniques that allow the acquisition of single or multiple images during a breath hold are still in the process of development [79–81]. Although images can be obtained using these techniques, the images tend have poor soft-tissue contrast. MRI holds a distinct advantage over CT in three areas. The most obvious is the ability of MRI to reconstruct images in sagittal or coronal planes. Because of the MR characteristics of flowing blood, MRI is particularly sensitive to vascular invasion by tumor without the need for contrast. Less obvious, and sometimes more difficult to appreciate, is MRI's ability to distinguish different tissues based on T1 and T2 spin characteristics and relaxation phenomena.

There have been several studies conducted comparing the relative merits of CT and MRI in the staging of bronchogenic carcinoma [82–85]. These studies agree that MRI offers no obvious advantage over conventional CT. Furthermore, a combined interpretation of MRI with CT does not appear to improve the accuracy of either study interpreted alone. There is a suggestion that MRI may be more sensitive than CT in diagnosing the presence or extent of chest wall invasion in pancoast-type tumors [86,87]. As with CT, effacement of the extrapleural fat plane is a sensitive indicator of early chest wall involvement. It also may be useful in demonstrating mediastinal invasion [88], particularly vascular invasion by tumor.

In general, MRI is quite similar to CT in its ability to detect and define mediastinal lymph nodes [80,81,89,90]. This finding is no more or less than expected if size is the sole criterion for evaluating lymph nodes. T1 and T2 spin characteristics have been evaluated and found to have no discriminating value [91,92]. Nor does the addition of gadolinium-DTPA serve as a useful adjunct [93]. MRI is more accurate than CT in diagnosing the presence of hilar lymphadenopathy [94,95]. Because rapid flow of blood causes little MR signal, only the walls of pulmonary vessels are visible. Enlarged hilar nodes are easily detected and differentiated from adjacent vascular structures.

MRI can distinguish between a lung mass and consolidation secondary to bronchial obstruction [96,97].

In practice, the additional information gleaned from MRI has been disappointing. Only rarely has this information influenced the decision to proceed to thoracotomy or otherwise.

Transesophageal ultrasonography

Air in the lung presents a physical barrier to examination by ultrasonography. However, this factor can be used to advantage when assessing mediastinal infiltration (T4 status). The pulmonary arteries, aorta, left atrium, pulmonary veins, superior vena cava, and esophagus can be evaluated by transesophageal endoscopic ultrasonography (E-EUS). When used in patients with CT evidence of mediastinal invasion, E-EUS was 77% sensitive and 81% specific, with an accuracy of 80% [110]. E-EUS was particularly sensitive to involvement of the superior vena cava, descending thoracic aorta, and esophagus (table 6).

Mediastinoscopy

Scalene lymph node biopsy in patients with carcinoma of the bronchus was first advocated by Daniels in 1949 [123] and extended to the include the mediastinum by Harken in 1954 [124]. Cervical mediastinoscopy, a more refined procedure with access to many more lymph node stations, was

Table 6. Ultrasonic criteria for mediastinal infiltration

Grade 0	Existence of a hyperechoic area between the tumor mass and mediastinum
Grade I	Tumor mass in direct contact with the mediastinum, which appears normal in structure, accompanied by movement of the tumor mass on respiration
Grade II	Partial disappearance of the laminar structures and changes in the mediastinum, with no relative movement of the tumor mass with respiration
Grade III	Tumor invasion within the lumen of the mediastinal vasculature

described by Carlens six years later [125]. This procedure was rapidly and widely accepted because of its high specificity. Poor diagnostic yield in some patients prompted Chamberlain to introduce anterior mediastinotomy [126]. These procedures are well tolerated by patients. In a large review of 3742 procedures, complications occurred in 1.6% and mortality was 0.08% [127]. There is a wide range of diagnostic yields from routine mediastinoscopy. In patients with small cell cancer, mediastinoscopy is productive in over 70%, but in patients with squamous cell cancers the procedure is positive in less than 20%. Overall, the diagnostic yield from routine mediastinoscopy is less than 30%.

Patients with left upper lobe tumors represent a special case. Nodes in the anterior mediastinum, subaortic fossa, and posterior subcarinal region are not accessible to cervical mediastinoscopy. It has been shown that in patients with left upper lobe tumors with negative cervical mediastinoscopy, left anterior mediastinotomy will prove positive in 36% of cases [128]. In a recent study critically examining the role of mediastinoscopy in 619 patients, sensitivity was 71%, specificity was 100%, accuracy was 92.4%, and negative predictive value was 90.6% [129]. The use of 'extended mediastinoscopy' has been reintroduced and popularized by Ginsberg [130,131]. Using blunt dissection, a plane is developed in the 'innominate triangle' formed by the left common carotid, innominate vein, and innominate artery. Para-aortic and subaortic fossa, previously inaccessible to cervical mediastinoscopy, are now available without the need for mediastinotomy.

Mediastinal assessment is not limited to assessment of N status. There are few studies recording the accuracy of T status. The original description of anterior mediastinotomy limits the dissection to the extrapleural component of mediastinal disease. It is a simple matter to incise the pleura and examine the pulmonary hilum and structure anterior to it. In our study, the sensitivity of mediastinal exploration in the detection of mediastinal invasion was only 46% [73]. While this figure rose to 71% for upper-lobe tumors, it fell to only 17% for lower-lobe lesions. However, surgical assessment of mediastinal invasion is not without its limitations. These figures are understandable given the anatomical restrictions of mediastinal exploration. Tumors of the left upper lobe or lower lobe that have reached the left main bronchus should be assessed by simultaneous mediastinoscopy and anterior mediastinotomy. We advocate bimanual palpation of the mediastinum to assess the presence of tumour or metastasis not accessible to direct inspection (figure 9).

Because of safety considerations, clinicians have been reluctant to perform mediastinoscopy as a repeat procedure or in patients with superior vena cava obstruction (SVCO). Provided that the operator is sufficiently experienced with the technique, mediastinoscopy is not contraindicated in these patients. We have performed mediastinoscopy in patients in both categories without an increase in attendant morbidity [132] and have been supported by others [133–136].

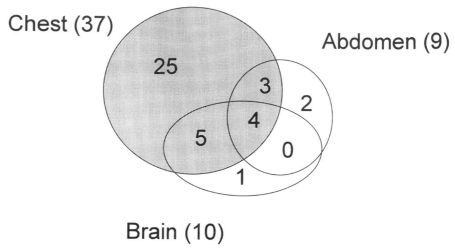

Chest (37)   Abdomen (9)

25   3   2   4   5   0   1

Brain (10)

Figure 8. Computed tomography identification of nonresectable chest and metastatic disease by region (*n* = 114).

There remains wide variation in the application of mediastinoscopy to the staging of patients with carcinoma of the bronchus. The source of debate centers on the use of mediastinoscopy in patients in whom there is no demonstrable evidence of extrapulmonary disease from noninvasive investigations. In a survey of thoracic surgical practive in the U.K. [137], 10% performed routine mediastinoscopy and 88% performed mediastinoscopy if nodes were enlarged on CT. However, only 41% performed routine CT examination of the thorax!

Regardless of how extensive a mediastinal exploration one undertakes, there are mediastinal lymph node stations accessible to thoracotomy alone, namely, the para-aortic, posterior subcarinal, and para-esophageal lymph node stations, as well as nodes within the inferior pulmonary ligament (stations 6,7,8, and 9). These lymph nodes are all within reach of the thoracoscope, as are nodes higher in the mediastinum. Careful consideration will need to be given to the prospect of thoracoscopy replacing conventional mediastinoscopy as the invasive procedure of choice in the staging of patients with lung cancer. Since the specificity of both procedures will be 100%, the basis for comparison will lie in the sensitivity, morbidity, and cost effectiveness of the two techniques. We must not miss the opportunity to perform careful prospective randomized trials before the playing field is muddied by overenthusiasm for a scientifically unproven technique.

Metastases to distant sites

Autopsy studies have characterized the pattern of metastatic disease in patients dying of lung cancer. Favored sites are liver (30%–40%), adrenal

244

glands (18%–38%), brain (15%–48%), bone (19%–33%), and kidney (16%–23%) [98]. The pattern of relapse in patients that have undergone 'curative' resection is similar to those who have inoperable disease at the time of presentation [99,100]. Local recurrence is infrequent. The major reason for relapse is our failure to identify subclinical metastases present at the time of preoperative evaluation.

The advent of whole-body CT scanning raised the hope that this technique would identify such occult metastases and save futile resection. CT has been shown to be superior to isotope liver scans and ultrasound at detecting liver secondaries [101] and superior to brain isotope scans in detecting cerebral secondaries [102]. The yield of CT brain scans depends upon the presence or absence of nonspecific clinical features suggestive of occult metastases [103]. In the presence of neurological symptoms or signs, 16% of brain scans were positive.

Reports suggest that 10%–25% [104–106] of patients with lung cancer have adrenal abnormalities on CT. In the majority of these, the adrenal was only one of a number of metastatic lesions. An adrenal metastasis was the only contraindication to surgery in less than 5% of patients. CT cannot distinguish benign from malignant adrenal masses, and at least 60% of these are due to adenomas [107]. Specific features on CT that suggest malignancy are low attenuation, size greater than 2 cm, and failure to enhance with contrast medium [108]. When in doubt, it is wise to continue to press for histological confirmation of any CT abnormality that constitutes an isolated contraindication to surgery.

It is clear from these studies that the yield of abnormal CT scans of brain, chest, and abdomen undertaken prior to thoracotomy is disappointingly low and falls far short of the numbers of occult metastases expected from autopsy and relapse studies. We performed a study [109] in 114 patients with non-small cell lung cancer, assessing the yield of routine CT scans of brain, chest, and abdomen. Fifteen patients were found to have extrathoracic metastatic disease. Of these, 12 had enlarged mediastinal lymph nodes and were shown to have N2 disease at mediastinoscopy. Only one isolated brain metastasis was identified. Similarly, only two patients had isolated abdominal metastatic disease (figure 8).

In view of the disturbing pattern of relapse in patients undergoing surgical resection, a more sensitive means of determining subclinical and micro-metastatic disease is sorely needed.

Isotope scans

In many patients, clinical, organ-specific signs and symptoms may suggest the presence of metastases and direct the clinician to the relevant investigation. Nonspecific clinical features such as weight loss, abnormal liver function, and unexplained anemia have been associated with occult metastatic disease [111], and isotope scans can yield worthwhile results [112]. Nuclear

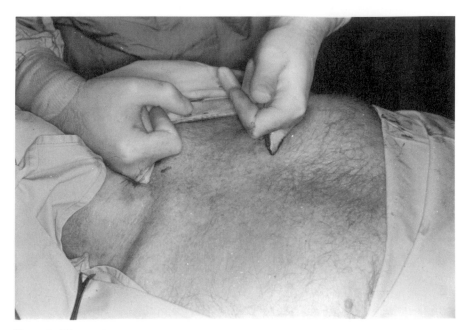

Figure 9. Bimanual examination of the subaortic fossa in a man with left upper lobe carcinoma of the bronchus.

medicine covers a wide range of diagnostic techniques. Many have been an important part of routine staging protocols for lung cancer in the past. Some are no longer routine, because they have been superseded by more accurate imaging modalities. The fact that patients ultimately relapse with distant metastases gives testimony to the generally poor sensitivity of these examinations [113]. How best can we utilize nuclear isotope scans to improve the accuracy of diagnostic and staging protocols? Which isotope scans should be used, and which patients should be scanned?

Bone scintigraphy with $^{99}Tc^m$ is a test that combines high sensitivity for detection of focal skeletal abnormalities with poor specificity for lung cancer. Approximately 15% of asymptomatic patients will have a positive bone scan [114]. We have demonstrated that the figure falls to less than 2% in patients with no other evidence for extrapulmonary disease. In patients with symptoms of bone pain or tenderness, bone scans are positive in nearly 88% [115]. Generally, less than half of patients with scintigraphic evidence of bony metastases have raised serum alkaline phosphatase levels; in the majority of these patients, the level was within 10% of the upper limit of the normal range.

The bone scan should not be interpreted in isolation when determining the existence of metastatic disease. When bone scintigraphy is combined with additional planar or tomographic projections, it becomes a much more powerful means of discrimination. High false-positive rates occur when bone scans are reported without the benefit of other imaging [116]. If strict criteria are adhered to and appropriate further radiology is obtained, the incidence of false-positive examinations should be zero [117,118]. False negatives are well documented, occurring in nearly 15% [119].

Gallium-67 has a high affinity for lung cancer cells. However, it also has a high affinity for inflammatory cells. In addition to lung cancer, abnormal foci of gallium accumulation may be present in patients with acute infections, sarcoidosis, Hodgkin's disease, lymphoma, etc. In general, the resolution of gallium scanning in optimal circumstances requires a lesion of at least 2 cm for detection. It cannot, therefore, effectively screen for lung cancer. There are proponents of Gallium scanning as a means of assessing the mediastinum metastatic disease [120–122], but the recommendations from these studies have been contradictory. A major drawback is the inability of gallium scanning to differentiate between hilar and mediastinal disease. The present limitations associated with this mode of imaging make it an unattractive means of staging lung cancer.

Thoracotomy

The investigation upon which treatment ultimately rests is thoracotomy. The clinical evaluative phase is known to be inaccurate [138]. Patients with proven M1 and N2 disease have been excluded from surgical intervention. Although not common practice, intraoperative assessment of mediastinal lymph nodes is arguably more important than any other means of determining N status. Intraoperative mediastinal node dissection has given added insight to the limitations of clinical staging protocols [139]. Despite rigorous screening, unsuspected N2 disease occurs in up to 26% [140,141] of our patients. Malignant infiltration of mediastinal lymph nodes assessed by naked-eye appearances has been shown to have a sensitivity of 71% and a specificity of 94% [141]. The positive and negative predictive values were 64% and 96%, respectively. Decisions regarding the extent of resection (exploration only, lobectomy, or pneumonectomy) should be made on the grounds of firm histological confirmation of the naked-eye appearances.

Conclusions

Despite remarkable technological improvements, we are no closer to accurate clinical staging of lung cancer than we were 20 years ago. Provision of representative tissue for histological examination is the only standard presently acceptable as the basis for treatment decisions. There is evidence to support the view that screening is worthwhile in patients with lung cancer, if only the at-risk population could be identified effectively. Recognition of premalignant changes in exfoliated sputum cells seems a promising area of investigation. Staging investigations must be individualized to each patient. The staging protocol should be structured so that the simplest and least invasive tests are performed early. Costly or invasive investigations should be requested only when surgical intervention is a serious proposition. Staging investigations are presently insufficiently sensitive to exclude patients with occult micrometastatic disease. The repeated scenario of adequate local control at operation, followed by disease relapse at distant sites, serves to underscore the inadequacies of current staging protocols. No solution to this problem lies on the horizon.

Those technologies that are currently being developed each have important financial implications, and are unlikely to be widely available for some time. Thoracotomy remains the ultimate diagnostic and staging tool, and patients must be offered surgical exploration in borderline cases.

References

1. Shure D, Fedullo PF. 1984. The role of transcarinal needle aspiration in the staging of bronchogenic carcinoma. Chest 86:693–698.
2. Westcott JL. 1980. Percutaneous transthoracic needle aspiration of localized pulmonary lesions: Results in 422 patients. Radiology 137:31–35.
3. Weisbrod GL. 1990. Transthoracic percutaneous lung biopsy. Radiol Clin North Am 28:647–655.
4. Brett GZ. 1969. Earlier diagnosis and survival in lung cancer. Br Med J 4:260–262.
5. Nash FA, Morgan JM, Tomkins JG. 1968. South London Lung Cancer Study. Br Med J 2:715–21.
6. Melamed MR, Flehinger BJ, Zaman MB, Heelan RT, Perchick WA, Martini N. 1984. Screening for early lung cancer. Results of the Memorial Sloan-Kettering study in New York. Chest 86:44–53.
7. Tockman MS. 1986. Survival and mortality from lung cancer in a screened population. The Johns Hopkins Study. Chest 89(suppl):324s–325s.
8. Flehinger BJ, Kimmel M, Melamed MR. 1992. The effect of surgical treatment on survival from early lung cancer. Chest 101:1013–1018.
9. Rodenhuis S, Van de Wetering ML, Mooi WJ, Evers SJ, Van Zandwijk N, Bos JL. 1987. Mutational activation of the K-ras oncogene. A possible factor in carcinoma of the lung. N Engl J Med 317:929–935.
10. Slebos RJC, Kibbelar RE, Dalsio O, Kooistra A, Stam J, Meifier CJLM, Wagenaar SS, Van dee Schueren R, Van Zandwijk N, Mooi WJ, Bos JL, Rodenhuis S. 1990. K-ras oncogene activation as a prognostic marker in adenocarcinoma of the lung. N Engl J Med 323:561–565.
11. Nigro JM, Baker SJ, Preisinger AC, Hessop JM, Hostetter R, Cleary K, Bigner SJ, Davidson N, Baylin S, Devilee P, Glover T, Collins FS, Weston A, Modali R, Harris CC, Vogelstein B. 1989. Mutations in p53 gene occur in diverse human tumour types. Nature 342:705–708.

12. Iggo R, Gatter K, Bartek J, Lane D, Harris A. 1990. Increased expression of mutant forms of p53 oncogene in primary lung cancer. Lancet 335:675–679.
13. Chiba I, Takahashi T, Nau M, D'Amico D, Curiel DT, Mitsudomi T, Buchhagen DL, Carbone D, Piantadosi S, Koga H, Reissman PT, Slamon DJ, Holmes EC, Minna JD. 1990. Mutations in the p53 gene are frequent in primary, resected non-small cell lung cancer. Oncogene 5:1603–1610.
14. Little C, Nau M, Carney D, Gazdar A, Minna JD. 1983. Amplification and expression of the c-myc oncogene in human lung cancer cell lines. Nature 306:194–196.
15. Takahashi T, Obata Y, Sekido Y, Hida T, Ueda R, Watanabe H, Ariyoshi Y, Sugiura T. 1989. Expression and amplification of the myc gene family in small cell lung cancer and its relation to biological characteristics. Cancer Res 49:2683–2688.
16. Schneider P, Hung MC, Chiocca SM, Manning J, Zhao X, Fang K, Roth JA. 1989. Differential expression of c-erb-B2 gene in human small cell and non-small cell lung cancer. Cancer Res 49:4968–4971.
17. Harbour JW, Lai SL, Wahng-Peng J, Gazdar AD, Minna JD, Kaye FJ. 1989. Abnormalities in structure and expression of the human retinoblastoma anti-oncogene. Science 243:937–940.
18. Brauch H, Johnson B, Hovis J, Yano T, Gazdar A, Pettengil OS, Graziano S, Sorenson GD, Poisz BJ, Minna JD. 1987. Molecular analysis of the short arm chromosome 3 in small cell and non-small cell carcinoma of the lung. N Engl J Med 317:1109–1113.
19. Rapp U, Huleihel M, Pawson T. 1988. Role of raf oncogenes in lung carcinogenesis. Lung Cancer 4:162–167.
20. Schutte J, Nau M, Birrer MJ, Thomas F, Gazdar A, Minna JD. 1988. Constitutive expression of multiple mRNA forms of the c-jun oncogene in human lung cancer cell lines. Proc Am Assoc Cancer Res 29:455.
21. Keiffer P, Bepler G, Kubassch M, Havemann K. 1987. Amplification and expression of protooncogenes in human small cell lung cancer lines. Cancer Res 47:6236–6242.
22. Vlasbloem H, Schultze Kool LJ. 1988. AMBER: A scanning multiple beam equalization system for chest radiography. Radiology 169:29–34.
23. Wandtke JC, Plewes DB, McFaul JA. 1989. Comparison of scanning equalization and conventional chest radiography. Radiology 172:641–645.
24. Schultze Kool LJ, Busscher DLT, Vlasbloem H, Hermans J, Merwe PC, Algra PR, Herstel W. 1989. Advanced multiple-beam equalization in chest radiology: A simulated nodule detection study. Radiology 169:35–39.
25. Comstock GW, Vaughan RH, Montgomery G. 1956. Outcome of solitary pulmonary nodules discovered in an x-ray screening program. N Engl J Med 254:1018–1022.
26. Cummings SR, Lillington GA, Richard RJ. 1986. Estimating the probability of malignancy in solitary pulmonary nodules: A Bayesian approach. Am Rev Respir Dis 134:449–452.
27. Weiss W. 1974. Tumour doubling time and survival of men with bronchogenic carcinoma. Chest 65:3–8.
28. Sagel SS, Ferguson TB, Forrest JV, Roper CL, Weldon CS. 1978. Percutaneous transthoracic aspiration needle biopsy. Ann Thorac Surg 26:399–405.
29. Kallender WA, Seissler W, Klotz E, Vock P. 1990. Spiral volumetric CT with single-breath-hold technique, continuous transport, and continuous scanner rotation. Radiology 176:181–183.
30. Dedrick CG. 1984. The solitary pulmonary nodule and staging of lung cancer. Clin Chest Med 5:345–363.
31. Siegelman SS, Zerhoni EA, Leo FP. 1980. CT of the solitary pulmonary nodule. AJR 135:1–13.
32. Godwin JD, Speckman JM, Fram EK. 1982. Distinguishing benign from malignant nodules by CT. Radiology 144:349–351.
33. Huston J, Muhm JR. 1989. Solitary pulmonary nodules: Evaluation with a reference phantom. Radiology 170:653–656.

34. Mahoney MC, Shipley RT, Corcoran HL, Dickson MA. 1990. CT demonstration of calcification in carcinoma of the lung. AJR 154:255–258.
35. Tonami N, Shuke N, Yokoyama K, Seki H, Takayama T, Kinuya S, Nakajima K, Aburano T, Hisada K, Watanabe Y. 1989. Thallium-201 single photon emission computed tomography in the evaluation of lung cancer. J Nucl Med 30:997–1004.
36. Gupta NC, Frank AR, Dewan NA, Redepenning LS, Rothberg ML, Maillard JA, Phalen JJ, Sunderland JJ, Frick MP. 1992. Solitary pulmonary nodule: Detection of malignancy with 2-(fluoro-18)-fluoro-2-deoxy-D-glucose. Radiology 184:441–444.
37. Tonami N, Yokoyama K, Taki J, Hisada K, Watanabe Y, Takashima T, Nonomura A. 1991. Thallium-201 SPECT depicts radiologically occult lung cancer. J Nucl Med 32:2284–2285.
38. Harmer EM. 1968. TNM Classification of Malignant Tumours. Union Internationale Contre Le Cancer: Geneva, pp. 41–45.
39. Staging of Lung Cancer. 1979. American Joint Committee for Cancer Staging and End Results Reporting: Task Force on Lung Cancer: Chicago, IL.
40. Mountain CF. 1986. A new international staging system for lung cancer. Chest 15:236–241.
41. Liewald F, Hatz R, Storck M, Orend KH, Weiss M, Wulf G, Valet G, Sunder-Plassmann L. 1992. Prognostic value of deoxyribonucleic acid aneuploidy in primary non-small cell lung carcinomas and their metastases. J Thorac Cardiovasc Surg 104:1476–1482.
42. Frankfurt OS, Slocum HK, Rustum YM. 1984. Flow cytometry analysis of DNA-aneuploidy in primary and metastatic human solid tumours. Cytometry 5:71–80.
43. Volm M, Mattern J, Vogt-Schaden M, Wayss K. 1987. Flow cytometric analysis of primary lung carcinomas and their lymph node metastases. Anticancer Res 7:71–76.
44. Liotta LA, Saidel G, Kleinerman J. 1974. Quantitative relationships of intravascular tumour cells, tumour vessels, and pulmonary metastases following tumour implantation. Cancer Res 34:997–1004.
45. Liotta LA, Saidel G, Kleinerman J. 1976. The significance of haematogenous tumour cell clumps in the metastatic process. Cancer Res 36:889–894.
46. Macchiarini P, Fontanini G, Hardin JM, Pingitore R, Angeletti CA. 1992. Most peripheral, node-negative, non-small cell lung cancers have low proliferative rates and no intratumoral and peritumoral blood and lymphatic vessel invasion. J Thorac Cardiovasc Surg 104:892–899.
47. Glazer HS, Kaiser LR, Anderson D. 1989. Indeterminate mediastinal invastion in bronchogenic carcinoma: CT evaluation. Radiology 173:37–42.
48. Yokoi K, Mori K, Miyazawa N, Saito Y, Okuyama M, Sasagawa M. 1991. Tumour invasion of the chest wall and mediastinum in lung cancer: Evaluation with pneumothorax CT. Radiology 181:147–152.
49. Piehler JM, Pairolero PC, Weiland LH. 1982. Bronchogenic carcinoma with chest wall invasion: Factors affecting survival following en bloc resection. Ann Thorac Surg 34:684–691.
50. Paulson D. 1975. Carcinomas in the superior pulmonary sulcus. J Thorac Cardiovasc Surg 70:1095–1102.
51. Nakahara K, Ohno K, Matsumura A. 1989. Extended operation for lung cancer involving the aortic arch and superior vena cava. J Thorac Cardiovasc Surg 97:326–432.
52. Pearson FG, Nelems JM, Henderson RD. 1972. The role of mediastinoscopy in the selection of treatment for bronchial carcinoma with involvement of superior mediastinal lymph nodes. J Thorac Cardiovasc Surg 64:382–390.
53. Faber LP, Kittle CF, Warren WH. 1989. Preoperative chemotherapy and irradiation for stage IIIA non-small cell lung cancer. Ann Thorac Surg 47:669–677.
54. Rusch VW, Albain KS, Crowley JJ, Rice TW, Lonchyna V, McKenna R, Livingston RB, Griffen BR, Benfield JR. 1993. Surgical resection of stage IIIA and stage IIIB non-small cell lung cancer after concurrent induction chemotherapy. J Thorac Cardiovasc Surg 105:97–106.

55. Schnyder PA, Gamsu G. 1981. CT of the pretracheal retrocaval space. AJR 136:303–308.
56. Kerr W, Walker W, Cameron EJ, Lamb R. 1992. Lymph node metastasis in carcinoma of the bronchus. Thorax 46:337–339.
57. Friedman PJ, Feigin DS, Liston SE. 1984. Sensitivity of chest radiography, computed tomography, and gallium scanning to metastases of lung carcinoma. Cancer 54:1300–1306.
58. Ekhom S, Albrechtsson U, Kugelberg J. 1980. Computed tomography in preoperative staging of bronchogenic carcinoma. J Comput Assist Tomogr 4:763–765.
59. Fernando HC, Goldstraw P. 1990. The accuracy of clinical evaluative intrathoracic staging in lung cancer as assessed by postsurgical pathologic staging. Cancer 65:2503–2506.
60. Martini N, Flehinger BJ. 1987. The role of surgery in N2 lung cancer. Surg Clin North Am 67:5–17.
61. American Thoracic Society. 1983. Clinical staging of primary lung cancer. Am Rev Respir Dis 127:659–669.
62. Naruke T, Suemasu K, Ishikawa S. 1978. Lymph node mapping and curability at various levels of metastasis in resected lung cancer. J Thorac Cardiovasc Surg 76:833–839.
63. Faling LF, Pugatch RD, Jung-Legg Y. 1981. Computed tomographic scanning of the mediastinum in the staging of bronchogenic carcinoma. Am Rev Respir Dis 124:690–695.
64. Osborne DR, Korobkin M, Ravin CE. 1982. Comparison of plain radiography and computed tomography in detecting intrathoracic lymph node metastases from lung carcinoma. Radiology 142:157–161.
65. Lewis JW, Madrazo BL, Gross. 1982. The value of radiographic and computed tomography in the staging of lung carcinoma. Ann Thorac Surg 34:553–558.
66. Webb WR, Gamsu G, Glazer G. 1981. Computed tomography of the normal pulmonary hilum I. J Comput Assist Tomogr 5:476–484.
67. Webb WR, Gamsu G, Glazer G. 1981. Computed tomography of the abnormal pulmonary hilum II. J Comput Assist Tomogr 5:485–490.
68. Daly BD, Faling LJ, Bite G. 1987. Mediastinal lymph node evaluation by computed tomography in lung cancer. J Thorac Cardiovasc Surg 94:664–672.
69. Thoads AC, Thomas JH, Hermreck AS. 1986. Comparative studies of computerized tomography and mediastinoscopy for the staging of bronchogenic carcinoma. Am J Surg 152:587–593.
70. Modinin C, Passariello R, Iascone C. 1982. TNM staging in lung cancer: Role of computed tomography. J Thorac Cardiovasc Surg 84:569–574.
71. Baron RL, Levitt RG, Sagel SS. 1982. Computed tomography in the preoperative evaluation of bronchogenic carcinoma. Radiology 145:727–732.
72. Friedman PJ, Feigin DS, Liston SE. 1984. Sensitivity of chest radiography, computed tomography, and gallium scanning to metastases of lung carcinoma. Cancer 54:1300–1306.
73. Goldstraw P, Kurzer M, Edwards D. 1983. Preoperative staging of lung cancer: Accuracy of computed tomography versus mediastinoscopy. Thorax 38:10–15.
74. Crowe JK, Brown LR, Muhm JR. 1978. Computed tomography of the mediastinum. Radiology 128:75–87.
75. Goldstraw P. 1991. Pretreatment minimal staging. Lung Cancer 7:21–26.
76. Gross BH, Glazer GM, Orringer MB, Spizarny DL, Flint A. 1988. Bronchogenic carcinoma metastatic to normal sized lymph nodes: Frequency and significance. Radiology 166:71–74.
77. Izbicki JR, Thetter O, Kreusser T, Passlick B, Trupka A, Haussinger K, Woeckel W, Kenn RW, Wilker DK, Limmer J, Schweiberer L. 1992. Accuracy of computed tomographic scan for staging bronchial carcinoma. A prospective study. J Thorac Cardiovasc Surg 104:413–420.
78. McLoud TC, Bourgouin PM, Greenberg RW, Kosiuk JP, Templeton PA, Shepard JO, Moore EH, Wain JC, Mathisen DJ, Grillo HC. 1992. Bronchogenic carcinoma: Analysis of staging in the mediastinum with CT by correlative lymph node mapping and sampling. Radiology 182:319–323.
79. Spritzer C, Gamsu G, Sotzman HD. 1989. Magnetic resonance imaging of the thorax:

251

Techniques, current applications, and future directins. J Thorac Imaging 4:1–7.

80. Stern RL, Johnson GA, Ravin CE. 1990. Magnetic resonance imaging of the thoracic cavity using a paused 3DFT acquisition technique. Magn Reson Imaging 8:747–750.

81. Weinreb JC, Naidich DP. 1991. Thoracic magnetic resonance imaging. Clin Chest Med 12:33–41.

82. Webb WR. 1989. The role of magnetic resonance imaging in the assessment of patients with lung cancer: A comparison with computed tomography. J Thorac Imaging 4:65–71.

83. Grenier P, Dubray B, Careete MF. 1989. Preoperative thoracic staging of lung cancer: CT and MR evaluation. Diagn Intern Radiol 1:23–27.

84. Laurent F, Drouillard J, Dorcier F. 1988. Bronchogenic carcinoma staging: CT vs MR imaging. Assessment with surgery. Eur J Cardiothorac Surg 2:31–36.

85. Musset D, Grenier P, Carrete MF. 1986. Primary lung cancer staging: Prospective comparative study of MR imaging with CT. Radiology 160:607–611.

86. Heelen RT, Demas BE, Caravelli JF. 1989. Superior sulcus tumours: CT and MR imaging. Radiology 171:125–130.

87. Haggar AM, Pearlberg JL, Froehlich JW. 1987. Chest wall invasion by carcinoma of the lung: Detection by MR imaging. AJR 148:1177–1182.

88. Kameda K, Adachi S, Kono M. 1988. Detection of T-factor in lung cancer using magnetic resonance and computed tomography. J Thorac Imaging 3:73–77.

89. Batra P, Brown K, Collins JD. 1988. Evaluation of intrathoracic extent of lung cancer by plain chest radiography, computed tomography, and magnetic resonance imaging. Am Rev Respir Dis 137:1456–1461.

90. Poon PY, Bronskill MJ, Henkelman RM. 1987. Mediastinal lymph node metastases from bronchogenic carcinoma: Detection with MR imaging and CT. Radiology 162:651–657.

91. de Geer G, Webb MR, Sollitto R. 1986. MR characteristics of benign lymph node enlargement in sarcoidosis and Castleman's Disease. Eur J Radiol 6:145–159.

92. Glazer GM, Orringer MB, Chenevert TL. 1988. Mediastinal lymph nodes: Relaxation time/pathological correlation and implications in staging of lung cancer with MR imaging. Radiology 168:429–435.

93. Kono M, Sako M, Adachi S. 1989. MR imaging in the assessment of lung cancer patients: Primary lung cancer staging, evaluation of therapeutic effect, and diagnosis of recurrent tumour. Hoshasen Gakai Zasshi 7:55–61.

94. Glazer GM, Gross BH, Aisen AM. 1985. Imaging of the pulmonary hilum: A prospective comparative study in patients with lung cancer. AJR 145:245–251.

95. Webb WR. 1986. Magnetic resonance imaging of the hila and mediastinum. Cardiovasc Intervent Radiol 8:306–311.

96. Bourgouin PM, McCloud TC, Fitzgibbon JE. 1991. Differentiation of bronchogenic carcinoma from post-obstructive pneumonitis by magnetic resonance imaging: Histopathologic correlation. J Thorac Imaging 6:22–28.

97. Shioya S, Haida M, Ono Y. 1988. Lung cancer: Differentiation of tumour, necrosis, and atelectasis by means of T1 and T2 values measured in vitro. Radiology 167:105–111.

98. Abrams HL, Spiro R, Goldstein N. 1950. Metastases in carcinoma. Analysis of 1000 cases. Cancer 41:74–85.

99. Matthews MJ, Kanhouwa S, Pickren J. 1973. Frequency of residual and metastatic tumours in patients undergoing curative surgical resection for lung cancer. Cancer Chem Rep 4:63–67.

100. Winstanley DP. 1968. Fruitless resections (abstract). Thorax 23:327.

101. Snow JH, Goldstein HM, Wallace S. 1979. Comparison of scintigraphy, sonography and computed tomography in the evaluation of hepatic neoplasms. AJR 132:915–918.

102. Lusins JO, Chayes Z, Nakagawa H. 1980. Computed tomography and radionuclide brain scanning: Comparison in evaluating metastatic lesions to the brain. NY Stat J Med 80:185–189.

103. Hooper RG, Tenholder MF, Underwood GH. 1984. Computed tomography scanning of the brain in the initial staging of bronchogenic carcinoma. Chest 85:774–776.

104. Nielson ME, Heaston DK, Dunnock NR. 1982. Preoperative CT evaluation of the adrenal glands in non-small cell bronchogenic carcinoma. AJR 139:317–320.

105. Chapman GS, Kumar D, Redmond J. 1982. Upper abdominal CT scanning in staging non-oat cell lung carcinoma (letter). N Engl J Med 315:189.

106. Sandler MA, Pearlberg KL, Madrazo BL. 1982. Computed tomographic evaluation of the adrenal gland in the preoperative assessment of bronchogenic carcinoma. Radiology 145:733–736.

107. Oliver TW, Bernardino ME, Miller JI, Mansour K, Greene D, Davis WA. 1984. Isolated adrenal masses in non-small cell bronchogenic carcinoma. Radiology 153:217–218.

108. Gillams A, Roberts CM, Shaw P, Spiro SG, Goldstraw P. 1992. The value of CT scanning and percutaneous fine needle aspiration of adrenal masses in biopsy-proven lung cancer. Clin Radiol 46:18–22.

109. Grant D, Edwards D, Goldstraw P. 1988. Computed tomography of the brain, chest, and abdomen in the preoperative assessment of non-small cell lung cancer. Thorax 43:883–886.

110. Sakio H, Yagamuchi Y. 1989. Trans-esophageal endoscopic ultrasonography in lung cancer involving mediastinal organs in the assessment of resectability. J Jpn Assoc Thorac Surg 37:650–657.

111. Hooper RG, Beechler CR, Johnson MC. 1978. Radioisotope scanning in the initial staging of bronchogenic carcinoma. Am Rev Respir Dis 188:279–286.

112. Ramsdell JW, Peters RM, Taylor AT. 1977. Multiorgan scans for staging lung cancer: Correlation with clinical evaluation. J Thorac Cardiovasc Surg 73:653–659.

113. Immerman SC, Vanecko RM, Fry WA. 1981. Site of recurrence in stage I and II carcinoma of the lung resected for cure. Ann Thorac Surg 32:23–27.

114. Kelly RJ, Cowan RJ, Ferree CB, Raben M, Maynard CD. 1979. Efficacy of radionuclide scanning in patients with lung cancer. JAMA 242:2855–2857.

115. White DM, McMahon LJ, Denny WF. 1982. Usefulness outcome in evaluating the utility of nuclear scans of the bone, brain, and liver in bronchogenic carcinoma patients. Am J Med Sci 283:114–118.

116. Kunkler IH, Merrick MV, Roger A. 1985. Bone scintigraphy in breast cancer. Clin Radiol 36:279–282.

117. Williams SJ, Green M, Kerr IH. 1975. Detection of bone metastases in carcinoma of the bronchus. Br Med J 274:1004–1006.

118. Donato AT, Ammerman EG, Sullesta O. 1979. Bone scanning in the evaluation of patients with lung cancer. Ann Thorac Surg 27:300–304.

119. Merrick MV, Merrick JM. 1986. Bone scintigraphy in lung cancer: A reappraisal. Br J Radiol 59:1185–1194.

120. DeMeester TR, Golomb HM, Kirschner P. 1979. The role of gallium-67 scanning in the clinical staging of patients with carcinoma of the lung. Ann Thorac Surg 28:451–455.

121. Alazraki NO, Ramsdell JW, Taylor A. 1978. Reliability of gallium scan chest radiography compared to mediastinoscopy for evaluating mediastinal spread of lung cancer. Am Rev Respir Dis 117:415–419.

122. Waxman AD, Julien PJ, Brachman MB. 1984. Gallium scintigraphy in bronchogenic carcinoma: the effect of tumour location on sensitivity and specificity. Chest 86:178–183.

123. Daniels AS. 1949. A method of biopsy useful in diagnosing certain intrathoracic diseases. Dis Chest 16:360–364.

124. Harken DE, Black H, Clauus R. 1954. Simple cervical mediastinal exploration for tissue diagnosis of intrathoracic disease. N Engl J Med 251:1041–1045.

125. Carlens E. 1959. Mediastinotomy: A method for inspection and tissue biopsy in the superior mediastinum. Dis Chest 36:343–347.

126. McNeil TM, Chamberlain JM. 1966. Diagnostic anterior mediastinotomy. Ann Thorac Surg 2:532–539.

127. Foster ED, Munro DD, Dobell ARC. 1972. Mediastinoscopy: a review of anatomical relationships and complications. Ann Thorac Surg 13:273–281.

128. Bowen TE, Zajtchuk R, Green DC. 1978. Value of anterior mediastinoscopy in broncho-genic carcinoma of the left upper lobe. J Thorac Cardiovasc Surg 76:269–274.
129. Funatsu T, Matsubara Y, Hatakenaka R, Koaba S, Yasuda Y, Ikeda S. 1992. The role of mediastinoscopic biopsy in preoperative assessment of lung cancer. J Thorac Cardiovasc Surg 104:1688–1695.
130. Specht VG. 1965. Erweiteite mediastinoskopie. Thoraxchirurgie 13:401–407.
131. Ginsberg RJ, Rice TW, Goldberg M, Waters PF, Schmocker BJ. 1987. Extended cervical mediastinoscopy. J Thorac Cardiovasc Surg 94:673–678.
132. Pugsley W, Kay PH, Goldstraw P. 1989. Diagnostic mediastinoscopy in superior vena caval obstruction. Thorax 44:339.
133. Lewis RJ, Sisler GE, Mckensie JW. 1981. Mediastinoscopy in advanced superior vena cava obstruction. Ann Thorac Surg 32:458–463.
134. Palva T, Palva A, Karja J. 1975. Re-mediastinoscopy. Arch Otolaryngol 101:748–752.
135. Lewis RJ, Sisler GE, Mckensie JW. 1984. Repeat mediastinoscopy. Ann Thorac Surg 37:147–152.
136. Meersschaut D, Vermassen F, Brutel de la Riviera A, Knaepen PJ, Van den Bosch JM, Vanderschueren R. 1992. Repeat mediastinoscopy in the assessment of new and recurrent lung neoplasm. Ann Thorac Surg 53:120–122.
137. Tsang GMK, Watson DCT. 1992. The practice of cardiothoracic surgeons in the peri-operative staging of non-small cell lung cancer. Thorax 47:3–5.
138. Fernando HC, Goldstraw P. 1990. The accuracy of clinical evaluative intrathoracic staging in lung cancer as assessed by postsurgical pathologic staging. Cancer 65:2503–2506.
139. Goldstraw P. 1991. Pretreatment minimal staging. Lung Cancer 6:186–190.
140. Goldstraw P, Mannam GC, Kaplan DK, Michail P. In press. Surgical management of NSCLC with ipsilateral mediastinal lymph node metastasis. J Thorac Cardiovasc Surg.
141. Gaer JAR, Goldstraw P. 1990. Intraoperative assessment of nodal staging at thoracotomy for carcinoma of the bronchus. Eur J Cardiothorac Surg 4:207–210.

254

12. The role of chest irradiation in small cell lung cancer

Rodrigo Arriagada, Jean-Pierre Pignon, and Thierry Le Chevalier

Introduction

Chest irradiation was the main treatment of small cell lung cancer (SCLC) before the 1970s; long-term survival was poor (below 5% at five years). From then on, chemotherapy began to be widely used for the treatment of SCLC. The high response rates yielded with chemotherapy gave rise to a controversy over the inclusion of chest irradiation in combination regimens; many physicians discarded its use in their therapeutic schedules, claiming that local radiotherapy barely offered a benefit, if any, and significantly increased treatment-related toxicity. When used alone, chemotherapy was able to achieve a moderate gain in long-term survival (approximately 8% at five years). However, it became obvious that even in the best series of patients treated with chemotherapy alone, thoracic local control remained a major problem, since more than 50% of chest recurrences continued to be observed after complete remission. A review of randomized trials showed that chest irradiation decreased the risk of thoracic recurrences and promised a gain in long-term survival of approximately 5% to 10% in limited disease [1–3]. This gain in long-term survival was recently confirmed by a comprehensive meta-analysis of 13 unconfounded randomized trials [4].

The demonstrated benefit in terms of overall survival supports the general use of combined radiotherapy and chemotherapy approaches as the standard treatment of limited SCLC. In this chapter, we will discuss treatment parameters in an attempt to delineate questions to be tested in future trials.

Chest irradiation and local failures

It is widely recognized that chest irradiation decreases the local failure rate. Chemotherapy alone may obtain up to 50% of complete responses; however, approximately half of these patients will develop local recurrences in the first two years of follow-up. Combined radio-chemotherapy approaches may obtain a complete response in up to 80% of patients, and in approximately one third of them disease will recur within two years [5].

Heine H. Hansen, (ed), Hansen: Lung Cancer.
© 1994 Kluwer Academic Publishers. ISBN 0-7923-2835-3. All rights reserved.

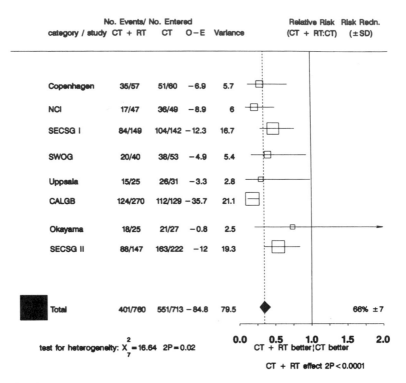

category / study	No. Events/ No. Entered		O−E	Variance	Relative Risk (CT + RT:CT)	Risk Redn. (±SD)
	CT + RT	CT				
Copenhagen	35/57	51/60	−6.9	5.7		
NCI	17/47	36/49	−8.9	6		
SECSG I	84/149	104/142	−12.3	16.7		
SWOG	20/40	38/53	−4.9	5.4		
Uppsala	15/25	26/31	−3.3	2.8		
CALGB	124/270	112/129	−35.7	21.1		
Okayama	18/25	21/27	−0.8	2.5		
SECSG II	88/147	163/222	−12	19.3		
Total	401/760	551/713	−84.8	79.5		66% ±7

test for heterogeneity: $X^2_7 = 16.64$ 2P = 0.02

0.0   0.5   1.0   1.5   2.0
CT + RT better ¦ CT better

CT + RT effect 2P < 0.0001

Figure 1. Literature-based review evaluating the effect of thoracic radiotherapy on the thoracic recurrence rate.

It was possible to estimate the effect of radiotherapy in eight published randomized trials comparing chemotherapy alone to the combination of chest irradiation and chemotherapy. The review of literature-based data including 1473 patients [6–12] is shown in figure 1. The overall odds ratio for the two-year local failure is 0.32 (0.26–0.40), indicating that the risk of local failure may be decreased threefold with the adjunction of chest irradiation; this effect is highly significant ($p < 10^{-5}$). Such results should be cautiously interpreted, since both the method used and publication bias may lead to an overestimation of the treatment effect [13,14].

Chest irradiation and overall survival

The effect of chest irradiation on survival remained controversial until the early 1990s, when a comprehensive meta-analysis based on individual data was performed on a series of 2140 patients with limited SCLC [4]. This study included 13 unconfounded randomized trials comparing chemotherapy alone to the combination of chest irradiation and chemotherapy. The overall

256

Table 1. Relative risks of deaths with chemotherapy and radiotherapy (CT + RT) compared to chemotherapy alone (CT), by radiotherapy–chemotherapy type of combination (sequential versus nonsequential)

Category/trial	No. dead/no. entered		O−E	Variance	Relative risk (95% CI)
	CT + RT	CT			
Sequential					
Sydney [15]	44/45	48/49	−8.2	21.7	0.68 (0.45–1.04)
London [16]	59/63	74/75	−7.9	32.5	0.78 (0.56–1.10)
SWOG [9]	43/47	46/56	4.0	21.6	1.20 (0.79–1.83)
SAKK [17]	35/36	32/34	0.6	16.6	1.04 (0.64–1.68)
Uppsala [10]	22/26	31/31	−4.5	12.5	0.70 (0.40–1.22)
ECOG [18]					
Okayama [12]	22/28	27/28	−4.8	12.0	0.67 (0.38–1.18)
GETCB [19]	14/19	12/17	1.0	6.4	1.18 (0.54–2.55)
Subtotal	361/395	391/423	−27.1	183.2	0.86 (0.75–1.00)
Nonsequential					
Copenhagen [6]	69/69	74/76	11.2	34.0	1.39 (0.99–1.95)
NCI [7]	46/48	46/49	−8.9	21.3	0.66 (0.43–1.01)
SECSG I [8]	123/153	111/142	−12.1	56.4	0.81 (0.62–1.05)
CALGB [11]	257/292	128/134	−20.0	75.9	0.77 (0.61–0.96)
SECSG II [8]	116/154	140/168	−10.4	63.1	0.85 (0.66–1.09)
Subtotal	611/716	499/569	−40.2	250.7	0.85 (0.75–0.96)
Total	972/1111	890/992	−67.3	433.9	0.86 (0.78–0.94)

The relative risk (RR) for individual trials and the pooled RR are given with their 95% confidence interval (CI; see [4] for details about statistical methods. The two chemotherapy plus radiotherapy arms of the CALGB trial (early chemotherapy plus radiotherapy, late chemotherapy plus radiotherapy) were grouped together for the analysis. For the ECOG trial, the RR is not shown because this trial has not been published, but it contributed to the overall RR. The test for heterogeneity was not significant ($x^2_{12} = 16.95$, $p = 0.15$), nor was the test for interaction ($x^2 = 0.02$, $p = 0.9$). The test for over all treatment effect was significant ($x^2 = 10.42$, $p = 0.001$).

results showed a reduction of 14% in mortality ($p = 0.001$) in favor of the combined approach, as shown in table 1. Until then, and because there was a mixture of 'positive' and 'negative' results, a controversy persisted regarding the true effect of chest irradiation on survival. The effect on mortality was translated into a 5.4% increase in the three-year survival rate (14.3% versus 8.9%). Radiotherapy afforded a greater benefit in patients under 55 years of age [4]. The overall effect observed represents a mean effect for the trials conducted from 1976 to 1988. It is worthwhile to note that 15 years elapsed between the initation of the first trial [6] and the acquisition of a definite answer. This time lag clearly illustrates the necessity of analyzing large numbers of patients when a moderate effect on survival is expected. Small and even moderately large trials do not have enough statistical power to detect such a difference.

It is likely that a major benefit could be obtained if treatment variables were optimal. To date, we are still unaware of which is the optimal combination. In our series [5], we recently demonstrated that chest recurrence is still the first main cause of failure. Chest irradiation and combined radiochemotherapy are composite parameters, and the analysis of their effects can be equivocal. Seven fundamental aspects have to be taken into account: 1) treatment toxicity; 2) volumes to be treated; 3) total tumor dose; 4) fraction size; 5) early versus late radiotherapy; 6) sequential versus nonsequential approaches; and 7) the quality of radiotherapy delivery.

Treatment toxicity

It should be borne in mind that a therapeutic gain will be offset by an increase in lethal toxicity. Toxic effects on normal tissues have always been the limiting factor in any therapeutic strategy whose aim is to eradicate malignant disease. Unfortunately, reports on toxicity are very heterogeneous, and it is difficult to have a clear idea of its intensity and extent. Combinations of CT and RT can produce severe and even life-threatening complications. We have chosen to report results in SCLC under the heading of causes of death unrelated to cancer, including deaths not directly related to treatment toxicity [2]. This procedure eliminates bias due to medical

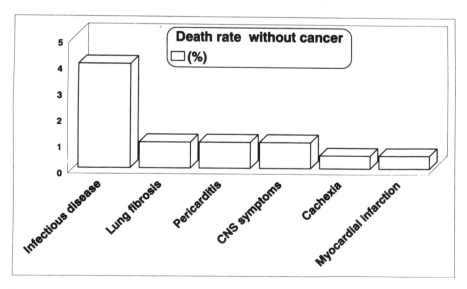

Figure 2. Alternating radiotherapy–chemotherapy protocols in limited small cell lung cancer (IGR and cooperating centers): death rates without cancer.

258

interpretation that can artificially reduce the rate of so-called lethal toxicity. For example, figure 2 shows the overall rate of death unrelated to cancer (8%) in 202 patients with limited SCLC treated at the Institut Gustave-Roussy and cooperative centers as developed below.

Severe complications have mainly been observed in the tissues located within the irradiated volume. It would be safer to avoid the administration of drugs such as bleomycin and doxorubicin, which are associated with an elective toxic effect on such tissues. However, other treatment parameters are closely associated with these interactions, and they will be discussed below.

Target tumor volume

The standard recommendation [20,21] is to treat the original tumor volume, i.e., before chemotherapy, with a 1.5–2 cm free-margin. However, this recommendation is only supported by retrospective studies. Only one prospective randomized trial, including 191 patients, focused on this subject [9]. The overall intrathoracic recurrence rate was 32% in the 'wide volume radiotherapy' arm compared to 28% in the 'reduced volume radiotherapy' arm; this difference was not significant. On the other hand, three retrospective studies on a total of 159 patients [22–24] showed that the use of inadequate portals could cause a two- to threefold increase in intrathoracic recurrences. This significant adverse effect could be related to major protocol variations, since the recurrence rates were over 50%. These data are summarized in table 2. Our own data [25] showed no increase in the local

Table 2. Intrathoracic recurrences according to tumor coverage

Author	n	Intrathoracic recurrence (%)	P value
Mantyla [22]			
— Original tumor volume	28	18	0.003
— Reduced tumor volume	24	58	
Perez [23]			
— Adequate portals	40	33	0.02
— Inadequate portals	13	69	
White [24]			
— Fully evaluable or minor variations	38	34	0.04
— Major protocols variations	16	69	
Kies [9]			
— Wide volume RT	93	32	N.S.
— Reduced volume RT	98	28	
Arriagada [25]			
— Adequate coverage	12	33	0.86
— Inadequate coverage	50	36	

relapse rate in the event of inadequate coverage — strictly defined — of the initial tumor: 36% versus 33% in the case of adequate coverage. This finding is in agreement with the results of the above-mentioned randomized trial, and it would suggest that tumor shrinkage after chemotherapy is sufficient to allow the tumor to be completely encompassed by 'inadequate' fields. We should not hastily conclude, however, that small fields should be recommended for the treatment of these patients. Retrospective series clearly indicate that very limited fields do not improve local control compared to treatments with chemotherapy alone. Three further arguments should be taken into account: 1) the difficulties encountered when attempting to define what adequate coverage means, 2) the relatively small number of patients included in these studies, and 3) the fact that the most frequent site of relapse was found inside the fields when the irradiation encompassed the initial tumor volume [25]. This finding is possibly indicative of an insufficient dose level [26,27].

The use of progressively shrinking fields could be proposed, but this technique has not been evaluated prospectively. The amount of the surrounding lung that should be treated after chemotherapy is important, inasmuch as it is closely linked to treatment toxicity and treatment failure. Further randomized and a priori well-defined studies, using strict definitions of initial and reduced tumor volumes specified by the individual investigators, are necessary to settle this issue.

Total radiation dose

The optimal radiation dose level remains an enigma, and only one randomized trial has been conducted on this subject [26]. The dose levels compared were low versus moderate: 25 Gy in 10 fractions over two weeks and 37.5 Gy in 15 fractions over three weeks. The authors concluded that the use of a higher dose seemed to delay rather than prevent thoracic recurrence. All other data are only provided by retrospective studies, and a summary is shown in table 3. Clearly, a total radiation dose of below 40 Gy will control local disease less effectively, but nothing can be affirmed regarding the effect of moderate (40–50 Gy) versus high dose (≥60 Gy) chest irradiation. In table 3, wide variations can also be observed in the local failure rate at each dose level. These variations are probably related to different definitions of local failure in each center: 1) recurrence after complete remission versus overall local failure, 2) overall failure versus first site of failure, or 3) methodology used to report the results: total, censored or competing event approaches [5]. Our own data [5,25] did not show a significant difference in long-term local control in four consecutive alternating radiochemotherapy protocols that delivered a total radiation dose ranging from 45 Gy to 65 Gy. However, it should be underlined that this was also a retrospective analysis based on a limited number of patients and that radiotherapy was delivered in three split courses. Clearly, there is room for a

Table 3. Total tumor dose delivered by thoracic radiotherapy in small cell lung cancer and overall local failure

Total tumor dose (Gy)		Overall local failure (%)
<40	[21]	79–100
40	[7,21,28]	23–43
45[a]	[5,21,29–32]	16–39
50	[21]	30
≥55[b]	[5]	33
60–65[b]	[5]	32

[a] Includes accelerated fractionation.
[b] Using alternating schedules.

randomized trial testing a moderate versus a high total radiation dose, for example, 40 Gy versus 65 Gy or the biological equivalent using nonconventional fractionation.

Fractionation schedule

Conventional fractionation, defined as 5 fractions of 2 Gy per week, allows a total radiation dose of as high as 70 Gy to be delivered in a limited mediastinal volume. The fraction size used in the 13 randomized trials included in the meta-analysis [4] varied between 2 and 4 Gy. A large fraction size could possibly account for the increased toxicity reported in some of these trials. The fraction size can be reduced and repeated a few hours later on the same day, and this procedure is termed hyperfractionated irradiation. With such a schedule, the overall treatment time remains the same, but the total dose is slightly higher. The Radiation Therapy Oncology Group (RTOG) has conducted trials in non-SCLC using fractions of 1.2 Gy twice daily and increasing the total dose up to 79 Gy in a limited volume [33]. The rationale for the use of this type of schedule has been extensively developed in the relevant literature [34,35], and is based on the premise that healthy normal tissue can be relatively spared while higher radiation doses can be delivered to tumor cells. This approach can be particularly interesting in 'pure' SCLC, as demonstrated by Mitchell et al. [36] with the survival curves obtained from cell cultures. Looney et al. [37] studied the possibility of integrating multifractionated radiotherapy in an alternating radiochemotherapy schedule in the rat hepatoma 3924A and concluded that a probable benefit could be gained for cure.

Some clinical studies have been conducted in limited SCLC [38,39–41]. The results are still preliminary but encouraging. The studies of Turrisi and Johnson are summarized in table 4. In the three studies, accelerated fractionation (1.5 Gy twice daily) was used, allowing 45 Gy to be delivered

Table 4. Pilot studies on concurrent bifractionated RT and CT in limited small cell lung cancer

Author	n	Chemotherapy	Dose RT (Gy/fraction)	Two-yr survival (%)
Turrisi [41]	32	Etoposide–cisplatin	45/30	48
Johnson [40]	38	Etoposide–cisplatin	45/30	65
ECOG [42]	41	Etoposide–cisplatin	45/30	36

in three weeks with the concurrent administration of etoposide and cisplatinum. In our experience [43], 29 patients were treated by an alternating radiochemotherapy schedule in which the first course of chest irradiation was given with accelerated hyperfractionation using reduced fields without treating the spinal cord. This first course consisted of a dose of 21 Gy given in fractions of 1.4 Gy three times daily. The results were not different from those observed with our previous protocols, but we registered a higher, although nonsignificant, incidence of death unrelated to cancer and probably related to treatment toxicity [5]. Two patients died with sepsis or infectious disease, one with heart failure, one with renal failure, and one with lung fibrosis [43]. There are two possible explanations for this toxicity: 1) a higher initial dose of cisplatinum (150 mg/m^2 given over five days); 2) a four-hour time gap between the three daily fractions. Currently, a time gap equal to or above six hours is recommended to permit the repair of sublethal lesions in normal tissues [35]. It should be noted that small changes may have an unexpected impact on toxicity, and this complicates the evaluation of different combined schedules. For instance, for the first four patients in this series, we used a dose of 25 Gy in the first multifractionated course. Three of the patients developed early and unusually severe esophagitis. By simply reducing the dose down to 21 Gy (16% of the multifractionated course dose and 6% of the total radiation dose), the ocurrence and intensity of the mucosa reaction reverted to previous levels.

Accelerated multifractionated radiotherapy is an interesting approach in the management of SCLC. However, its integration in combined schedules should be carefully planned and evaluated in prospective studies exploring toxicity, since small changes in treatment parameters may have an unexpected impact on early and late toxicity. A large randomized trial conducted by the ECOG is exploring this question [42].

Timing of chest irradiation

There are at least two theoretical reasons to prefer early chest irradiation to late irradiation. The first is the emergence of chemoresistant cells, and the second is tumor repopulation during treatment. If chemotherapy and chest irradiation have to be given sequentially and at full doses, the consequence

Table 5. Relative risks of deaths with CT + RT compared to CT, by radiotherapy timing (60 days or less versus more than 60)

Category/trial	No. dead/no. entered		O−E	Variance	Relative risk (95% CI)
	CT + RT	CT			
Early RT					
Seven trials	619/721	647/730	−41.0	307.5	0.88 (0.78−0.98)
Late RT					
Seven trials	353/390	371/396	−37.2	172.3	0.81 (0.69−0.94)
Total	972/1111	1018/1126	−78.2	479.8	0.85 (0.78−0.93)

Early trials included Copenhagen [6], NCI [7], SECSG I and II [8], CALGB [11], ECOG [18], and Okayama [12]. Late RT trials included Sydney [15], London [16], SWOG [9], SAKK [17], Upsala [10], CALGB [11], and GETCB [19]. The CALGB trial was included both in the comparison between early CT + RT versus CT and in the comparison of late CT + RT versus CT. This fact explains the change in the p value of the overall treatment effect. The test for heterogeneity was not significant ($x^2_{13} = 18.68$, $p = 0.13$), nor was the test for interaction ($x^2 = 0.76$, $p = 0.38$). The test for overall treatment effect was significant ($x^2 = 12.76$, $p = 0.0004$).

of this protracted administration may be a high level of tumor repopulation [35,44]. Occult distant metastases will continue to proliferate if the delivery of cytotoxic drugs is delayed. For example, if the tumor doubling time is 30 days, a delay of two months would permit a fourfold increase in the volume of metastases [44]. Chest irradiation cannot be delayed for too long because chemotherapy used alone often has a limited effect on bulky tumors and can even elicit the development of radioresistance. In view of the uncertainty regarding the extent of repopulation, the shortest delay between the two treatment modalities is advisable.

The indirect comparisons made in the SCLC meta-analysis [4] did not provide a definite answer to whether a preference should be given to early or late radiotherapy as shown in table 5. However, three randomized studies have directly tested this question [11,45,46]. The National Cancer Institute of Canada (NCIC) trial showed a significant difference ($p = 0.016$) in favor of early radiotherapy [45]. In the CALGB trial [11], there was a slight difference in favor of late radiotherapy, which may be explained by the nondelivery of full chemotherapy doses in the early chest irradiation arm due to increased acute toxicity. This finding suggests that initial full doses of chemotherapy may have an influence on survival observed in our experience [47−49]. The Danish trial [46] did not show a significant difference. For the time being, we consider that the use of early radiotherapy should be favored, but further research is needed to support this attitude.

We have previously analyzed theoretical and clinical reasons to prefer concurrent or alternating combinations to sequential delivery of both modalities [1,44,50]. The main advantage of concurrent combinations is that it is possible to deliver radiotherapy early and without intervals between both modalities. The National Cancer Institute (NCI) trial [7] reported a high incidence of complications and lethal toxicities in spite of the survival benefit obtained with the combined treatment. For a while, these results were a reference to avoid concurrent combinations. However, the high rate of complications, mainly esophageal reactions or strictures, may have been due to the use of a moderate concentrated radiation schedule (fractions of 2.66 Gy five times a week) and the administration of doxorubicin. These two factors were avoided in the two concurrent arms of the CALGB and the NCIC trials, and the toxicity observed seemed acceptable. In addition, some reports of pilot studies with similar schedules have demonstrated the feasibility of this kind of combination [40–42,51,52].

The alternating approach has been defined as 'combined modality therapy in which radiotherapy is given on days of the chemotherapy cycle in which no chemotherpay is administered, without any delay in chemotherapy beyond that which would occur if chemotherapy were being given alone' [1]. It was developed to reconcile the needs for early administration of both agents and for sequential delivery of each modality without a long interruption [44]. This alternating regimen is consistent with experimental data reported by Looney et al. [53] using a rat hepatoma model. Many experiments combining radiotherapy and cyclophosphamide have allowed an optimal schedule to be defined: alternating courses of cyclophosphamide with three courses of radiotherapy with an interval of seven days between each treatment modality. This treatment obtained a cure rate of 60% compared to 0% when the animals were treated by each single modality. The clinical investigation was developed simultaneously in the Institute Gustave-Roussy (IGR). The use of three split courses of chest irradiation in these schedules is open to criticism because of a decreased tumor effect due to tumor repopulation between the rest periods. This criticism is true for tumors responding poorly to cytotoxic agents, but, in SCLC, interdigitated chemotherapy probably precludes tumor repopulation between radiotherapy courses. The details of the therapeutic schedule have been previously published [54,55]. Chest irradiation started one week after completion of the second chemotherapy course and was given for 12 days with a rest of one week between both modalities. Three courses of chest irradiation alternated with chemotherapy, which was continued up to a total of six courses. A complete assessment including fiber-optic bronchoscopy was performed at the end of the induction to assess the response. The first pilot trial started in May 1980 at the IGR, and these studies were later extended to four cooperating centers. The summarized description of these trials, which included a total of 202 patients,

Table 6. Summary of alternating radiotherapy–chemotherapy protocols conducted at the IGR and cooperating centers

Protocol	002 (1980–81)	004 (1982–84)	006 (1985–86)	010 (1987–88)
Number of patients	28	81	64	29
Cyclophosphamide (mg/m^2)	300 × 4	300 × 4	300 × 3	300 × 4
Doxorubicin d1 (mg/m^2)	40	40	40	40
Etoposide (mg/m^2)	75 × 3	75 × 3	100 × 3	75 × 5
Methotrexate (mg/m^2)	400	—	—	—
Cisplatinum (mg/m^2)	—	100	120	30 × 5
Thoracic Rt (Gy)	15–15–15	20–20–15	20–20–25	21[a]–20–20
PCI (Gy)[b]	30	30	24[c]	24[c]
Maintenance CT (number of cycles)	12	8	6	0

[a] Multifractionated RT given by reduced radiation fields.
[b] Fractions of 3 Gy.
[c] Randomized for complete responders.

Table 7. Results of alternating radiotherapy and chemotherapy in limited small cell lung cancer (202 patients)

Protocol	002	004	006	010
Complete response rate (%)	86	78	69	79
Two-year RFS (%)	32	25	22	26
Two-year local control rate (%)	57	61	53	62
Two-year metastasis rate (%)	32	36	37	24
Death unrelated to cancer (%)	4	6	8	18

is shown in table 6. The main results are summarized in table 7. The five-year overall survival rate is 16%.

The alternation of radiotherapy–chemotherapy schedules is an interesting area of research worth developing in the coming years. The reproducibility of such schedules has been proven in different French centers, and they have been included in prospective trials. It must be recalled that this approach was also used in one of the randomized trials, which demonstrated a significant advantage with the combined approach [8].

Even if concurrent or alternating approaches promise a therapeutic gain, no randomized trial has been published comparing these combinations to sequential ones. The indirect comparisons effectuated in the SCLC meta-analysis [4] did not provide a definite answer when trials using sequential timing were compared to those using alternating or concurrent (nonsequential) schedules, as shown in table 1. However, direct comparisons within the framework of randomized trials should be preferred. One ongoing EORTC trial is comparing an alternating to a sequential combined radiochemotherapy schedule; the direct comparison between concurrent and alternating radio chemotherapy combinations is being explored by a French GETCB study. A very large number of patients will probably be needed to detect a significant difference between these schedules.

Quality of chest irradiation

All previous considerations are only valid if the quality of radiotherapy delivery is good. Poor-quality radiotherapy may overshadow benefits and increase toxicity. Modern megavoltage radiotherapy standards include 1) an unequivocal definition of the volumes to be treated, 2) an unequivocal definition of the tumor dose, 3) prechemotherapy simulator film and CT-scan-based planning, 4) optimal beam arrangement to cover the previous defined volume and to protect critical organs, 5) computer dosimetry to describe dose distribution, 6) checking of films in the treatment machine to ensure treatment reproducibility. Of course, these standards should be used in the randomized trials aimed at defining optimal treatment schedules.

Discussion

Progress in improving survival in limited SCLC has been slow during the last two decades. The change in standard treatment from chest irradiation alone to chemotherapy alone in the 1970s increased the five-year survival rate from roughly 5% to 10%. The combination of radiotherapy and chemotherapy in the 1980s yielded an additional benefit of 5%. These moderate effects on survival should be tested in randomized trials with a large number of patients. Small or medium-sized trials can result in equivocal answers or provide a mixture of 'positive' and 'negative' results; most of these contradictions may be due to statistical variations. Comprehensive meta-analyses using individual data may provide a solution to this problem [56]. A case in point is the study that evaluated the role of chest irradiation in limited SCLC [4]. One of the main merits of this study was to contradict the contention that meta-analysis is not a feasible means of evaluating the treatment effect in lung cancer [57]. It also showed the advantages of meta-analyses based on individual data rather than on a review of the literature [14]. The above-mentioned study [4], summarized in table 1, concluded that chest irradiation affords a survival benefit of 5% to 6% at three years; this is the mean effect of 13 randomized trials comprising more than 2000 patients. The next step will be to determine the optimal combined radiochemotherapy schedule. One question has been answered, but many others are now emerging, since the combined approaches are multiparametric. It is inherent to scientific knowledge that each step forward generates new problems that are ever increasing in depth [58].

For the time being, we are not able to define the optimal combination

266

required to treat limited SCLC. However, we think that the most appropriate treatment for this disease is chemotherapy containing etoposide–cisplatin, and probably cyclophosphamide, with chest irradiation at a minimal total dose of 50 Gy with a conventional fractionation schedule or its radiobiological equivalent. This chest irradiation should be delivered without a delay in chemotherapy using a concurrent or alternating combined schedule.

In this chapter, we have discussed some aspects of what optimal chest irradiation and what the timing of optimal radiochemotherapy could be. It is interesting to note that we are looking for moderate effects. However, hundreds of patients are needed to test differences between two treatment attitudes. It would be useless to compare very similar treatments, considering the number of patients required; years of research would be lost with this type of strategy. Treatments with rather extreme differences should be investigated (e.g., moderate versus high radiation doses, conventional versus unconventional fractionation, sequential versus nonsequential schedules) in order to test the validity of our hypotheses. It is in the interest of our patients that we should investigate the new questions raised, so as to optimize the management of SCLC with combined modalities, by conducting large randomized trials in the next few years.

Acknowledgments

The authors wish to thank all trialists who collaborated in the meta-analysis on the role of chest irradiation in limited small cell lung cancer [4]. They also thank the Centre Hospitalier Intercommunal de Créteil, the Hôpital A. Béclère, and the Fondation Bergonié participants in the IGR SCLC protocols, Mrs. M. Tarayre for data collecting, Mrs. G. Feris for secretarial assistance, and Ms. L. Saint Ange for editing the manuscript. The IGR SCLC 010 protocol was partially supported by the research grants INSERM/CNAMTS No. 883063 and ECC No. ST-A-000309.

References

1. Arriagada R, Bertino JR, Bleehen NM, Brodin O, Feld R, Goldie JH, Hansen HH, Ihde DC, Le Chevalier T, Souhami RL, workshop participants. 1988. Consensus report on combined radiotherapy and chemotherapy modalities in lung cancer. In Treatment Modalities in Lung Cancer: Vol. 41: Antibiotic Chemotherapy. Karger: Basel, pp. 232–241.
2. Arriagada R, Pignon JP, Le Chevalier T. 1989. Thoracic radiotherapy in small cell lung cancer: rationale for timing and fractionation. Lung Cancer 5:237–247.
3. Payne D, Arriagada R, Dombernowsky P, Evans WK, Giaccone G, Holsti L, Johnson D, Mc Vie G, Sculier JP, Smyth J. 1989. The role of thoracic radiation therapy in small cell carcinoma of the lung: a consensus report. Lung Cancer 5:135–138.
4. Pignon JP, Arriagada R, Ihde DC, Johnson DH, Perry MC, Souhami RL, Brodin O, Joss RA, Kies MS, Lebeau B, Onoshi T, Österlind K, Tattersall MHN, Wagner H. 1992. A

meta-analysis of thoracic radiotherapy for small cell lung cancer. N Engl J Med 327:1618–1624.

5. Arriagada R, Kramar A, Le Chevalier T, De Cremoux H, for the French Cancer Centers' Lung Group. 1992. Competing events determining relapse-free survival in limited small-cell lung carcinoma. J Clin Oncol 10:447–451.

6. Österlind K, Hansen HH, Hansen HS, Dombernowsky P, Hansen M, Rorth M. 1986. Chemotherapy versus chemotherapy plus irradiation in limited small cell lung cancer. Results of a controlled trial with 5 years follow-up. Br J Cancer 54:7–17.

7. Bunn PA Jr, Lichter AS, Makuch RW, Cohen MH, Veach SR, Matthews MJ, Anderson AJ, Edison M, Glatstein E, Minna JD, Ihde DC. 1987. Chemotherapy alone or chemotherapy with chest radiation therapy in limited stage small cell lung cancer: a prospective randomized trial. Ann Intern Med 106:655–662.

8. Birch R, Omura GA, Greco FA, Perez CA. 1986. Patterns of failure in combined chemotherapy and radiotherapy for limited small cell lung cancer: Southeastern Cancer Study Group experience. In Conference on the Interaction of Radiation Therapy and Chemotherapy, RE Wittes and CN Coleman (eds.). NCI Monogr 6:265–270.

9. Kies MS, Mira JC, Livingston RB, Crowley JJ, Chen TT, Pazdur R, Grozea PN, Rikvin SE, Coltman CA, Ward JH, Livingston RB. 1987. Multimodal therapy for limited small cell lung cancer. A randomized study of induction combination chemotherapy with or without thoracic radiation in complete responders; and with widefield versus reduced volume radiation in partial responders. J Clin Oncol 5:592–600.

10. Nou E, Brodin O, Bergh JA. 1988. A randomized study of radiation treatment in small cell bronchial carcinoma treated with two types of four-drug chemotherapy regimens. Cancer 62:1079–1090.

11. Perry MC, Eaton WL, Propert KJ, Ware JH, Zimmer B, Chahinian AP, Skarin A, Carey RW, Kreisman H, Faulkner C, Comis R, Green MR. 1987. Chemotherapy with or without radiation therapy in limited small cell carcinoma of the lung. N Engl J Med 316:912–918.

12. Onoshi T, Hiraki S, Kimura I. 1987. Randomized trial of chemotherapy alone or with chest irradiation in limited stage small cell lung cancer. In Cancer Chemotherapy: Challenges for the Future, K Kimura, K Ota, RB Herberman, and H Takita (eds.). Amsterdam, Excerpta Medica: Amsterdam, pp. 186–191.

13. Stewart LA, Parmar MKB. 1993. Meta-analysis of the literature or of individual patient data: is there a difference? Lancet 341:418–422.

14. Pignon JP, Arriagada R. 1993. Meta-analysis (letter). Lancet 341:964–965.

15. Rosenthal MA, Tattersall MHN, Fox RM, Woods RL, Brodie GN. 1991. Adjuvant thoracic radiotherapy in small cell lung cancer: ten-year follow-up of a randomized study. Lung Cancer 7:235–241.

16. Souhami RL, Geddes DM, Spiro SG, Harper PG, Tobias JS, Mantell BS, Fearon F, Bradbury I. 1984. Radiotherapy in small cell cancer of the lung treated with combination chemotherapy: a controlled trial. Br Med J 288:1643–1646.

17. Joss R, Alberto P, Bleher E, Kapansi Y, Cavalli F. 1985. Combined modality treatment of small cell lung cancer: randomized comparison of three induction chemotherapies followed by maintenance chemotherapy with or without radiotherapy to the chest (abstract). In Proceedings Fourth World Conference on Lung Cancer, Toronto, p. 141.

18. Creech R, Richter M, Finkelstein D. 1988. Combination chemotherapy with or without consolidation radiation therapy for regional small cell carcinoma of the lung (abstract). Proc Am Soc Clin Oncol 7:196.

19. Lebeau B, Chastang C, Brechot JM. 1991. Small cell lung cancer: negative results of a randomized clinical trial on delayed thoracic radiotherapy administered to complete responders patients (abstract). Lung Cancer 7(Suppl):94.

20. Bleehen NM. 1986. Radiotherapy for small cell lung cancer. Chest 89:268S–276S.

21. Choi NC. 1983. Reassessment of the role of radiation therapy relative to other treatments in small-cell carcinoma of the lung. In Thoracic Oncology, NC Choi and HC Grillo (eds.). Raven Press: New York, pp. 233–256.

22. Mantyla M, Nuranen A. 1985. The treatment volume in radiation therapy of small cell lung cancer (Abstract 473). IV World Conference of Lung Cancer, Toronto, p. 34.
23. Perez CA, Krauss S, Bartolucci AA, Durant JR, Lowerbraun S, Salter MM, Storaasli J, Kellermeyer R, Comas F, and the Southeastern Cancer Group Study. 1981. Thoracic and elective brain irradiation with concomitant or delayed multiagent chemotherapy in the treatment of localized small cell carcinoma of the lung: a randomized prospective study by the Southeastern Cancer Study Group. Cancer 47:2407–2413.
24. White JE, Chen T, MacCracken J, Kennedy P, Seydel MG, Hartman G, Mira J, Khan J, Durrance FY, Skinner O. 1982. The influence of radiation therapy quality control on survival, response and sites of relapse in oat cell carcinoma of the lung. Preliminary report of a Southwest Oncology Group Study. Cancer 50:1084–1090.
25. Arriagada R, Pellae-Cosset B, Cueto Ladron de Guevara J, El Bakry H, Benna F, Martin M, de Cremoux H, Baldeyrou P, Cerrina ML, Le Chevalier T. 1991. Alternating radiotherapy and chemotherapy schedules in limited small cell lung cancer: analysis of local chest recurrences. Radiother Oncol 20:91–98.
26. Coy P, Hodson BM, Payne D, Evans WK, Feld R, Macdonald AS, Osoba D, Pater JL. 1987. The effect of dose of thoracic irradiation on recurrence in patients with limited stage small cell lung cancer. Initial results of a Canadian Multicenter randomized trial. Int J Radiat Oncol Biol Phys 14:219–226.
27. Perez CA, Bauer M, Edelstein S, Gillespie BW, Birch R. 1986. Impact of tumor control on survival in carcinoma of the lung treated with irradiation. Int J Radiat Oncol Biol Phys 12:539–547.
28. Perez CA, Einhorn L, Oldham RK, Greco FA, Cohen HJ, Silberman H, Krauss S, Hornback N, Comas F, Omura G, Salter M, Keller JW, Mclaren J, Kellermeyer R, Storaasli J, Birch R, Dandy M. 1984. Randomized trial of radiotherapy to the thorax in limited small-cell carcinoma of the lung treated with multiagent chemotherapy and elective brain irradiation: a preliminary report. J Clin Oncol 2:1200–1208.
29. Einhorn LH, Crawford J, Birch R, Omura G, Johnson DH, Greco FA. 1988. Cisplatin plus etoposide consolidation following cyclophosphamide, doxorubicin, and vincristine in limited small-cell lung cancer. J Clin Oncol 6:451–456.
30. McCracken JD, Janaki LM, Crowley JJ, Taylor SA, Shankir Giri PG, Weiss GB, Gordon W, Baker LH, Mansouri A, Kuebler JP. 1990. Concurrent chemotherapy/radiotherapy for limited small-cell lung carcinoma: A Southwest Oncology Group Study. J Clin Oncol 8:892–898.
31. Shank B, Scher H, Hilaris BS, Pinsky C, Martin M, Wittes RE. 1985. Increased survival with high-dose multifield radiotherapy and intensive chemotherapy in limited small cell carcinoma of the lung. Cancer 56:2771–2778.
32. Turrisi AT, Glover DJ. 1990. Thoracic radiotherapy variables: influence on local control in small cell lung cancer limited disease. Int J Radiat Oncol Biol Phys 19:1473–1479.
33. Cox JD, Azarnia N, Byhart RW, Shin KH, Emami B, Pajak TF. 1990. A randomized phase I/II trial of hyperfractionated radiation therapy with total doses of 60.6 Gy to 79.2 Gy: possible survival benefit with ≥69.6 Gy in favorable patients with stage III non-small cell lung carcinoma: report of Radiation Therapy Oncology Group 83–11. J Clin Oncol 8:1543–1555.
34. Tubiana M. 1988. Repopulation in human tumors. A biological background for fractionation in radiotherapy. Acta Oncol 27:83–88.
35. Withers HR, Taylor JMG, Maciejewski B. 1988. The hazard of accelerated tumor clonogen repopulation during radiotherapy. Acta Oncol 27:131–146.
36. Mitchell JB, Morstyn G, Russo A, Carney DN. 1985. In vitro radiobiology of human lung cancer. Cancer Treat Symp 2:3–10.
37. Looney WB, Hopkins HA. 1988. The integration of multifractionated radiotherapy into combined chemotherapeutic-radiotherapeutic approaches to lung cancer treatment. In Treatment Modalities in Lung Cancer, R Arriagada and T Le Chevalier (eds.). Karger: Basel. Antibiot Chemother 41:176–183.

38. Choi NC, Propert K, Carey R, Eaton W, Leone LA, Silberfarb P, Green M. 1987. Accelerated radiotherapy followed by chemotherapy for locally recurrent small-cell carcinoma of the lung. A phase II study of Cancer and Leukemia Group B. Int J Radiat Oncol Biol Phys 13:263–266.
39. Hodson DI, Malaker K, Meikle AL, Levitt M. 1984. Pilot studies of superfractionated radiotherapy and combination chemotherapy in limited oat cell carcinoma of the bronchus. Int J Radiat Oncol Biol Phys 10:1941–1945.
40. Johnson BE, Grayson J, Woods E, Gazdar AF, Anderson M, Lesar M, Linnoila I, Minna JD, Glatstein E, Ihde DC. 1989. Limited stage small cell lung cancer treated with concurrent etoposide/cisplatin plus bid chest radiotherapy. Proc Am Soc Clin Oncol 8:228.
41. Turrisi AT, Glover DJ, Mason BA. 1988. A preliminary report: concurrent twice-daily radiotherapy plus platinum-etoposide chemotherapy for limited small cell lung cancer. Int J Radiat Oncol Biol Phys 15:183–187.
42. Turrisi AT, Wagner H, Glover D, Mason B, Oken M, Bonomi P. 1990. Limited small cell lung cancer: concurrent bid thoracic radiotherapy with platinum-etoposide: an ECOG study (abstract). Proc Am Soc Clin Oncol 9:230.
43. Arriagada R, Pellae-Cosset B, Baldeyrou P, Monet I, Ruffie P, Hanzen C, Tarayre M, Le Chevalier T. 1991. Initial high dose chemotherapy and multifractionated radiotherapy in limited small cell lung cancer (abstract). Lung Cancer 7(Suppl):159.
44. Tubiana M, Arriagada R, Cosset JM. 1985. Sequencing of drugs and radiation. The integrated alternating regimen. Cancer 55:2131–2139.
45. Murray N, Coy P, Pater JL, Hodson I, Arnold A, Zee BC, Kostashuk EC, Evans WK, Dixon P, Sudura A, Feld R, Levitt M, Wierbicki R, Ayoub J, Maroun JA, Wilson KS. 1993. Importance of timing for thoracic irradiation in the combined modality treatment of limited-stage small cell lung cancer. J Clin Oncol 11:336–344.
46. Nielsen OS, Fode K, Bentzen SM, Schultz HP, Steenholdt S, Palshof T. 1991. Timing of radiotherapy and chemotherapy in limited stage small cell lung cancer. Final analysis (abstract). Eur J Cancer 2(Suppl):S182.
47. Arriagada R, De The H, Le Chevalier T, Thomas F, Ruffie P, De Cremoux H, Martin M, Duroux P, Dewar JA, Sancho-Garnier H. 1989. Limited small cell lung cancer: a possible prognostic impact of initial chemotherapy doses. Bull Cancer 76:605–615.
48. De Vathaire F, Arriagada R, De The H, Tarayre M, Ruffie P, Chomy P, De Cremoux H, Sancho-Garnier H, Le Chevalier T. 1993. Dose intensity of initial chemotherapy may have an impact on survival in limited small cell lung carcinoma. Lung Cancer 8:301–308.
49. Arriagada R, Le Chevalier T, Pignon JP, Riviere A, Monnet I, Chomy P, Tuchais C, Tarayre M, Ruffie P. 1993. Initial chemotherapy doses and survival in limited small cell lung cancer. N Eng J Med 329:1848–1852.
50. Arriagada R, Cosset JM, Le Chevalier T, Tubiana M. 1990. The value of adjunctive radiotherapy when chemotherapy is the major curative method. Int J Radiat Oncol Biol Phys 19:1279–1284.
51. Kwiatkowski DJ, Propert KJ, Carey RW, Choi N, Green M. 1987. A phase II trial of cyclophosphamide, etoposide and cisplatin with combined chest and brain radiotherapy in limited small-cell-lung cancer: a Cancer and Leukemia Group B Study. J Clin Oncol 5:1874–1879.
52. Murray N, Shah A, Brown E, Kostashuk E, Laukkanen E, Goldie J, Band P, Van den Hoek J, Murphy K, Sparling T, Noble M. 1986. Alternating chemotherapy and thoracic radiotherapy with concurrent Cisplatin-Etoposide for limited-stage small cell carcinoma of the lung. Semin Oncol 13:24–30.
53. Looney WB. 1988. Special lecture: alternating chemotherapy and radiotherapy. NCI Monogr 6:85–94.
54. Arriagada R, Le Chevalier T, Baldeyrou P, Pico JL, Ruffie P, Martin M, El Bakry HM, Duroux P, Bignon J, Lenfant B, Hayat M, Rouesse JG, Sancho-Garnier H, Tubiana M. 1985. Alternating radiotherapy and chemotherapy schedules in small cell lung cancer, limited disease. Int J Radiat Oncol Biol Phys 11:1461–1467.

270

55. Le Chevalier T, Arriagada R, De The H, De Cremoux H, Martin M, Baldeyrou P, Ruffie P, Benna F, Cerrina ML, Sancho-Garnier H, Hayat M. 1988. Combination of chemotherapy and radiotherapy in limited small cell lung carcinoma: Results of alternating schedule in 109 patients. NCI Monogr 6:335–338.
56. Early Breast Cancer Trialists' Collaborative Group. 1990. Treatment of early breast cancer, Vol. 1. Worldwide evidence 1985–1990. Oxford Medical Publications: Oxford.
57. Nicolucci A, Grilli R, Alexanian AA, Apolone G, Torri V, Liberati A. 1989. Quality, evolution, and clinical implications of randomized, controlled trials on the treatment of lung cancer. A lost opportunity for meta-analysis. JAMA 262:2101–2107.
58. Popper KR. 1989. Conjectures and Refutations. The Growth of Scientific Knowledge (5th ed.). Routledge Publishers: London.

13. The role of hematopoietic growth factors in small cell lung cancer: a review

Véronique N. Trillet-Lenoir

Introduction

Small cell lung cancer (SCLC) is the model of a highly chémosensitive although still noncurable tumor. Very high response rates, including 30% to 50% complete responses, result in a less than 10% long-term disease-free survivalship. Therefore, many attempts have been made in order to optimize the administration of chemotherapy in this setting, but the therapeutic results seem to have reached a plateau roughly one decade ago. The availability of hematopoietic growth factors may offer the opportunity to test new concepts and to define new therapeutic goals with the use of chemotherapy in SCLC.

Hematopoietic growth factors in cancer treatment

Introduction

The control of hematopoietic stem cell renewal, commitment, proliferation, and differentiation is ensured by a complex regulatory network involving both stimulating and inhibiting mediators. Colony stimulating factors (CSFs) have been identified because of their ability to stimulate the growth of various colonies of differenciated blood cells in in vitro semisolid cultures of bone marrow cells [1]. Purification techniques led to the discovery of four major distinct human CSFs with overlapping effects on the stem cells of the granulocyte-macrophage lineage: multi-CSF interleukin 3 (IL3), Granulocyte Macrophage-CSF (GM-CSF), Granulocyte-CSF (G-CSF) and Macrophage-CSF (M-CSF). Figure 1 shows the respective target cells of each of the four main human CSFs. During the last decade, the genes encoding for these cytokines have been identified, allowing the production of recombinant CSF [2–6]. This has allowed precise identification of the structural features of the CSFs, which appeared to be glycoproteins of various molecular weights and conformations (see table 1). Specific membrane receptors are detectable on the cell surface of target hematopoïetic cells, and have been cloned and

Heine H. Hansen, (ed), Hansen: Lung Cancer.
© 1994 Kluwer Academic Publishers. ISBN 0-7923-2835-3. All rights reserved.

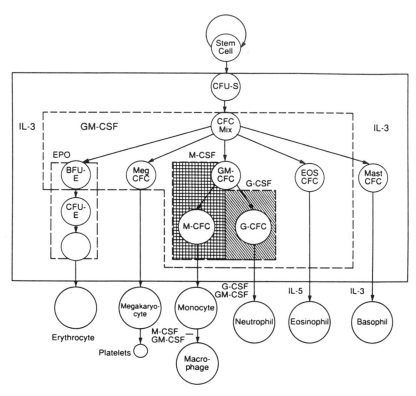

Figure 1. Regulation of hematopoietic cell development by hematopoietic growth factors. Reproduced from [84].

Table 1. The human colony-stimulating factors

Factor	Acronym	Molecular weight of core protein	Molecular weight of glycosylated protein	Chromosomal location of gene
Granulocyte-macrophage colony stimulating factor	GM-CSF	14,700	18,000–30,000	5q21–q31
Granulocyte colony stimulating factor	G-CSF	18,600	20,000	17q21–q32
Macrophage colony stimulating factor	M-CSF	21,000 (×2 dimer)	70,000–90,000	5q33.1
Multipotential colony stimulating factor (interleukin-3)	Multi-CSF (IL-3)	15,400	15,000–30,000	5q21–q31

Reproduced from [5].

274

identified. Above all, the availability of recombinant CSF has permitted testing of their potential clinical use, that is, their ability to stimulate hematopoiesis in vivo. This ability was initially demonstrated in hamsters [7] and primates [8,9] before the clinical trials started in humans [1,10,11]. Preliminary phase I/II trials in cancer patients have demonstrated a dramatic increase in the number of circulating granulocytes as a result of the use of G-CSF [12] or GM-CSF [13] in patients with either cancer or acquired immunodeficiency syndrome.

Clinical use

Effects on hematopoiesis. Within 30 minutes of administration of either G-CSF or GM-CSF, a transient decrease in peripheral blood neutrophils is observed, which is thought to be due to endothelial margination. A substantial dose-dependant increase above normal level occurs 5 to 6 hours later that is related to peripheral demargination, accelerated cell proliferation, and stimulation of bone marrow release. The effects on white cells counts differ between G-CSF, which is essentially responsable for an increase in neutrophils, and GM-CSF, which also affects eosinophils, monocytes, and macrophages counts. The cell counts usually fall to normal 24 to 48 hours after withdrawal of the growth factor administration.

Endogenous G-CSF levels are increased during neutropenia, while GM-CSF and IL3 are not [14]. The latter compounds are probably only released at the site of infection and involved in the prolonged attraction of the neutrophils [15]. In fact, the functional capacities of G-CSF released neutrophils appear very similar to those of normal cells, whereas GM-CSF treatment might be associated with a substantial reduction in the phagocytic and chemotactic functions [16]. These differences are probably related to different mechanisms of actions: while GM-CSF acts by shortening the committed progenitor cell half-life [17], G-CSF is more directly involved in the proliferation of more mature cells.

Toxicity. G-CSF administration is associated with very few adverse effects. Musculoskeletal pain in the medullary areas (mainly pelvis, back and inferior limbs) is observed in roughly 15% of the patients [18]. Transient increases in lactate dehydrogenase, alkaline phosphatases, transaminases, and uric acid have been described, as well as a decrease in serum cholesterol.

GM-CSF administration may induce bone pain as well as fever and, at least at high dosages, a capillary leak syndrome including multivisceral fluid retention and hypotension. However, GM-CSF appears to be extremely well-tolerated in children [19].

Clinical applications. Such a strong capacity to induce the stimulation of myelopoiesis has been extensively tested on chemotherapy-induced neutropenia [20], the duration and deepness of which are known to be strongly

275

related to the infectious risk in cancer patients [21,22]. So far, the only available published data from closed clinical trials concern the use of G-CSF and GM-CSF.

Using recombinant intravenous (IV) G-CSF at doses ranging from 1 to $60 \mu g/kg$, prior to melphalan $25 \, mg/m^2$ given as a single-drug chemotherapy, Morstyn et al. [23] demonstrated a dose-dependent rise in circulating neutrophils up to $80 \, 10^9/l$. The same team later on described the subcutaneous route as equally effective for G-CSF [24]. In this latter study, they concluded that administration of G-CSF prior to chemotherapy did not reduce the duration of neutropenia, and that a single dose of $10 \mu g/kg/$ day given after chemotherapy for seven days was sufficient to abrogate melphalan-related neutropenia. Antman et al. [25] used escalating doses of GM-CSF following a combination of Doxorubicin $20 \, mg/m^2/day$, Ifosfamide $2500 \, mg/m^2/day$, and Dacarbazine $300 \, mg/m^2/day$ for three days continuous infusion, in a series of 16 patients with metastatic sarcomas. As a control, the second course was given without GM-CSF support. In addition to a significant increase in leukocyte and granulocyte counts, these authors were able to demonstrate a significantly less severe and prolonged neutropenia after the first cycle compared to the second one. The maximum recommended dosage of GM-CSF was $32 \mu g/kg/day$ because of limiting capillary toxicity.

The potential benefit of G-CSF and GM-CSF on hematopoietic adverse effects of high-dose myeloablative chemotherapy regimen followed by autologous bone marrow transplantation rescue has also been studied. In the trial performed at Duke University [26], GM-CSF was given in adjunction to a combination of cyclophosphamide $1875 \, mg/m^2/day$ for three days, cisplatin $165 \, mg/m^2$ for four days, and carmustine $600 \, mg/m^2$ on one day. Chemotherapy was immediately followed by the reinfusion of a previously cryopreserved bone marrow, and GM-CSF was started three hours later and delivered as a 14-day continuous IV infusion at escalating doses ranging from 2 to $32 \mu g/kg/day$. Dose increases of GM-CSF were limited by the development of fluid retention. Leukocyte-count recovery was accelerated when compared to the data from a series of historical controls [26]. These results have been confirmed in a randomized double-blinded placebo-controlled trial using high doses of various chemotherapeutic agents (including cyclophosphamide, etoposide, carmustin, cytarabine, and hydroxyurea) with or without total body irradiation and followed by autologous bone marrow transplantation for lymphoid neoplasia [27]. One hundred and twenty-eight patients were randomly assigned to receive either GM-CSF $250 \mu g/m^2/day$ or a placebo, starting from graft and during 21 days through a two-hour daily IV infusion. The neutrophil recovery to $0.5 \, 10^9/l$ was shortened by seven days in the GM-CSF treated group, which resulted in significantly fewer infections, days of antibiotics (from 27 to 24), and days of hospitalization (from 33 to 27). A similar reduction of the neutropenic period associated with high doses of oral busulphan ($4 \, mg/kg/day$ for four days) and cyclophosphamide (60 mg/kg/day for two days) followed by autologous bone marrow rescue was demonstrated on a series of 15 patients by the Royal Melbourne Hospital team using continuous subcutaneous G-CSF (starting 20 µg/kg/day and gradually decreasing based on the neutrophils counts). The delay to neutrophil recovery ($0.5 \ 10^9/l$) was shortened (to mean day 11 versus day 20) compared to an historical control group of 18 patients, as were the number of days of antibiotic treatment (from 18 to 11) and severe mucositis [28].

The capacity of the CSFs to mobilize hematopoietic cells progenitors into the peripheral blood is also of potential clinical usefulness. The harvest of such recruited cells may be obtained by leukopheresis and their reinfusion after separation, and cryoconservation may be performed in adjunction to (and possibly instead of) marrow cells reinfusion. Using such a technique, both granulocytic and platelet reconstitution may be substantially accelerated, as demonstrated by Gianni and coworkers [29]. In this series of seven patients, peripheral blood stem cells (PBSCs) were recruited after GM-CSF administration at the dose of 5.5 µg/day continuous IV infusion for 14 days. Intensive chemotherapy consisted of high doses of vincristin, methotrexate, etoposide, melphalan, and total body irradiation. Myeloablative treatment was followed by the reinfusion of GM-CSF-recruited stem cells plus bone marrow cells, and additional GM-CSF was started 24 hours later at the previously described dosage during 10 to 11 days. The mean times to $0.5 \ 10^9/l$ neutrophils and $50 \ 10^9/l$ platelets were 9 days and 10 days, respectively. The comparison with a control group of seven patients receiving simultaneously the same treatment program without GM-CSF showed a substantial reduction in the severity of mucositis.

Such an accelerated hematopoietic recovery after high doses busulphan (4 mg/kg/day per os for 4 days) plus cyclophosphamide (60 mg/kg/day IV for two days) was demonstrated by the previously cited Australian group using autologous bone marrow plus G-CSF-mobilized PBSC reinfusion followed by G-CSF at a dose of 12 µg/kg/day for six days. The neutrophils as well as the platelet counts recovered significantly faster ($50 \ 10^9/l$ platelet counts reached with a median of 15 days versus 39, $p = 0.0006$) than in a nonrandomized control group receiving the same treatment apart from the reinfusion of PBSCs [30].

Hematopoietic growth factors and small cell lung cancer

Standard induction treatment of SCLC consists in the use of a combined chemotherapy regimen, with marrow aplasia being the main and limiting toxicity. Lethal infectious complications of combination chemotherapy occur in 5% of the patients, and life-threatening sepsis is observed in 13% [31]. Febrile neutropenia often results in dose reductions and/or delays associated with a substantial risk of compromising the treatment results. Therefore,

SCLC has often been chosen as a tumor model to test the potential clinical consequences of the previously described effects of hematopoietic growth factors on chemotherapy-induced neutropenia. In addition, in vitro data had raised the question of a potential facilitating effect of G-CSF and GM-CSF on SCLC cell proliferation. Investigations into the clinical use of hematopoietic growth factors in the treatment of SCLC therefore required the setting of large, carefully designed prospective clinical trials.

Effects on neutropenia and neutropenia-related complications

Nonrandomized trials. In 1987, Bronchud et al. [32] initiated a phase I/II study on 12 patients with SCLC. In the phase I part of the study, no toxicity was seen with continuous infusion G-CSF given at escalating doses of, respectively, 1, 5, 10, 20, and 40 µg/kg/day. G-CSF administration resulted in a rapid increase in the neutrophil counts at all five dosages without any detectable effect on platelets, monocytes, eosinophils, or lymphocytes. In the phase II part of the study, starting one week later, patients received cytotoxic chemotherapy consisting in ifosfamide $5 g/m^2$, mesna $8 g/m^2$, and doxorubicin $50 mg/m^2$ on day one and Etoposide $120 mg/m^2$ on days 1 to 3, every three weeks. G-CSF was given for 14 days starting on day 4, on alternate cycles of chemotherapy and at the same dosage as in the phase I part for a given patient. With each patient taken as his own control, G-CSF considerably reduced the period of neutropenia and allowed the absolute neutrophils count to return to normal two weeks after the start of chemotherapy. Furthermore, while six severe infectious complications occured during the cycles without G-CSF, none were observed during G-CSF treatment.

A similar study was repeated in SCLC using GM-CSF at doses ranging from 50 to $500 µg/m^2$/day as a single subcutaneous injection on odd or even cycles of the same chemotherapy as in Bronchud's trial. A significant reduction ($p = 0.04$) in the duration of neutropenia was observed during cycles followed by GM-CSF. However, in this study, GM-CSF failed to determine any difference on the incidence of febrile neutropenic episodes [16]. This failure might be due either to a preferential mobilization of immature nonfunctional stem cells by GM-CSF or to the ability of GM-CSF to increase the neutrophils' half-life rather than their production.

Different dose schedules of subcutaneous GM-CSF were also evaluated in combination with carboplatin $100 mg/m^2$ and etoposide $120 mg/m^2$ given for three days in 18 patients with SCLC. A dose of $15 µg/kg/day$ starting on day 4 and given for a maximum of 14 days was considered optimal to reduce the incidence of neutropenia by half, as compared to a historical control [33].

Randomized trials. Two large, randomized, placebo-controlled clinical trials have been conducted, one in the United States on 199 patients [34] and one in Europe on 129 patients [18], to demonstrate the potential ability of G-

Table 2. Reduction in the incidence of febrile neutropenia in two randomized trials comparing G-CSF versus placebo after chemotherapy for SCLC [18,34]

	Placebo		G-CSF	
	U.S. trial	European trial	U.S.trial	European trial
N	104	64	95	65
FN (%) cycle 1	55	41	30	20
FN (%) overall	77	53	40	26

FN = Febrile neutropenia.

CSF to reduce the infectious risk and associated complications of conventional CDE chemotherapy in limited and extensive SCLC. In both studies, treatment consisted of six cycles of chemotherapy (cyclophosphamide $1 \, g/m^2$ on day 1, doxorubicin $50 \, mg/m^2$ on day 1, and etoposide $120 \, mg/m^2$ on day 1 to 3) repeated every three weeks. Before starting treatment, patients were randomly assigned to receive after each course of chemotherapy either G-CSF at the dose of $230 \, \mu g/m^2$ or a placebo administered daily and subcutaneously from day 4 to day 17 (or until the postnadir neutrophil count exceeded $10 \times 10^9/l$ after day 12). In both studies, the incidence of neutropenic fever (defined as the simultaneous observation of fever $\geqslant 38.2°C$ and absolute neutrophil count $<1.0 \times 10^9/l$) is significantly reduced in the G-CSF arm. The percentage reduction is similar in both trials — roughly 50% after the first course — as well as when considering overall cycles, as shown in table 2. The median duration of neutropenia and the median neutrophil nadir observed after the first cycle are also significantly reduced in both studies. Consequently, there is a significant decrease of the requirement for parenteral antibiotics use and re-hospitalizations due to infectious problems, expressed as mean number of days of treatment [34] or as percentages of patients treated [18]. For instance, in the European trial, the requirement for IV antibiotics was 58% versus 37% ($p < 0.02$) and the need for rehospitalizations 58% versus 39%. The incidence of culture-confirmed infections was 33% in the placebo arm and 20% in the G-CSF arm.

The preliminary results of a third non-placebo-controlled randomized study on 39 SCLC patients receiving CODE (cisplatin, vincristin, doxorubicin, and etoposide) chemotherapy alone or followed by G-CSF $50 \, \mu g/m^2/day$ also showed a significant reduction in the duration of leukopenia from 10 to 2 days [35]. According to Crawford [15], an interim analysis on the first 62 enrolled patients would show even a higher difference in the incidence of neutropenic events than in the previously cited studies (77% versus 37% in the G-CSF arm).

As far as GM-CSF is concerned, the potential reduction of infectious consequences of cytotoxic chemotherapy for SCLC was questioned in two German trials. In the non-randomized study by Drings et al. [36],

$250\,\mu g/m^2$ subcutaneous GM-CSF reduced the neutropenic period following a combined treatment with ifosfamide, vincristin, and doxorubicin and lowered the incidence of infections requiring antibiotics. Additional data come from the preliminary results of a large, randomized, controlled German trial on 148 patients planned to receive six courses of chemotherapy given every 21 days [37]. The treatment consists of cyclophosphamide $1\,g/m^2$ on day 1, doxorubicin $40\,mg/m^2$ on day 1, and etoposide $80\,mg/m^2$ on days 1 to 3 randomly followed by 0, 10, or $20\,\mu g/m^2$ GM-CSF administered subcutaneously from day 4 to day 13. After the first cycle, there is a significant reduction in the median neutrophil nadir and in the duration of neutropenia in the GM-CSF treated arms compared to the placebo arm. However, these data are still preliminary and need to be reconsidered at the end of the trial, since the ability of GM-CSF to have any impact on the infectious consequences of chemotherapy-induced neutropenia has recently been questioned in the above described study by Gurney et al. [16].

Absence of negative impact on response and survival after conventional chemotherapy

The presence of specific receptors to G-CSF [38], GM-CSF [39], and IL3 [40] has been identified on the cell surface of SCLC cell lines, although this finding has not been confirmed by all authors [41]. Furthermore, various histologic types of lung cancers have been shown to produce CSFs [42–44], including SCLC cell lines [45]. Therefore, the clinical use of these hematopoietic growth factors has raised the question of their potential proliferative effect on the tumor cells, which might negatively influence tumor response and survival. In vitro data are very controversial concerning the potential stimulatory effects of the three major CSFs on SCLC clonal tumor growth [39,40,45–47]. This crucial question had to be clearly solved in cautiously designed randomized controlled trials.

Despite the choice of identical treatment modalities and judgment criteria, the two randomized, fully published studies using G-CSF differ by a major modification in the study design performed in the European trial. Whereas any occurrence of neutropenic fever resulted in treatment unblinding and discontinuation of placebo treatment in both studies, the North American trial used a crossover method that allowed the placebo-treated patients to receive G-CSF at this time, while in the European trial, G-CSF was continued only in the G-CSF arm. For this reason, more than 75% of the patients received G-CSF for at least one cycle in the U.S. trial, a situation that does not allow any conclusions regarding the above-mentioned potential negative effects of G-CSF. The European study brings an additional comparison of the antitumor effect of chemotherapy between the two arms and shows no statistical difference between response rates or survival data. Therefore, no negative effect of G-CSF administration towards the antitumoral effects of chemotherapy was shown. Interestingly, while no significant difference was detected between the two groups in terms of response, the response duration and survival would appear superior for the G-CSF arm in the Japanese study [15]. However, these preliminary results on 62 patients have to be confirmed with longer follow-up.

Overall, such results suggest a significant benefit of hematopoietic growth factors in terms of quality of life and safety for patients with SCLC who are receiving conventional chemotherapy. However, we know from Bunn et al. [48,49] that a randomized phase III study trial comparing concurrent chemotherapy (cisplatin $25 \, mg/m^2$ plus etoposide $60 \, mg/m^2$ on days 1 to 3) and chest radiotherapy with or without GM-CSF for limited-stage SCLC had to be stopped after a planned interim analysis: lower response rates (63 versus 80%) and increased toxicity were observed in the GM-CSF arm, including seven episodes of acute pulmonary toxicity versus none. Patients treated with GM-CSF presented reduction in granulocytopenia, but they had 'more infections, more febrile days and a significantly increased granulocytopenia.' Although the precise mechanisms of such an increased toxicity are not yet elucidated, much caution is recommended in the use of GM-CSF in combination with radiotherapy.

Optimal dose-on-time delivery of chemotherapy

Significant differences in the percentages of chemotherapy dose reductions and delays are seen between the G-CSF and the placebo arm in the above-described European trial. In fact, the rules for dosing and timing chemotherapy were based on the occurrence of a neutropenic fever during the previous cycle. The significant reduction of this complication allows G-CSF to decrease the percentage of patients receiving at least one course reduced by more than 15%, from 61% to 37%, and the percentage of patients undergoing at least one delay of more than two days from 47% to 29%. As a consequence, the calculation of dose intensities actually received for each of the three neoplastic drugs shows a slight increase (roughly 10%) in favor of the G-CSF arm. However, as we have shown, such a small increase in dose intensity did not influence response rates or survival curves in this trial. The preliminary results of the ongoing Japanese randomized study showed that the 18 patients receiving G-CSF were more likely to receive the planned treatment on schedule than the 14 patients without G-CSF support (83% versus 57%).

In the German trial with GM-CSF [37], full-dose chemotherapy can be administered during the four first cycles in a significantly higher percentage of patients receiving the growth factor as compared to the placebo group. The dose intensity of cyclophosphamide, as well as of the entire combination, is increased by 10%.

Favaretto et al. [50] have compared in a nonrandom fashion a group of 21 patients (A) with SCLC receiving cisplatin $60 \, mg/m^2$ day 1, etopside $120 \, mg/m^2$ days 1 to 3, and epidoxorubicin at escalating dosages every 21 days and a further group of 20 patients receiving the same treatment combined with GM-CSF 10 μg/m^2 from days 4 to 14. The maximum tolerated dose (MTD) of epidoxorubicin was 60 mg/m^2 in group A and 70 mg/m^2 in group B. The percentage of planned received cycles was 72% in group A and 89% in group B, and the percentage of dose-reduced cycles was 14% in group A and 2% in group B. Consequently, the relative dose intensity of chemotherapy was increased by 26% for cisplatin and etoposide and 56% for epidoxorubicin in group B compared to group A. Furthermore, the complete response rate was significantly increased in group B, a finding that has to be validated in a randomized phase III trial.

Such an improvement in dose-on-time administration of chemotherapy programs should be prospectively tested for its potential ability to improve the therapeutic results in SCLC as well as in other tumor models in which the same effect of hematopoietic growth factors has been demonstrated. In bladder cancer, for instance, Gabrilove et al. [51] have shown the ability of G-CSF to significantly increase (from 29% to 100%) the percentage of patients qualified to receive M-VAC chemotherapy (methotrexate, vinblastin, doxorubicin, and cisplatin) on day 14 as planned in the treatment program. In patients with malignant lymphomas treated by VAPEC-B chemotherapy (vincristin, doxorubicin, prednisolone, etoposide and cyclophosphamide), the number of patients requiring dose delays is significantly reduced (by half) in the G-CSF group as compared to a control group, as well as the median duration of cycles delays (from 8 to 0 days) and the percentage of patients having at least one dose reduction (from 33% to 10%). Here again, these results led to a 10% increase of dose intensities of doxorubicin, etoposide, and cyclophosphamide [52].

Dose escalation and dose intensity

Because the emergence of very efficient mechanisms of drug resistance appears to be the main obstacle to the curability of SCLC, many attempts have been made to try to circumvent chemoresistance by escalating the doses. Therefore, the concept of a dose–response relationship in SCLC has been extensively tested. A number of randomized studies comparing conventional chemotherapy given at various doses have been published [53–56]. Although most groups have shown a significant improvement in complete response rates, only two have found a significant increase in survival. We must note, however, that both these studies compared low versus standard doses rather than standard versus high doses. The potential impact of intensive chemotherapy has been tested using high myeloablative regimens followed by autologous bone marrow transplantation rescue given as induction therapy [57] or as consolidation in sensitive tumors [58]. These two nonrandomized pilot trials resulted in very promising response rates and survival durations. However, because inclusion in such aggressive therapeutic programs requires a very strict selection of patients, these data had to be confirmed by larger randomized trials. Therefore, Humblet et al. [59] further designed a randomized trial comparing late intensification with high-dose chemotherapy followed by autologous bone marrow transplantation to conventional maintenance therapy in patients responding to induction treatment. Although both the complete remission rate and relapse-free survival were significantly increased, these authors failed to show any significant difference in overall survival, partly because of a very high lethal toxicity. In fact, SCLC is usually seen in a population of aged patients with past history of tobacco smoking and related compromised cardiovascular and pulmonary function, and only a fraction of these patients are suitable for clinical trials based on highly hematotoxic treatments.

Neither the U.S. nor the European randomized trial comparing G-CSF versus placebo was designed to test any dose intensification. Assessment of response and survival was performed to look for any possible negative impact of G-CSF, but the planned dose intensities were initially similar in both arms. Slight differences in dose intensities were only due to the ability of the growth factor to improve the dose-on-time delivery. In no case could these differences be considered as relevant dose modifications.

The availability of hematopoietic growth factors has enabled the design of new dose-escalation studies in SCLC. Luikart et al. [60] have performed a phase I/II study with escalating doses of carboplatin and etoposide and have shown that the MTD has not been reached in three patients receiving carboplatin $125 \, mg/m^2$ plus etoposide $200 \, mg/m^2$ both given on days 1 to 3 every 21 days if adjuvant GM-CSF was administered at a dose of $5 \, \mu g/kg$ twice daily from days 4 to 18. Interestingly, the same drug dosages and even lower dose intensities were much less tolerable when GM-CSF was given as a unique dose of 20 or $10 \, \mu g/kg/day$. Fujita et al. [61] have used G-CSF ($2 \, \mu g/kg/day$ subcutaneously from days 4 to 17) to perform another trial using a fixed dose of etoposide ($100 \, mg/m^2 \times 3$) in combination with escalated doses of carboplatin (from 400 to $700 \, mg/m^2$). The limiting toxicity appears to be thrombopenia, but the MTD has still not been reached at $650 \, mg/m^2$, and the trial is still ongoing. Masuda and co-workers [62] have administered high doses of etoposide ($500 \, mg/m^2/day$ for three days) and cisplatin (80 to $120 \, mg/m^2$ day 1) to 20 patients with recurring SCLC, five of whom additionally received $50 \, \mu g/m^2/day$ subcutaneous G-CSF daily until the resolution of leukopenia. The overall results on 18 evaluable patients were not considered as superior to standard doses of chemotherapy in this setting, since the overall response rate was 50% and the median survival 20 weeks. There were two treatment-related deaths, and G-CSF did not help to shorten the duration of severe neutropenia. By contrast, a combination of high doses of cisplatin and etoposide ($35 \, mg/m^2$ and $200 \, mg/m^2$, respectively) given for three days every 21 days with GM-CSF $10 \, \mu g/m^2$ from days 4 to 13 was considered as infeasible because of limiting hematopoietic toxicity in the six first patients, and none of the planned dose escalations was performed

283

[63]. Dose escalations have successfully been performed using cyclophospha-mide $2.5\,g/m^2$/day for two days plus etoposide $500\,mg/m^2$ for three days plus cisplatin $50\,mg/m^2$ for three days followed by GM-CSF at various dosages ranging from 250 to $1000\,\mu g/m^2$. GM-CSF shortened the duration of neutro-penia, but hematopoietic toxicity remained severe [64].

During the last 10 years, the knowledge of the dose–response relationship has improved, and the importance of timing has been emphasized. The concept of *dose intensity*, that is, the dose of a given drug per units of time, generally expressed as mg/m^2/week, has emerged from the work by Hryniuk et al. [65].

The above-cited phase II and phase III studies have demonstrated the remarkable ability of G-CSF [18,32,34] and GM-CSF [25] to allow acce-lerated neutrophil-count recovery after cytotoxic chemotherapy. Since the adjunction of hematopoietic growth factors allows the timing of sequential chemotherapy to become a potentially adjustable parameter, their use pro-vides new ways to explore the relationships between dose intensity and therapeutic results in solid tumors such as SCLC. Accelerated chemotherapy with the support of hematopoietic growth factors allows a substantial potential increase in dose intensity without dose-per-cure escalation, and various time intervals between two consecutive chemotherapy cycles are currently been tested by many groups. In fact, such an approach requires carefully designed feasibility trials, since both hematologic and nonhema-tologic side effects may result from dose intensification. For instance, high doses of doxorubicin (up to $150\,mg/m^2$) may be administered every two weeks with G-CSF (instead of every three weeks without) in patients with advanced breast and ovarian cancer, and the response rates are encouraging. However, there is a significant epithelial toxicity [66].

Ardizzoni et al. [67] have recently published the results of a phase II trial testing the ability of GM-CSF $10\,\mu g/kg$/day for 10 days to allow administra-tion of a CDE-derived chemotherapy every two weeks instead of every three weeks in SCLC. Using such a timing, the theoretical dose-intensity increase is 50%. However, only 6 out of the 15 tested patients were able to complete the six planned courses of chemotherapy with an effective dose intensity ranging from 87% to 97% of the theoretical dose intensity. Among the remaining nine patients, the main reason for prematurely stopping chemotherapy was thrombocytopenia. Thirteen patients received at least four courses of chemotherapy with a median percentage of dose intensity actually received to planned intensity of 96%. Interestingly, the median ratio of achieved dose intensity in these 13 patients compared to a conven-tional three-week regimen is 1.44 (range 1.21–1.54).

We are currently performing a similar feasibility trial using slightly higher dosages of doxorubicin and etoposide in combination with ifosfamide fol-lowed by G-CSF $5\,\mu g/m^2$ for 10 days and administered every two weeks instead of every three weeks. Another study is ongoing in England using the same dosages of CDE as in the European randomized trial, with G-CSF support at a fixed dose of 300 µg/day to reduce intervals between cycles from three to two weeks (J. Green, personal communication).

If these trials confirm that the toxicity on the megacaryocytic lineage is limiting, further exploration of dose intensity based on variations of the timing rather than the dose per cure might require the use of platelet-specific growth factors such as IL3 [68] or IL1 [69] or the use of PBSCs. The procedures to collect and store hematopoietic growth-factor-recruited stem cells to be reinfused after myeloablative chemotherapy have already been tested in a range of malignancies, including SCLC [70]. Repeated courses of high doses of cyclophosphamide ($2.5\,g/m^2$/day $\times$ 2), etoposide ($300\,mg/m^2$/day $\times$ 3), and cisplatin ($50\,mg/m^2$/day $\times$ 3) have been made possible by the use of sequential harvesting and reinfusion of PBSCs in SCLC [71]. A pilot study using such an accelerated chemotherapy with PBSCs in selected patients with SCLC is underway in Europe (S. Leyvraz, personal communication).

Unsolved questions

Although the potential usefulness of hematopietic growth factors, especially G-CSF and GM-CSF, has been extensively tested during the past few years, many points still need to be clarified.

Optimal doses, schedules, and administration routes are still to be determined. A dose−effect relationship has been shown for the increase in leukocyte counts, although it remains unclear whether dose escalation has any clinical impact on the neutropenia-related consequences of chemotherapy. As far as G-CSF is concerned, some authors have claimed that a G-CSF dose of $50\,µg/m^2$/day for 14 days was adequate for moderately myeloablative regimen given to patients with lung cancer, including 11 previously treated SCLC patients receiving cisplatin ($80\,mg/m^2$ day 1) and etoposide ($300\,mg/m^2$ day 1) alternating with cyclophosphamide ($1\,g/m^2$ day 1), doxorubicin ($40\,mg/m^2$ day 1), and vincristin ($1\,mg/m^2$ day 1) [72]. On the other hand, the minimal effective dose seems to be $100\,µg/m^2$ for patients with high-grade lymphomas [73]. As already mentioned, twice-daily doses of GM-CSF might increase its efficiency [60]. Optimal schedules remain to be defined for both G-CSF and GM-CSF. For the latter compound, most studies favor a $250\,µg/m^2$ or $5\,µg/kg$ twice a day administration on days 4 to 11 or 4 to 14 after chemotherapy [49,74]. Whether or not a fixed dose should be given without considering the patients' body areas is being questioned for G-CSF in the ongoing British trial. If the content of a single vial could be universally used, the ambulatory management of the compound would be greatly improved. The subcutaneous route is widely used in adults, since it induces greater and more prolonged effects on neutropenia than the IV route.

The effects on other hematopoietic lineages appear to be different for G-

CSF and GM-CSF. As far as G-CSF is concerned, no difference in the percentage of thrombopenias or the mean platelets nadirs could be shown both in the North American and in the European randomized trial on SCLC. There are some arguments in favor of a potential substantial effect of GM-CSF on platelets [19,75] that have been demonstrated in some [76], but not all [37], randomized studies.

Because of the high cost of recombinant growth factors, and despite the proven ability of G-CSF to significantly reduce the incidence of neutropenia-related infectious complications, one has to make sure that this benefit remains superior to the use of a prophylactic antibiotic treatment. At least two large randomized trials addressing this question in patients receiving conventional chemotherapy are underway in North America and Canada [15] as well as in the EORTC [76]. A Spanish group has recently shown that the addition of G-CSF or GM-CSF to standard antibiotic therapy was associated with a significant decrease in morbidity as well as in treatment cost in a randomized trial [77].

Repeated courses of myelotoxic chemotherapy rescued by recombinant CSF might induce hematopoietic stem cells depletion, thus resulting in 'bone marrow exhaustion.' This result has been demonstrated in bone marrow cells from mice treated for six cycles with cyclophosphamide followed by GM-CSF [78]. No available data testing this hypothesis can be obtained from the above-cited randomized trials, in which the significantly lower neutrophil nadirs during cycle 6 as compared to cycle 1 were attributed to significantly less frequent dose reductions in the G-CSF arm as compared to the placebo arm. Only clinical studies based on sequential chemotherapy without dose reductions will be able to answer the question of potential long-term damage to the stem cell compartment due to the repeated use of CSFs in humans. Interestingly, this adverse effect might be prevented by prechemotherapy treatment with IL1 [78,79].

There are some reports in the literature concerning a potential antitumor effect of GM-CSF, possibly mediated through the macrophage system [80]. Of particular interest in lung cancer is the fact that GM-CSF induces both expression of messenger RNA and secretion of tumor necrosis factor, interleukin 1, and interleukin 6 in alveolar macrophages and blood monocytes from the patients [81].

It seems that future improvement in the clinical use of CSFs will come from various combinations of these compounds and other cytokins. The synergistic effects of IL3 and GM-CSF upon progenitor cells have already been demonstrated in primates, and the fusion protein PIXY 321 [82] is currently being tested in humans. Multipotent cells might be even more stimulated by the combined use of IL6, IL3, and GM-CSF, for instance, or by the stem cell factor. However, very cautious and systematic assessment of any potential proliferative effect in tumor stem cells will have to be performed at each step of this fascinating cascade of new therapeutic compounds [83].

Last but not least, one must keep in mind that the most relevant aim of the use of hematopoietic growth factors should be a substantial benefit for survival. A new opportunity to test the dose-intensity concept in SCLC has been given to the oncologic community. So far, most of the clinical trials described above have been conducted on too few patients to draw any firm conclusions about the ability of hematopoietic growth factors to increase significantly the dose intensities and to test their potential benefit on survival. Whatever the method to escalate the doses is — increased dosages, accelerated treatments, use of growth factors' recruited PBSCs, autologous bone marrow transplantation — future studies should focus on potentially relevant increases in dose intensities. Any feasible dose-intense treatment should then be translated into a large enough randomized trial to be able to answer the crucial question of any effect on survival in SCLC.

References

1. Metcalf D. 1991. Control of granulocytes and macrophages: molecular, cellular and clinical aspects. Science 254:529–533.
2. Clark SC, Kamen R. 1987. The human hematopoietic colony-stimulating factors. Science 236:1229–1237.
3. Metcalf D. 1989. Peptide regulatory factors. Lancet i:825–827.
4. Platzer E. 1989. Human hemopoietic growth factor. Eur J Haematol 42:1–15.
5. Metcalf D. 1990. The colony stimulating factors. Cancer 65(10):2185–2195.
6. Demetri GD, Griffin JD. 1991. Granulocyte colony-stimulating factor and its receptor. Blood 78(11):2791–2808.
7. Cohen AM, Zsebo KM, Inoue H, Hines D, Boone TC, Chazin VR, Tsai L, Rich T, Souza LM. 1987. In vivo stimulation of granulopoiesis by recombinant human granulocyte colony-stimulating factor. Proc Natl Acad Sci USA 84:2484–2488.
8. Donahue RE, Wang EA, Stone DK, Kamen R, Wong GG, Sehgal PK, Nathan DG, Clark SC. 1986. Stimulation of haematopoiesis in primates by continuous infusion of recombinant GM-CSF. Nature 321:872–875.
9. Welte K, Bonilla MA, Gillio AP, Boone TC, Potter GK, Gabrilove JL, Moore AS, O'Reilly RJ, Souza LM. 1987. Recombinant human granulocyte colony-stimulating factor. J Exp Med 165:941–948.
10. Laver J, Moore AS. 1989. Clinical use of recombinant human hematopoietic growth factors. J Natl Cancer 81:1370–1382.
11. Devereux S, Linch DC. 1989. Clinical significance of the haemopoietic growth factors. Br J Cancer 59:2–5.
12. Dührsen U, Villeval JL, Boyd J, Kannourakis G, Morstyn G, Metcalf D. 1988. Effects of recombinant human granulocyte colony-stimulating factor on hematopoietic progenitor cells in cancer patients. Blood 72(6):2074–2081.
13. Groopman JE, Mitsuyasu RT, DeLeo MJ, Oette DH, Golde DW. 1987. Effect of recombinant human granulocyte-macrophage colony stimulating factor on myelopoiesis in acquired immunodeficiency syndrom. N Engl J Med 317:593–598.
14. Kawano Y, Takaue Y, Saito S, Sato J, Shimizu T, Suzue T, Hirao A, Okamoto Y, Abe T, Watanabe T, Kuroda Y, Kimura F, Motoyoshi K, Asano S. 1993. Granulocyte colony-stimulating factor (CSF), macrophage-CFS, granulocyte-macrophage-CSF, interleukin-3, and interleukin-6 levels in sera from children undergoing blood stem cell autografts. Blood 81(3):856–860.

15. Crawford J, Green MR. 1992. The role of colony stimulating factors as an adjunct to lung cancer chemotherapy: a commentary. Lung Cancer 8:153–158.
16. Gurney H, Anderson H, Radford J, Potter MR, Swindell R, Steward W, Kamthan A, Chang J, Weiner J, Thatcher N, Crowther D. 1992. Infection risk in patients with small cell lung cancer receiving intensive chemotherapy and recombinant human granulocyte-macrophage colony-simulating factor. Eur J Cancer 28(1):105–112.
17. Lord BL, Gurney H, Chang J, Thatcher N, Crowther D, Dexter TM. 1993. Haemopoietic cells kinetics in humans treated with rGM-CSF. Int J Cancer 50:26–31.
18. Trillet-Lenoir V, Green J, Manegold C, Von Pawel J, Gatzemeier U, Lebeau B, Depierre A, Johnson P, Decoster G, Tomita D, Ewen C. 1993. Recombinant granulocyte colony stimulating factor reduces the infectious complications of cytotoxic chemotherapy. Eur J Cancer 29A(3):319–324.
19. Furman WL, Fairclough DL, Huhn RD, Pratt CB, Stute N, Petros WP, Evans WE, Bowman LC, Douglass EC, Santana VM, Meyer WH, Crist WM. 1991. Therapeutic effects and pharmacokinetics of recombinant human granulocyte-macrophage colony-stimulating factor in childhood cancer patients receiving myelosuppressive chemotherapy. J Clin Oncol 9(6):1022–1028.
20. Groopman JE, Molina JM, Scadden DT. 1989. Hematopoietic growth factors. N Engl J Med 321(21):1449–1459.
21. Bodey GP, Buckley M, Sathe YS, Freireich EJ. 1966. Quantitative relationships between circulating leucocytes and infection in patients with acute leukemia. Ann Int Med 64(2): 328–340.
22. Pizzo PA. 1984. Granulocytopenia and cancer therapy. Cancer 54(11):2649–2661.
23. Morstyn G, Souza LM, Keech J, Sheridan W, Campbell L, Alton NK, Green M, Metcalf D, Fox R. 1988. Effect of granulocyte colony stimulating factor on neutropenia induced by cytotoxic chemotherapy. Lancet i:667–672.
24. Morstyn G, Campbell L, Lieschke G, Layton JE, Maher D, O'Connor M, Green M, Sheridan W, Vincent M, Alton K, Souza L, McGrath K, Fox RM. 1989. Treatment of chemotherapy-induced neutropenia by subcutaneously administered granulocyte colony-stimulating factor with optimization of dose and duration of therapy. J Clin Oncol 7(10): 1554–1562.
25. Antman KS, Griffin JD, Elias A, Socinski MA, Ryan L, Cannistraa SA, Oette D, Whitley M, Frei E, Schnipper LE. 1988. Effect of recombinant human granulocyte-macrophage colony-stimulating factor on chemotherapy-induced myelosuppression. N Engl J Med 319(10):593–598.
26. Brandt SJ, Peters WP, Atwater SK, Kurtzberg J, Borowitz MJ, Jones RB, Shpall EJ, Bast RC, Gilbert CJ, Oette DH. 1988. Effect of recombinant human granulocyte-macrophage colony-stimulating factor on hematopoietic reconstitution after high dose chemotherapy and autologous bone marrow transplantation. N Engl J Med 318(14):869–876.
27. Nemunaitis J, Rabinowe SN, Singer JW, Bierman PJ, Vose JM, Freedman AS, Onetto N, Gillis S, Oette D, Gold M, Buckner D, Hansen JA, Ritz J, Appelbaum FR, Armitage JO, Nadler LM. 1991. Recombinant human GM-CSF after autologous bone marrow transplantation for lymphoid cancer. N Engl J Med 324:1773–1778.
28. Sheridan WP, Morstyn G, Wolf M, Dodds A, Lusk J, Maher D, Layton JE, Green MD, Souza L, Fox RM. 1989. Granulocyte colony stimulating factor and neutrophil recovery after high-dose chemotherapy and autologous bone marrow transplantation. Lancet 2:891–895.
29. Gianni AM, Siena S, Bregni M, Tarella C, Stern AC, Piler A, Bonadonna G. 1989. Granulocyte-macrophage colony stimulating factor to harvest circulating haemopoietic stem cells for autotransplantation. Lancet 2:580–585.
30. Sheridan WP, Glenn Begley C, Juttner CA, Szer J, Bik To L, Maher D, McGrath KM, Morstyn G, Fox RM. 1992. Effect of peripheral-blood progenitor cells mobilised by filgrastim (G-CSF) on platelet recovery after high-dose chemotherapy. Lancet 339(14): 640–644.

288

31. Radford JA, Ryder WD, Dodwell D, Anderson H, Thatcher N. 1993. Predicting septic complications of chemotherapy: an analysis of 382 patients treated for small cell lung cancer without dose reduction after major sepsis. Eur J Cancer 29(1):81–86.

32. Bronchud MH, Scarffe JH, Thatcher N, Crowther D, Souza LM, Alton NK, Testa NG, Dexter TM. 1987. Phase I/II study of recombinant human granulocyte colony-stimulating factor in patients receiving intensive chemotherapy for small cell lung cancer. Br J Cancer 56:809–813.

33. Morstyn G, Stuart-Harris R, Bishop J, Raghavan D, Kefford R, Lieschke G, Bonnem E, Olver I, Green M, Rallings M, Fox R. 1989. Optimal scheduling of granulocyte macrophage colony-stimulating factor (GM-CSF) for the abrogation of chemotherapy induced neutropenia in small cell lung cancer. Proc Am Soc Clin Oncol 8:A850.

34. Crawford J, Ozer H, Stoller R, Johnson D, Lyman G, Tabbara I, Kris M, Grous J, Picozzi V, Rausch G, Smith R, Gradishar W, Yahanda A, Vincent M, Stewart M, Glaspy J. 1991. Reduction by granulocyte colony-stimulating factor of fever and neutropenia induced by chemotherapy in patients with small cell lung cancer. N Engl J Med 325:164–170.

35. Masuda N, Fukuoka M, Negoro N, Takada M, Nakagawa K, Kodama N, Kawahara M, Furuse K. 1991. CODE chemotherapy with or without recombinant human granulocyte colony-stimulating factor in extensive stage small cell lung cancer. Proc Am Soc Clin Oncol 10:A873.

36. Drings P, Fisher JR. 1990. Biology and clinical use of GM-CSF in lung cancer. Lung 168:1059–1068.

37. Hamm JT, Schiller JH, Oken MM, Gallmeier WM, Rusthoven J, Israel R. 1991. Granulocyte-macrophage colony stimulating factor (GM-CSF) in small cell carcinoma of the lung (SCLC): preliminary analysis of a randomised controlled trial. Proc Am Soc Clin Oncol 10:A878.

38. Avalos BR, Gasson JC, Hedvat C, Quan SG, Baldwin GC, Weisbart RH, Williams RE, Golde DW, Di Persio JF. 1990. Human granulocyte colony-stimulating factor: biologic activities and receptor characterization on hematopoietic cells and small cell lung cancer cell lines. Blood 75(4):851–857.

39. Baldwin GC, Gasson JC, Kaufman SE, Quan SG, Williams RE, Avalos BR, Gazdar AF, Golde DW, Di Persio JF. 1989. Nonhematopoietic tumor cells express functional GM-CSF receptors. Blood 73(4):1033–1037.

40. Vellenga E, Biesma B, Meyer C, Wagteveld L, Esselink GE, de Vries E. 1991. The effects of five hematopoietic growth factors on human small cell lung carcinoma cell lines: interleukin 3 enhances the proliferation in one of the eleven cell lines. Cancer Res 51:73–76.

41. Kuwaki T, Hosoi T, Hanazono Y, Tsumura H, Ishikawa F, Miyazono K, Miyagawa K, Takaku F. 1990. Distribution of human granulocyte colony stimulating factor receptors on hematopooietic and non-hematopoietic tumor cell lines. Jpn J Cancer Res 81:560–563.

42. Suda T, Miura Y, Mizoguchi H, Kubota K, Takaku F. 1980. A case of lung cancer associated with granulocytosis and production of colony-stimulating activity by the tumour. Br J Cancer 41:980–984.

43. Okabe T, Fujisawa M, Kudo H, Honma H, Ohsawa N, Takkaku F. 1984. Establishment of a human colony-stimulating-factor-producing cell line from an undifferentiated large cell carcinoma of the lung. Cancer 54:1024–1029.

44. Yamada T, Hirohashi S, Shimosato Y, Kodama T, Hayashi S, Ogura T, Gamou S, Shimizu N. 1985. Giant cell carcinomas of the lung producing colony-stimulating factor in vitro and in vivo. Jpn J Cancer Res 76:967–976.

45. Nakamura H, Sayami P, Hayata Y. 1992. Analysis of G-CSF producing lung cancer cell lines and non growth stimulatory effects of rhG-CSF on lung cancer cells in vitro and in vivo. Lung Cancer 8:141–152.

46. Salmon SE, Liu R. 1989. Effects of granulocyte-macrophage colony-stimulating factor on in vitro growth of human solid tumors. J Clin Oncol 7(9):1346–1350.

47. Twentyman PR, Wright KA. 1991. Failure of GM-CSF to influence the growth of small cell and non-small cell lung cancer cell lines in vitro. Eur J Cancer 27(1):6–8.

48. Bunn PA, Crowlet J, Hazuka M, Tolley R, Livingston R. 1992. The role of GM-CSF in limited stage SCLC: A randomized phase III study of the Southwest Oncology Group (SWOG). Proc Am Soc Clin Oncol 11:A974.

49. Bunn PA Jr, Kelly K. 1993. The role of GM-CSF in lung cancer: a review of the literature. Lung Cancer 9:45–58.

50. Favaretto A, Paccagnella A, Chiarion Sileni V, Ghiotto C, Comis S, Panozzo M, Ruffato R, Sartore F, Fiorentino MV. 1992. Correlation between GM-CSF administration and dose intensity (DI) of chemotherapy (CT) in SCLC. Proc Am Soc Clin Oncol 11: A1022.

51. Gabrilove JL, Jakubowski A, Howard Scher PD, Sternberg C, Wong G, Grous J, Yagoda A, Fain K, Moore MAS, Clarkson B, Oettgen HF, Alton K, Welte K, Souza L. 1988. Effect of granulocyte colony-stimulating factor on neutropenia and associated morbidity due to chemotherapy for transitional-cell carcinoma of the urothelium. N Engl J Med 318:1414–1422.

52. Pettengell R, Gurney H, Radford JA, Deakin DP, James R, Wilkinson PM, Kane K, Bentley J, Crowther D. 1992. Granulocyte colony-stimulating factor to prevent dose-limiting neutropenia in non-Hodgkin's lymphoma: a randomized controlled trial. Blood 80(6): 1430–1436.

53. Metha C, Vogl SE. 1982. High-dose cyclophosphamide in the induction chemotherapy of small cell lung cancer: minor improvements in rate of remission and survival. Proc Am Soc Cancer Res 23:A155.

54. Brower M, Ihde DC, Johnston-Early A, Bunn PA Jr, Cohen MH, Carney DN, Makuch RW, Matthews MJ, Radice PA, Minna JD. 1983. Treatment of extensive stage small cell bronchogenic carcinoma. Effects of variation in intensity of induction therapy. Am J Med 75:993–1000.

55. Figueredo AT, Hryniuk WM, Strautmanis I, Frank G, Rendells. 1985. Co-trimoxacole prophylaxis during high dose chemotherapy of small cell lung cancer. J Clin Oncol 3(1): 54–64.

56. Johnson DH, Einhorn LH, Birch R, Vollmer R, Perez C, Krauss S, Omura G, Greco FA, and the Southeastern Cancer Study Group. 1987. A randomized comparison of high-dose versus conventional-dose cyclophosphamide, doxorubicin and vincristin for extensive small cell lung cancer. A phase III trial of the Southern Cancer Study Group. J Clin Oncol 5(11):1731–1738.

57. Souhami RL, Harper PG, Linch D, Trask C, Goldstone AH, Tobias JS, Spiro SG, Geddes DM, Richards JDM. 1983. High dose cyclophosphamide with autologous marrow transplantation for small cell carcinoma of the bronchus. Cancer Chemother Pharmacol 10:205–207.

58. Spitzer G, Fahra P, Valdivieso M, Dicke K, Zander A, Vellekoop L, Murphy WK, Dhingra HM, Umsawasdi T, Chiuten D, Carr DT. 1986. High dose intensification therapy with autologous bone marrow support for limited small cell bronchogenic carcinoma. J Clin Oncol 4:4–13.

59. Humblet Y, Symann M, Bosly A, Delaunois L, Francis C, Machiels J, Beauduin M, Weynants P, Longueville J, Prignot J. 1987. Late intensification chemotherapy with autologous bone marrow transplantation in selected small cell carcinoma of the lung: a randomized study. J Clin Oncol 5:1864–1873.

60. Luikart SD, Macdonald M, Herzan D, Modeas C, Goutsou M, Clamon G, Maurer G, Perry MC, Green MR. 1991. Ability of daily or twice daily granulocyte-macrophage colony-stimulating factor (GM-CSF) to support dose escalation of etoposide (vp-16) and carboplatin (CBDCA) in extensive small cell lung cancer (SCLC). Proc Am Soc Clin Oncol 10:A825.

61. Fujita J, Kamei T, Ariyoshi Y, Ikegami H, Furuse K, Fukuoka M. 1993. Dose intensification study of carboplatin and etoposide with G-CSF in small cell lung cancer. Proc Am Soc Clin Oncol 12:A1101.

62. Masuda N, Fukuoka M, Matsui K, Negoro S, Takada M, Sakai N, Ryu S, Takifuji N, Ito

K, Kudoh S, Kusunoki Y. 1990. Evaluation of high dose etoposide combined with cisplatin for treating relapsed small cell lung cancer. Cancer 65:2635–2640.

63. Shepherd F, Rusthoven J, Goss P, Eisenhauer E. 1991. Phase I–II trial of high dose cisplating, etoposide and GM-CSF for small cell lung cancer (SCLC). Proc Am Soc Clin Oncol 10:A864.

64. Neidhart J, Stidley C, Ferguson J, Mangalik A, Andersson T, Oldham F. 1990. GM-CSF decreases duration of cytopenia in patients receiving dose intensive therapy with cyclophosphamide, etoposide and cisplatin. Proc Am Soc Clin Oncol 9:A753.

65. Hryniuk WM, Goodyear M. 1990. The calculation of received dose intensity. J Clin Oncol 8:1935–1937.

66. Bronchud MH, Howell A, Crowther D, Hopwood P, Souza L, Dexter TM. 1989. The use of granulocyte colony-stimulating factor to increase the intensity of treatment with doxorubicin in patients with advanced breast and ovarian cancer. Br J Cancer 60:121–125.

67. Ardizzoni A, Venturini M, Grino L, Sertoli MR, Bruzzi P, Pennucci MC, Mariani GL, Garrone O, Bracarda S, Rosso R, Van Zandwijk N. 1993. High dose-intensity chemotherapy, with accelerated cyclophosphamide-doxorubicin — etoposide and granulocyte-macrophage colony stimulating factor, in the treatment of small cell lung cancer. Eur J Cancer 29(5):687–692.

68. D'Hondt V, Canon JL, Humblet Y, Weynants P, Duprez P, Beauduin M, Dewitte M, Müll B, Symann M. 1992. Dose-dependant IL3 stimulation of thrombopoiesis and neutropoiesis in patients with small cell lung carcinoma (SCLC) before and after chemotherapy (CT): a placebo-controlled randomized phase II Study. Proc Am Soc Clin Oncol 11:A1321.

69. Smith JW, Longo DL, Alvord WG, Janik JE, Sharfman WH, Gause BL, Curti BD, Creekmore SP, Holmlund JT, Fenton RG, Sznol M, Miller LL, Shimizu M, Oppenheim JJ, Fiem SJ, Hursey JC, Powers GC, Urba WJ. 1993. The effects of treatment with interleukin-1 alpha on platelet recovery after high-dose carboplatin. N Engl J Med 328:756–751.

70. Ravagnani F, Siena S, Bregni M, Sciorelli G, Gianni AM, Pellegris G. 1990. Large scale collection of ciculating haematopoietic progenitors in cancer patients treated with high dose cyclophosphamide and recombinant human GM-CSF. Eur J Cancer 26(5):562–564.

71. Leyvraz S, Vuichard P, Grob JP, Scheider P, Ketterer N, von Fliedner V, Lejeune F, Bachmann F. 1993. Multiple sequential high-dose chemotherapy with r-MetHu G-CSF (filgrastim) and infusion of peripheral blood progenitor cells (PBPC) in patients with small cell lung cancer: a feasibility study. Proc Am Soc Clin Oncol 12:A1115.

72. Eguchi K, Shinkai T, Sasaki Y, Tamura T, Ohe Y, Nakagawa K, Fukuda M, Yamada K, Kojima A, Oshita F, Morita M, Suemasu K, Saijo N. 1990. Subcutaneous administration of recombinant human granulocyte colony-stimulating factor (KRN8601) in intensive chemotherapy for patients with advanced lung cancer. Jpn J Cancer Res 81:1168–1174.

73. Yoshida T, Nakamura S, Ohtake S, Okafuji K, Kobayashi K, Kondo K, Kanno M, Matano S, Matsuda T, Kanai M, Sugimoto R, Ogawa M, Takaku F. 1990. Effect of granulocyte colony-stimulating factor on neutropenia due to chemotherapy for non-Hodgkin's lymphoma. Cancer 66:1904–1909.

74. Bishop JF, Morstyn G, Stuart-Harris R, Matthews JP, Green M, Zalcberg J, Raghavan D, Fox R, Yuen K, Olver I, Zimet A, Kefford R. 1991. Dose and schedule of granulocyte macrophage colony stimulating factor (GM-CSF) carboplatin and etoposide in small cell lung cancer (SCLC). Proc Am Soc Clin Oncol 10:A820.

75. Appelbaum FR. 1989. The clinical use of haematopoietic growth factors. Semin Hematol 26(Suppl 3):7–14.

76. De Vries EGE, Biesma B, Willemse Pax HB, Mulder NH, Stern AC, Aalders JG, Vellenga E. 1991. A double-blind placebo-controlled study with granulocyte-macrophage colony-stimulating factor during chemotherapy for ovarian carcinoma. Cancer Res 51:116–122.

76. Van Zandwijk N. 1993. The experience of the EORTC Lung Cancer Cooperative Group (abstract). Proc 3rd International conference on small cell lung cancer, Ravenna, Italy, p. 97.

291

77. Mayordomo JI, Diaz-Puente MT, Lianes MP, Lopez-Brea M, Lopez E, Paz-Ares L, Hitt R, Alonso S, Sevilla I, Rivas I, Cortes-Funes H. 1993. Decreasing morbidity and cost of treating febrile neutropenia by adding G-CSF and GM-CSF to standard antibiotic therapy: results of a randomized trial. Proc Am Soc Clin Oncol 12:A1510.
78. Hornung RL, Longo DL. 1992. Hematopoietic stem cell depletion by restorative growth factor regimens during repeated high-dose cyclophosphamide therapy. Blood 80(1):77–83.
79. Moore MAS. 1992. Does stem cell exhaustion result from combining hematopoietic growth factors with chemotherapy? If so, how do we prevent it? Blood 80(1):3–7.
80. Thatcher N. 1992. Haematopoietic growth factors and lung cancer treatment. Thorax 47:119–126.
81. Thomassen MJ, Ahmad M, Barna BP, Antal J, Wiedemann HP, Meeker DP, Klein J, Bauer L, Gibson V, Andresen S, Bukowski RM. 1991. Induction of cytokine messenger RNA and secretion in alveolar macrophages and blood monocytes from patients with lung cancer receiving granulocyte-macrophage colony-stimulating factor therapy. Cancer Res 51:857–862.
82. Williams D, Park LS. 1991. Hematopoïetic effects of a granulocyte-macrophage colony stimulating factor/interleukin 3 fusion protein. Cancer 67(10):2705–2707.
83. Sekido Y, Takahashi T, Ueda R, Takahashi M, Suzuki H, Nishida K, Tsukamoto T, Hida T, Shimokata K, Zsebo KM, Takaheshi T. 1993. Recombinant human stem cell factor mediates chemotaxis of small-cell lung cancer cell lines aberrantly expressing the C-kit proto oncogene. Cancer Res 53(7):1709–1714.
84. Mertelsmann R. 1991. Hematopoietins: Biology, pathophysiology and potential as therapeutic agents, Ann Oncol 2:251–263.

292

14. Interferon and lung cancer

Karin V. Mattson, Anne M. Hand, and Paula K. Maasilta

The interferon system

Interferons are glycoproteins produced by many of the body's cells in response to foreign proteins such as viruses, microbes or tumors. There are three types of interferon (IFN): *alpha* (IFNα), produced by leukocytes; *beta* (IFNβ), produced by fibroblasts, macrophages and epithelial cells; and *gamma* (IFNγ), produced by activated T-lymphocytes and natural killer lymphocytes. There are at least 17 genes controlling the production of IFNα, but only one gene for IFNβ and one for IFNγ [1].

The anticancer effects of interferon

Interferons belong to a larger group of intercellular signaling molecules, or cytokines, which regulate cellular metabolism, proliferation and differentiation, as well as immune function, via complex interactions [1–3]. They interact with their target cells by first binding tightly to specific cell surface receptors: one for IFNα and IFNβ (class I IFNs) and a separate one for IFNγ (class II IFN) [4]. These transmembrane signals induce the synthesis of effector proteins, which mediate the various effects of interferon (figure 1).

The direct effects of interferon may be cytostatic or cytotoxic. Cell growth is slowed by modulation of the cellular levels of 2'5'oligoadenylate synthetase [5], or of the activity of cellular oncogenes [6], resulting in a longer cell cycle. Langdon et al. [7] have developed a small cell lung cancer (SCLC) cell line and xenograft that is 1000 times more sensitive to IFNα than other SCLC cell lines. IFNα seemed to cause the cells to accumulate in the G_0/G_1 phase of the cell cycle [8], inducing an antiproliferative effect. However, Bepler et al. [9] were not able to demonstrate that treatment with either IFNα or difluoromethylornithine, or a combination of the two, caused any accumulation of cells in a particular phase of the cell cycle.

Interferons may also deplete supplies of essential metabolites by, for example, inhibiting the induction of ornithine decarboxylase or inducing the synthesis of indolamine 2,3-dioxygenase [10,11].

IFNγ interacts synergistically with IFNα or IFNβ to increase lysis of

Heine H. Hansen, (ed), Hansen: Lung Cancer.

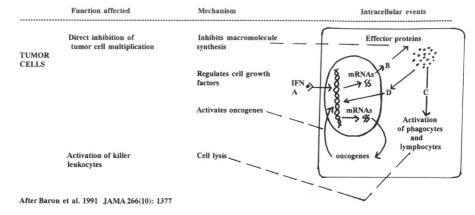

Function affected	Mechanism	Intracellular events

After Baron et al. 1991 JAMA 266(10): 1377

Figure 1: Mechanisms by which interferons (IFN) affect tumor cells. IFN reacts with cell receptors (A) to induce synthesis of effector proteins (B) that can activate immunocompetent cells (C) and inhibit cell macromolecule synthesis and regulate oncogenes (D).

malignant cells, a direct cytotoxic effect [12]. Interferon can also inhibit normal cells, such as those of the bone marrow [13], creating a mild myelotoxic effect.

All three types of interferon enhance the expression of cell surface antigens, such as MHC antigens and tumor necrosis factor (TNF) receptors, thereby rendering the tumor cells more recognizable to cytotoxic leukocytes or to TNF, a cytokine having potent cytostatic and cytotoxic effects. SCLC cells have low endogenous levels of class I antigen expression, in common with other tumors of neuroendocrine origin. For this reason, they may be able to escape immune surveillance and metastasize more easily in vivo. IFNα and IFNγ induce cell surface expression of the class I MHC antigens, HLA-A, -B, and -C, and β_2 microglobulin, by both SCLC and non-small cell lung cancer (NSCLC) cells [14]. IFNγ is also capable of inducing class II MHC antigens [14,15]. Funa et al. [16] were able to demonstrate that in patients with SCLC and midgut carcinoids, therapy using natural IFNα induced the tumor cells to express β_2 microglobulin. Crawford has shown that IFNγ activates the peripheral blood monocytes of patients with advanced NSCLC, as demonstrated by a 50% or greater increase in Fc receptor and β_2 microglobulin expression by these cells [17].

The possibility is being investigated that a change in interferon receptor status accounts for the antiproliferative effect, but studies by Jabbar and Twentyman [18] suggest that growth inhibition by IFNγ cannot be explained simply in terms of modulated receptor binding. Suarez-Pestena et al. [19] developed an IFNα-resistant SCLC cell line, which was also relatively resistant to IFNγ. They were not able to show any differences in the numbers of interferon binding sites, in growth rate, or in surface marker

294

expression that might have explained the resistance. They concluded that the resistance to interferon developed at the level of signal transduction. Interferons, especially IFNγ, also directly activate cytotoxic cells such as T-lymphocytes, macrophages, and NK cells [20], and may modulate antibody production. IFNγ has more immunomodulatory effects than IFNα or IFNβ, and also potentiates their effects. Interferons can also cause tumor cells to differentiate and therefore to become less malignant.

The immunomodulatory effects of inhaled IFNγ

Alveolar macrophages, like other phagocytes, generate oxygen-derived free radicals such as superoxide anions, hydrogen peroxide and hydroxyl radicals, which are thought to play an important role in the body's defense against tumors and micro-organisms. IFNγ increases the ability of phagocytes to generate oxygen radicals [21,22] and may thereby enhance their ability to kill tumor cells and micro-organisms.

In healthy volunteers, the inhalation of IFNγ activates alveolar macrophages without affecting the peripheral blood monocytes [23]. In rats, the inhalation of IFNγ enhanced the ability of alveolar macrophages to kill tumor cells and microorganisms [24], as well as interleukin-1 production and Ia antigen expression [25]. The functioning of systemic monocytes was also enhanced, without major systemic side effects [25]. The subcutaneous injection of IFNγ also enhanced peripheral monocyte activity, but in this case all patients develop systemic side effects [21].

The production of oxygen radicals by both the alveolar macrophages and the blood phagocytes of lung cancer patients has been evaluated using a chemoluminescence (CL) assay of the capacity of inhaled IFNγ to induce lysis of tumor cells and bacteria. The CL responses of the bronchoalveolar lavage fluid (BALF) cells of four of the eight patients who received IFNγ were greater after inhalation than before. The patients were described as 'high responders' to IFNγ. The response did not appear to depend on the dose of IFNγ given. The CL activity of BALF cells from low responders and nonresponders was also lower than that of the high responders prior to the inhalation. The poor response to both IFNγ and the CL stimuli used suggests that the patients were generally anergic. Kawatsu et al. [26] have demonstrate that BALF cells from individual lung cancer patients, particularly those who are anergic to skin tests, lack sensitivity to recombinant IFNγ. The possibility that skin testing and the CL response of BALF cells could provide a means of selecting patients who would respond to inhaled IFNγ warrants further study. The lack of cell response suggests that peripheral blood phagocytes were not activated in any of the patients who inhaled IFNγ. The CL responses of peripheral blood monocytes were increased in all patients, however, after subcutaneous injection of IFNγ. The responses of neutrophils was less clear-cut.

In vitro sensitivity studies in lung cancer cell lines

Tumor cells vary in their sensitivity to the different interferons [27,28], and this fact can be utilized therapeutically.

SCLC cell lines are divided, by growth characteristics and by biochemical, morphological and molecular biological features, into classic and variant lines [9,29]. Variant cell lines grow more aggressively in vitro and have a morphology more like the large cell anaplastic subtype of NSCLC. SCLC cells secrete many peptides, since they are of neuroendocrine origin; and they are also generally sensitive to radiotherapy and chemotherapy, but can be resistant to cytokines. It is possible that they are producing endogenous cytokines; these could modulate the cellular sensitivity to exogenous cytokine, by means of an autocrine loop. However, Lagadec et al. [30] were unable to find any mRNA of TNF, TGF-β, or interleukin-1β or -6 (IL-1β, or IL-6) in 10 SCLC cell lines resistant to these cytokines. In the same study, all 10 cell lines were sensitive to both NK and lymphokine-activated killer (LAK) cells, despite their resistance to most cytokines. This LAK cell sensitivity was enhanced by IFNγ, although IFNγ has been shown to protect other types of tumor cell from LAK cell lysis [31].

NSCLC cell lines are generally resistant to irradiation and chemotherapy, although some have recently been shown to express certain neuroendocrine markers in common with SCLC cell lines and to be relatively sensitive to chemotherapeutic agents [32].

Bepler et al. [9] showed that recombinant leukocyte IFNα inhibits the growth of variant but not classic SCLC cell lines. Of the three NSCLC cell lines studied, only one adenocarcinoma cell line was sensitive to the interferon. In the same study, it was found that the malignancy of the variant cell lines, as measured by their low population doubling times, was related to their sensitivity to IFNα. The growth-inhibiting effects of IFNα seen in this study did not appear to be related to changes in c-myc or N-myc oncogene expression or L-dopa decarboxylase activity.

In another study [33] of six SCLC cell lines and nine NSCLC cell lines, neither classic nor variant SCLC cell lines responded to alpha, beta or gamma interferons, whereas a majority of the NSCLC cell lines were inhibited by at least 30%. Other studies have reported on the significant antiproliferative effects of interferon on some, but not all, lung cancer cell lines [28,30,33,34].

Some interferon combinations, e.g., IFNα plus IFNγ and IFNβ$_{ser}$ plus IFNγ, have demonstrated additive or synergistic growth inhibition of NSCLC cells [28,33,35], but no such effect has been seen in the case of SCLC cells [30].

Given the relatively weak direct antitumor effects of interferon, and their many indirect biological effects, it would be reasonable to examine the possibility of using interferon to improve the effects of other therapies for lung cancer. A large amount of work has been done on the interactions of

296

chemotherapeutic agents and interferons on tumor cells in experimental systems (for review, see [36]). Interferons augment the activity of a wide variety of chemotherapeutic agents. This finding supports the view that the interaction occurs at many levels: the level of the cellular uptake of the drug; the intracellular drug metabolism; and the levels of cell cycle, genetic (oncogenes, p450, etc.), and immune system modulation. This hypothesis is supported by the fact that interferon–drug interactions are often synergistic, and the effects can be dependent on the relative scheduling of the individual agents.

In a pioneering study, Carmichael and his colleagues [37] demonstrated the potentiation of cisplatin and cyclophosphamide by recombinant and natural IFNα in human NSCLC xenografts [37]. This study provided the rationale behind many subsequent clinical studies of combinations of interferon and cisplatin-based chemotherapy for lung cancer.

Cole et al. [38] found that a doxorubicin-resistant SCLC cell line responded differently to IFNγ than had the sensitive parent cell line. The growth of the resistant cell line was not inhibited by IFNγ, nor was HLA antigen expression enhanced, in contrast to the results for the parent cell line. The responses to IFNα were the same for both cell lines, suggesting that multidrug resistance may be in some way linked to IFNγ rather than IFNα. However, in a study of three SCLC cell lines with similarly depressed HLA antigen expression levels [39], a variety of responses to chemotherapeutic agents and to irradiation were observed.

Experimental studies have shown that recombinant IFNα-2b enhances the sensitivity of SCLC cell lines to irradiation [40]. Interferons also markedly enhance the radiation response of mouse Swiss 3T3 cells [41]; the change in radiation response is due to a reduction in response threshold, rather than an ability to absorb sublethal doses of radiation by rapid repair of the DNA. Carncy ct al. [42] noticed a similar change in the response to radiation in SCLC cell lines established before and after chemotherapy. Cell lines established from relapsed tumors behaved more like NSCLC cell lines in that they expressed fewer antigenic markers and were relatively resistant to irradiation.

Chang and Zeng [43] demonstrated that interferon enhanced the inhibiting effect of radiation on cell growth in human hypernephroma tumor cells. This effect varied according to the dose of radiation and the exposure time to interferon. The authors suggest that the radiosensitizing effect of interferon was associated with increased blockage of the cell cycle in the G_2-M phase, but other studies of lung cancer cell lines have not supported their hypothesis [40].

Kardamakis et al. [40] suggested instead that the radiosensitizing effect of IFNα may depend on interference with the DNA repair process. Improved tumor response and survival in vivo have been noted following the administration of an interferon inducer at the same time as radiotherapy [44].

The relevance of in vitro sensitivity testing to the clinical situation has been questioned. Tsai et al. [45] were able to show that predictions of response to therapy and patient survival can be obtained from drug sensitivity tests on long-term lung cancer cell lines as well as on short- and medium-term lung cancer cell cultures [45]. Such systems may therefore have a role in assessing the effects of new chemotherapeutic agents, biological agents, and various combinations of agents [46], as well as in developing new treatment strategies.

Clinical studies

The results of clinical studies of interferons against NSCLC and SCLC have been disappointing with regard to tumor response, as defined by World Health Organization (WHO) or UICC criteria. This raises a question: should criteria other than tumor shrinkage, e.g., the maintenance of stable disease or the prolongation of disease-free interval, be used to measure the biological activity of interferon against solid tumors?

Very few of the earliest studies of the use of interferon against lung cancer were well defined with respect to protocol, patients or endpoints. Many were small studies that included patients who had received intensive treatment prior to interferon therapy and patients who had high tumor burdens. Both natural and recombinant alpha interferon, as well as recombinant gamma interferon, have been used, in doses ranging from 3 to 200 MU per day. Administration has been most commonly intramuscular, although subcutaneous and intravenous methods have also been used. The most common treatment schedules have been daily or three times per week, with scheduled protocol treatment duration rarely exceeding 12 weeks.

Acute and chronic toxicity was seen at all doses and schedules, causing the acute 'flu' syndrome as well as dose-limiting chronic fatigue, anorexia and weight loss. In most cases, the toxicity has been clinically manageable. Dose-limiting neurotoxicity was experienced by patients receiving higher doses of any type of IFNα, but never by those receiving IFNγ [47]. Dose-limiting cardiotoxicity was noted in one study of high-dose IFNγ [48].

Interferons as single agents against lung cancer

The results of the studies on NSCLC patients are summarized in table 1 [48–57]. Two early studies [50,51] reported no response (according to WHO criteria) to natural IFNα (3 MU im daily or TIW) in patients with previously-treated advanced epidermoid NSCLC. However, Stoopler reported significant increases in NK cell activity [50]. Grunberg [53] and Olesen [54] both used high-dose (50 MU im TIW) recombinant IFNα-2a against NSCLC. The Grunberg series included previously untreated patients, but only one out of 12 evaluable patients achieved a minimal response: 50% tumor shrinkage

298

Table 1. Activity of interferons as single agents against non-small cell lung cancer

Type	Dose/schedule	Patients	Histology	Toxicity	Response	Comments	Author [ref]
nIFNα	3 MU/d i.m. × 30 d	12	10 adeno 2 epiderm	Fever Malaise Anorexia	No tumor regression in 9 eval. patients	All previously treated; NK cell activity measured	Krown et al. [49]
nIFNα	3 MU/d i.m. × 30 d	14	9 adeno 2 epiderm		No tumor regression in 11 eval. patients	NK cell activity increased; all previously treated	Stoopler et al. [50]
nIFNα	3 MU/d i.m. TIW	38	20 adeno 13 epiderm 5 large-cell	Fever (90%) Granulocytopenia (29%)	37 eval. 1 PR 1 MR	—	Figlin et al. [51]
rIFNα-2a	20 MU/m²/d i.m. for 12 wks	8	2 adeno 3 epiderm 2 large-cell 1 bronchiolo-alveolar	Elevate transaminases Confusion Granulocytopenia	2 MR	No patient completed course due to toxicity or PD	Leavitt et al. [52]
rIFNα-2a	50 MU/m² i.m. TIW	12	6 adeno 3 epiderm 1 large 1 adeno-epiderm 1 undifferentiated	Significant cardiovascular toxicity	1 MR 6 SD 5 PD	—	Grunberg et al. [53]
rIFNα-2a	50 MU/m² i.m. TIW for 12 wks	13	All epiderm	Fatigue and anorexia Weight loss Liver toxicity	11 eval. 1 PR 6 NC 4 PD	Only one patient completed course without dose reduction	Olesen et al. [54]

Table 1. Continued

Type	Dose/schedule	Patients	Histology	Toxicity	Response	Comments	Author [ref]
nIFNα	6 MU/d i.m. 5/wk for 12 wks	13	9 epiderm 3 adeno 1 large-cell	Fatigue Weight loss	7 completed course: 4 SD 3 PD	Previously untreated pts	Niiranen et al. [55]
rIFNγ	2 mg/m² TIW for 12 wks	15	10 epiderm 3 adeno 2 large-cell	Cardio-toxicity: 3 pts withdrawn	No tumor response *At 4 wks* 1 MR 1 SD 1 PD *At 12 wks* 1 PR 6 SD	Did not interfere with subsequent therapy	Mattson et al. [48]
nIFNα	1–10 MU/d or TIW increasing to 20 MU/d by *inhalation*	10	Bronchiolo-alveolar	Only mild toxicity in most pts	*8 eval.* No tumor response 6 SD		Van Zandwijk et al. [56]
nIFNα	1–6 MU TID by aerosol *inhalation*	6	Bronchiolo-alveolar	Bronchial hyperactivity	No tumor response		Kinnula et al. [57]

lasting less than four weeks. The disease was stabilized in six other patients, but at the expense of significant cardiovascular toxicity. Olesen's series included patients who had developed resistance to earlier conventiond treatment. A partial response lasting 14 months was achieved by one of the 13 patients, and six other patients achieved stable disease for 14 to 20 weeks. This relatively long period without progression may suggest that interferon was having some biological effect, although no tumor shrinkage was apparent. All the patients in Olesen's study suffered severely from both acute and chronic toxicities; only one patient was able to complete the minimum scheduled 12 weeks of therapy without a reduction in the dose of interferon administered.

Niiranen et al. [55] gave natural IFNα to previously untreated patients for 12 weeks before proceeding to chemotherapy or radiotherapy. Twelve of the 13 patients achieved stable disease for at least one month during IFN monotherapy, but only seven patients were able to complete the 12-week course; of these, four had stable disease and three progressive disease.

Mattson [48] treated 15 patients suffering from previously untreated NSCLC with high-dose recombinant IFNγ ($2\,mg/m^2$ iv TIW). Seven patients were evaluable after 12 weeks: one had achieved a partial response and six had stable disease, suggesting that IFNγ may be more active than IFNα against NSCLC.

The single-agent studies made among patients with SCLC are summarized in table 2 [54,58–61]. In the early studies, higher doses of interferon were used than against NSCLC and were administered intravenously [58,60]. There have been at least four different studies that have investigated the use of interferon monotherapy in patients suffering from SCLC. In Olesen's study [54], 15 patients who had not responded to intensive chemotherapy were treated with $50\,MU/m^2$ of recombinant IFNα, given subcutaneously three times a week. No objective responses were seen, and only one patient completed the 12-week course without disease progression. In an earlier study [58], 10 SCLC patients who had received no prior treatment were given $50–100\,MU/m^2$ purified lymphoblastoid IFN by daily intravenous injection for five days, followed by $3\,MU/m^2$ given intramuscularly, three times a week for a further three weeks. No objective responses were seen. Two patients did not complete the therapy because of toxicity and disease progression, and another six patients showed progressive disease after the month of IFN therapy. In a second study from the same institution [61], no objective responses were observed to $28\,MU/m^2/day$ of recombinant IFNγ given by continuous intravenous infusion for five days, followed by $14\,MU/m^2$ given intravenously three times a week. In this study, IFN therapy stopped after one month if no response was seen, although four of the eight evaluable patients had stable disease at this point.

In contrast, the study of 15 patients with previously untreated limited disease by Mattson et al. [60] continued natural leukocyte IFNα monotherapy until disease progression. One partial response of 12 weeks duration was

Table 2. Activity of interferons as single agents against small-cell lung cancer

Type	Dose/schedule	Patients	Previous therapy	Toxicity	Response	Comments	Author [ref]
nIFNα (Ly)	50–100 MU/m²/d i.v. × 5 d, then 3 MU/m² i.m. TIW × 3 wks	10	None	Considerable	None	Patients previously untreated	Jones et al. [58]
rIFNα-2	50 MU/m²/d i.v. × 5 d	3	2 had received RT and CT	Fever Anorexia Malaise Confusion	None	Small study Only one patient had more than one course	Jackson et al. [59]
rIFNα-2	50 MU/m² i.m. TIW × 12 wks	17	All had progressed on combination CT	Fever Fatigue Leucopenia	None (15 eval.)	Only one patient completed course	Olesen et al. [54]
nIFNα (Le)	100–200 MU/m²/d c.i.v. for 5 d then 6 MU/m² i.m. TIW until progression	9	None	CNS dysfunction Anorexia Fatigue	3 MR/9	Subsequent RT and CT given in combination with IFN until PD	Mattson et al. [60]
nIFNα (Le)	6 MU/m²/d i.m. × 5 d then 6 MU/m² i.m. TIW until progression	6	None	CNS dysfunction Anorexia Fatigue	1/6	Subsequent RT and CT given in combination with IFN until PD	Mattson et al. [60]
rIFNγ	28 MU/m² 24 h i.v. × 5 d then 14 MU/m² TIW for 25 d	12	None	Fever Malaise Headache	None (8 eval.)	—	Newman et al. [61]

observed among six patients receiving low-dose IFNα alone (6 MU/m^2 sc TIW) until progression. Three minor responses of 20-, 25- and 42-weeks duration were seen among the nine patients placed under a high-dose regime of 800 MU over five days, followed by the low-dose regime until progression. The policy of continuing IFNα therapy until progression, i.e., much longer than in other studies, allowed the team to study the biological and toxic effects of IFNα monotherapy in more detail. They observed that disease stabilization developed gradually over 10 to 40 weeks and could be maintained for up to 40 weeks. This finding suggests that natural IFNα is active biologically against SCLC. The long duration of the interferon treatment would therefore appear to be more important than the dose used, and the maintenance of stable disease would appear to be as significant for survival as any shrinkage in the tumor. Interferon monotherapy is obviously not appropriate for patients with bulky SCLC tumors; but the results of single-agent studies, although not wholly consistent, suggest that interferon could be used in combination with other therapies to maintain the response already achieved or to enhance sensitivity to other therapies. This possibility is now being widely investigated in clinical trials.

Interferons combined with chemotherapy

Studies of experimental models of human lung cancer have suggested that interferon may significantly enhance the activity of some cytotoxic drugs [37,62].

Non-small cell lung cancer (table 3) [63–73]. Walsh carried out a phase I/II study of eight patients using a treatment regime of 5 MU/m^2 rIFNα-2b given subcutaneously three times a week, together with increasing weekly doses of cisplatin [63]. One partial response was achieved.

Schiller et al. [64] observed major responses in two patients suffering from adenocarcinoma who had received IFNβ and IFNγ immediately before cisplatin/etoposide chemotherapy. The subsequent phase II trial of IFN-β$_{ser}$ plus IFN-γ for six weeks, followed by cisplatin and etoposide, did not demonstrate any increase in the effectiveness of the chemotherapy, from pretreatment by these interferons, in patients with inoperable NSCLC. The patients in the combined interferon–chemotherapy arm achieved a partial response rate of 11% (2/18), but suffered more hematological toxicity from the chemotherapy; in the study arm in which chemotherapy was given alone, the partial response rate was 17% (3/18). The duration of response and overall survival were longer for patients in the combination arm, but the differences were not significant.

Bowman [66] performed a phase II trial giving cisplatin (100 mg/m^2 q 21 or 28) and recombinant IFNα-2 (3 or 5 MU TIW) to 68 patients suffering from NSCLC, following the observation of a significant enhancement of the effectiveness of cisplatin by human IFNα in three human NSCLC xenografts

Table 3. Activity of interferons combined with chemotherapy or other cytokines against non-small cell lung cancer

Type	IFN Dose/schedule	Chemotherapy & sequence	Patient no. histology	Response	Progression free interval	Survival	Author [ref]
rIFNα-2b	5 MU/m² sc TIW	5–30 mg/m²/wk P × 5 wks	8	1 PR/8			Walsh et al. [63]
rIFNγ	200 μg i.v. TIW	60 mg/m² P d1	CT (n = 19)		73 days	190 d	Schiller et al. [64]
rIFNβ ser	plus 30 MU i.v. TIW	120 mg/m² VP16 d 4, 6, 8	adeno 9, epith 6, large cell 4	3 PR			
		Alone or after 6 weeks IFN	IFN + CT (n = 18) adeno 10, epith 5, large cell 3	2 PR	140 days	246 d	
rIFNα-2b	5 MU/d i.m. ×8 d then 5 MU TIW	CAP q 28d alone or with IFN	154	CT alone OR = 10% CT + IFN OR = 22%		177 d 189 d	Rosso et al. [65]
rIFNα 2	3 MU sc TIW or 5 MU sc TIW	100 mg/m² P d1 q 28d or 100 mg/m² P d1 q 21d	n = 60 adeno 20, epiderm 24, large & others 16	5 PR 11 PR	Some pretreated mixture LD/ED		Bowman et al. [66]

	Dose	Chemotherapy	Patients	Response			Reference
rIFNα-2b	5 MU i.m. TIW minimum 2 mo	100 mg/m² P d 1, 8 q 28 d	30	4/30			Rosell et al. [67]
rIFNα-2b	3–5 MU i.m. d 1–7 q 28 d	CAP i.v. d4	n = 34 adeno 9 epiderm 17 large cell & others 8	n = 31 6 PR 18 SD 5 PD 2 ED	20 wks	37 wks 43 wks for responders	Ardizzoni et al. [68]
rIFNα-2a	9 MU TIW for 6 mo or unitl PD	100 mg/m² P d8 q 28 d	n = 100 epiderm 45 other NSCLC 55	n = 84 1 CR 27 PR 32 SD }33%	median 5.3 mo	median 6.4 mo, longer for stage III patients	Kataja [69]
rIFNα	9 MU i.m. 6, 30, 54 hrs	Bleomycin 15 mg/m² i.v.	13 previously treated	0/13	median 5 mo		Giaccone et al. [70]
rIFNα-2b	3 MU sc TIW × 12 wks	1.5 g/m² d1–5 I q 3 wks × 4	n = 45	2 CR 7 PR			Lind et al. [71]

Table 3. Continued

Type	IFN Dose/schedule	Chemotherapy & sequence	Patient no. histology	Response	Progression free interval	Survival	Author [ref]
rIFN	5 MU/m²/d i.m. × 3 d then 5 MU/m²/d BIW × 12	IL-2 18 MU/m²/d c.i.v. × 3 d then 2.4 MU/m²/d c.i.v. wk 2–5 8–9 11–12 or 3.6 MU/m²/d c.i.v. wk 2–5 8–9 11–12 without IFN	n = 11 6 5	None	9/11 pts <5 wks	median 7 mo	Jansen et al. [72]
rIFNα-2b	After CT 3 MU/d until PD then rIL-2 3 MU/m² BD × 5 d	P, V, Mitomycin C i.v. d1 q 3 wks × 2 cycles ↓ 20 PR, 4MR, 10 SD	n = 34 adeno 14 epiderm 19 large cell 1	n = 31 3 PR 4 SD 24 PD	median 27 wks	median 36 wks	Cellerino et al. [14]

P, platistin; VP16, etoposide; V, vincristine; I, ifosfamide; C, cyclophosphamide; A, adriamycin.

[37]. He achieved an overall response rate of 30% (in evaluable 60 patients), but for patients with epidermoid carcinoma, the partial response rate was 46% (11/24). They observed no increase in the renal, hematological or neurological toxicities associated with the chemotherapy for those patients also receiving interferon. Patients with epidermoid carcinoma who received 5 rather than 3 MU IFNα per dose tended to survive longer. There was no evidence that the higher doses exacerbated the toxicities associated with interferon therapy.

Rosso [65] achieved a response rate of 22% among 154 untreated NSCLC patients, using the cyclophosphamide/epirubicin/cisplatin regime with recombinant IFNα-2b (5 MU/day for seven days, then 5 MU TIW). However, Rosell's study [67] achieved a response rate of only 13% in 30 patients (3 stage IIIa, 7 stage IIIb, 20 stage IV) using a treatment regime of 5 MU recombinant IFNα-2b given intramuscularly three times a week for at least two months, together with cisplation on days 1 and 8, every 28 days. They concluded that interferon does not potentiate cisplatin in advanced NSCLC, but their study did not include any other treatment for comparison, nor were the patients selected at random. Interestingly, the tumors of the four patients whose disease responded demonstrated neuroendocrine markers such as NSE and Leu-7. Ardizzoni's trial of cisplatin-based chemotherapy (CAP) and recombinant IFNα-2a against advanced NSCLC was more encouraging [68]. A relatively long mean survival time of 37 weeks was achieved, and 32 out of the 34 patients had stage IV disease. The median survival for those responding to chemotherapy was 43 weeks.

A recent report [69] of a phase II study using recombinant IFNα-2a and cisplatin found that more patients with stage III NSCLC responded to the treatment than did the stage IV patients (47% as against 27%; 100 patients enrolled), and that the mean survival period of the former was longer. This result supports the experimental finding that interferon potentiates cisplatin [37].

Few studies have been performed using interferon with chemotherapeutic regimes other than those based on cisplatin. Giaccone [70] did not find that interferon enhanced the activity of bleomycin (15 mg/m^2) given intravenously against NSCLC, despite promising experimental results. However, Lind [71] was able to demonstrate that interferon potentiated the action of ifosfamide, a drug that has shown activity as a single agent against NSCLC. In a group of 45 patients with advanced NSCLC, they achieved two complete responses and seven partial responses, with only mild toxicity.

Recombinant IL-2 has shown activity against several solid tumors. Jansen designed a study [72] to investigate the effects of IL-2 combined with recombinant IFNα in 11 patients with advanced NSCLC. Five MU/m^2/day IFNα was administered intramuscularly for three days while IL-2 (18 MU/m^2/day) was given by continuous intravenous infusion on the same three days. After four days rest, this induction treatment was followed by either low-dose IL-2 and IFNα for 11 weeks, or high-dose IL-2 for 11 weeks. No

307

responses were documented, and 9 of the 11 patients developed progressive disease during the first five weeks of treatment. Cellerino [73] administered recombinant IL-2 subcutaneously and recombinant IFNα to patients who had achieved an objective response or stable disease after chemotherapy. The treatment was continued until progression or until it became too toxic. Only 10% of the patients showed any further improvement; the disease progressed in 77% of patients.

Small cell lung cancer (table 4) [74–78]. An effective therapy against SCLC has proved elusive; 50% of patients die within a year of diagnosis, despite a high initial response to induction chemotherapy. For patients who respond to induction therapy, long-term survival was improved in one study by the use of cytokine maintenance therapy. Mattson [75] has shown a significant prolongation of survival ($p = 0.03$, unpublished updated results) among patients receiving low-dose natural IFNα as a maintenance therapy for six months following induction therapy, over those patients receiving either maintenance chemotherapy or no maintenance therapy (420 patients accrued, 237 randomly allocated). However, in a similar trial using recombinant IFNγ maintenance therapy (4 MU/day for six months) for patients who had responded to chemotherapy, no such advantage was seen, and significant systemic toxicities were experienced in the interferon arm of the study (100 patients randomly allocated) [74]. Neither was recombinant IFNα-2a (3–9 MU/m^2) found to be an effective maintenance therapy for patients with limited SCLC, with respect to either the duration of remission or overall survival (281 patients accrued, 140 randomly allocated) [77]. Moreover, significant toxicity was experienced, and no patient was able to complete the scheduled 24 months of maintenance therapy. A trial is under way of carboplatin/etoposide/vincristine chemotherapy and radiotherapy against limited SCLC, followed by IFNα-2b maintenance therapy [76]. It will be interesting to study the results of such a long-term interferon maintenance therapy (2 MU/m^2/day sc for 30 days, then 3 MU/m^2 alternate days for eight months or until progression).

The next logical step in the development of combined therapies for SCLC is to start interferon therapy at the same time as chemotherapy. A three-arm phase III study was started in 1990, with recombinant IFNα-2a or natural leukocyte IFNα given concomitantly with six cycles of cisplatin/etoposide induction chemotherapy, and continued indefinitely or as long as it is tolerable, irrespective of other treatment changes [79]. Only chemotherapy is given to patients in the third (control) arm. The preliminary results from 98 patients accrued indicate that interferon can safely be administered with chemotherapy in this way, and that although patients receiving interferon and chemotherapy suffer more hematological toxicity, this is mild and clinically manageable. No differences in efficacy have been seen so far between the three arms. Antibodies have developed in 3 of 41 patients receiving recombinant IFNα-2a. No patients receiving natural IFNα have

Table 4. Activity of interferons combined with chemotherapy against SCLC

Type	IFN Dose/schedule	Chemotherapy & Sequence	Patient no. Histology	Response	Progression free interval	Survival	Author [ref]
rIFNγ	4 MU/d sc for 6 months or observation	induction CT/RT →CR	n = 51 SCLC / n = 49 SCLC		7 mo / 8 mo	13 mo / 19 mo	Jett et al. [74]
nIFNα	3 MU i.m. 5/wk for 1 mo 6 MU i.m. TIW for 5 mo	induction CT+RT →CR PR	n = 87 CT+RT only / n = 91 CT/RT+IFN SCLC		5 year survival 2% / 11%	10 mo / 11 mo	Mattson et al. [75]
rIFNα-2b	After CT/RT 2MU/m² sc d 1–30 then 3 MU sc alternate days for 8 mo or until PD or observation	4 cycles P+VP16+V then RT	107 enrolled limited SCLC	n = 29 Responders to CT + RT	Too early	Too early	Kohne-Wompner et al. [76]
rIFNα-2a	After CT/RT 3 MU/m² sc escalating to 9 MU/m² sc TIW for 2 yrs or observation	6 cycles P+VP16 +Chest RT	n = 140 Responders to CT + RT Limited SCLC		No difference between groups	12 mo / 13 mo	Kelly et al. [77]
IFNα	Induction 6 MU/m² d 1–3 q 21 d 6 cycles / Maintenance 5 MU/m² TIW 6 cycles	P+VP16 d 1–3 q 21 d 6 cycles / MEGACE 40 mg q i d 6 cycles	n = 36 Extensive SCLC / No prior treatment	33 eval. 3 CR 25 PR		46 wks IFN had no impact on survival	Glisson et al. [78]

P, cisplatin; VP16, etoposide; V, vincristine.

developed antibodies. The trial will continue until 100 patients are accrued to each arm. In another trial of etoposide/cisplatin chemotherapy and concomitant IFNα followed by IFN/MEGACE maintenance therapy for 36 patients, no survival advantage has been seen, although the treatment is being tolerated well and the response rate is high [80]. Neither of these studies is yet mature.

Interferons combined with radiotherapy

Interferon has been shown to have either radioprotective [80] or radiosensitizing potential [41,81–83], or no effect at all [84] when used in conjunction with radiation, depending on the type of interferon used and the system studied.

Holsti's study of SCLC patients [82] suggested that both high and low doses of parenteral natural IFNα enhance the effects of radiation on both the tumor and the lung, and that the effect may depend on the dose and/or the schedule of administration of both the interferon and the radiotherapy. Maasilta et al. [85] looked at the effect of natural IFNα and hyperfractionated radiotherapy applied together in the treatment of NSCLC. Twenty patients were randomly assigned to receive either radiotherapy or radiotherapy and concomitant natural IFNα given by inhalation (1.5 MU twice daily) and intramuscularly (3 MU once a day). No patient in either study arm achieved a complete response. Five patients in the radiotherapy arm and six in the radiotherapy/interferon arm experienced partial response; the corresponding numbers for stable disease were three and one. The side effects included influenza-like symptoms, anorexia, malaise and leukopenia, similar to those documented in studies using interferon alone [60]. Radiation pneumonitis appeared earlier and was more severe in the patients given both interferon and radiotherapy [82,86,87]. IFNα used in conjunction with radiotherapy has been reported to increase the risk of complications in several organs other than the lung [83,88,89].

These studies demonstrate that the optimal dosage and schedules for the administration of interferon with radiotherapy have not yet been established. The results of cell line studies have shown that interferon can potentiate radiation treatment; further well-designed studies are therefore to be encouraged. A particularly interesting approach is that of administering interferon by inhalation in conjunction with radiotherapy to ensure that the interferon reaches the target cells [85].

Inhaled interferons

Considerable ethical and practical problems arise in experimental studies using inhaled interferon on patients suffering from lung cancer. Patients are required to undergo frequent bronchoalveolar lavage, which causes them considerable discomfort. The studies which have been performed at the

Helsinki University Central Hospital [90–93] are therefore very small, but the results are important for the development of interferon therapy.

Pharmacokinetics. Only a small proportion, if any, of systemically administered interferon reaches the target cells in the respiratory tract [94]. Bocci et al. [95] showed that the concentration of interferon in pulmonary tumors is lower than that in plasma samples after intravenous administration of IFNα and IFNβ. They also showed that although the bulk of inhaled interferon reaching the bronchoalveolar region is absorbed, only a small percentage can be detected in the pulmonary venous circulation [96].

Experimental data suggest that there may be differences in the pharmacokinetics of natural and recombinant IFNα in the airways [96]. Data from the human studies undertaken in Helsinki (table 5) support this finding [90,91]. Only inhaled single doses greater than 60 MU of natural human IFNα gave measurable levels of circulating interferon and caused systemic side effects: a rise in temperature, headache and malaise [90]. Reversible bronchoconstriction was occasionally noted.

Measurable levels of serum interferon were only achieved using the highest dose of inhaled recombinant IFNα-2a, and even then only in one sample [91]. The side effects were less severe, but similar in character, to those seen after the inhalation of natural IFNα.

IFNβ was not detected in any serum samples taken after the inhalation of natural IFNβ over a dose range of 3 to 100 MU [93], nor did the patients experience any side effects. Inhaled IFNβ was better tolerated than other IFNs.

Patients inhaling recombinant IFNγ-1b over a dose range of 0.1–5.4 mg [92] experienced few, if any, clinical side effects. IFNγ was only detectable in serum on two occasions: 10 and 27 hours after inhalation of the maximum dose by one patient. The patient developed a fever reaction at the same time. None of the patients experienced the bronchoconstriction seen after the inhalation of IFNα.

IFNγ was detectable in bronchoalveolar lavage fluid (BALF) samples taken three hours after inhalation of 0.6 mg or more of IFNγ [92]. On the other hand, of the samples taken 27 hours after inhalation, IFNγ could still

Table 5. The pharmacokinetics and side effects of inhaled interferon

Interferon	Doses inhaled	Measurable serum IFN levels (inhaled IFN dose)	Systemic side effects	Broncho-constriction
IFNα-natural	1–120 MU	≥ 60 MU	Yes	Yes
-recombinant	18–216 MU	≥ 126 MU	Yes	Yes
IFNβ-natural	3–100 MU	Not seen	No	No
IFNγ-recombinant	0.1–5.4 mg	5.4 mg only	Yes (mild)	No

be detected only in those taken after the highest dose (5.4 mg). Even these were low, suggesting that most IFNγ is cleared from the alveoli within 27 hours of inhalation.

IFN was not detectable in BALF after subcutaneous injections of IFNγ. Neither did the alveolar macrophages exhibit increased CL response [97]. Circulating IFNγ was detected 3 to 12 hours after an injection of the highest dose, and all patients developed systemic side effects: transient fever, nausea, headache and flu-like symptoms. However, Jaffe et al. [23] did not report any side effects after inhaled IFNγ, and those seen in the Helsinki study were minor. This suggests that IFNγ does not easily penetrate the bronchioloalveolar epithelium. Inhaled alpha, beta and gamma IFNs differ in the extent to which they are absorbed from the airways and in the extent to which they cause bronchoconstriction.

Tumor response. In two clinical trials, there was no clear evidence that inhaled natural or recombinant IFNα was active against bronchioloalveolar carcinoma [56,57], although patients with metastatic renal cell carcinoma have been reported to respond to inhaled interleukin-2 [98]. Transbronchial intratumor interferon infiltration has been suggested as a more effective form of treatment for pulmonary malignancies whenever it is possible [99]. IFNγ does not easily penetrate the bronchioloalveolar epithelium either into the circulation or from the blood to the pulmonary alveolar spaces [92]. We therefore recommend further investigation into the administration of IFNγ by inhalation for the treatment of respiratory infections and malignancies. Treatment by inhalation can be further improved with more efficient nebulizers, better formulation of the solution, and more precise dosage.

It seems that at least by using inhaled recombinant IFNγ, we can activate oxygen-radical generation locally in lung tissue, and possibly potentiate lytic activity without systemic side effects. This activation could be exploited, for example, for patients who have difficulty tolerating the side effects associated with systemically administered IFN.

From this discussion, we believe it is apparent that interferons have a role to play in the treatment of both SCLC and NSCLC in combination with other therapies [51,54,61,100,101]. However, the use of the maximum tolerated dose may not be appropriate for biological response modifiers, especially when they are used in combined regimes. In contrast, it is possible that frequent long-term administration of small doses of interferon may deactivate the tumor cells. However, with more prolonged use of interferon, there have been reports of patients developing antibodies to IFNα [102,103]. Recombinant or lymphoblastoid IFNα treatment may cause the development of interferon-neutralizing antibodies, and any type of interferon may encourage the development of autoimmune antibodies such as antinuclear and antithyroid antibodies [103,104]. Neutralizing antibodies block the therapeutic effects of interferon altogether, while autoimmune antibodies only reduce their impact [105]. Neutralizing antibodies have only been

312

shown to develop against recombinant or lymphoblastoid IFNα, and appear to be specific to the type of IFNα. Progression of clinical disease caused by this problem can be overcome by changing the treatment from recombinant to natural IFNα, which does not apparently stimulate the production of antibodies. The switch to natural IFNα treatment causes the interferon-neutralizing antibody levels to diminish, and an objective response (or at least tumor stability) can be reestablished [104,106]. The possibility of neutralizing antibodies (13%–15% according to Öberg [104] and Smith [107]) and of autoimmune or binding antibodies (30% in the Öberg study [104]) must be considered where recombinant or leukocyte IFNα is to be used, and their levels monitored during prolonged administration. A report in 1992 [108] found the incidence of neutralizing antibodies to recombinant IFNα-2c to be much lower than that reported earlier for IFNα-2a and -2b: 0.87% among 346 patients who had received long-term interferon therapy. The authors suggest that there are many factors controlling the development of interferon antibodies: the molecular structure of the interferon, other antigens in the preparation, the method of administration, the therapeutic regime, the type of disease, and the immune status of the patient.

The combination of interferon with chemotherapy for lung cancer patients enhances the effects of chemotherapy and may prolong survival. We need to further assess the benefit of including interferon in well-defined prospective studies for which patients are selected according to precisely defined prognostic criteria. New drugs such as gemcitabine should also be tested in this type of study.

The endpoints for studies using biological response modifiers should be the duration of the progression-free period and overall survival, rather than tumor shrinkage. A successful therapy for an incurable disease is one that prolongs quality survival, and only minor side effects are experienced by patients undergoing interferon treatment.

Interferon and malignant mesothelioma

Malignant mesothelioma cell lines have been established at several centers [109,111], allowing the study of the biology of these cells in vitro, and in vivo using xenografts. Mesothelioma cells are generally sensitive to interferon, although the sensitivity to IFNγ in particular is variable [111–113]. These cells constitutively express class I HLA antigens, but not necessarily class II antigens [112], suggesting that therapy using IFNγ could be effective against malignant mesothelioma. Further experimental studies have shown that the sensitivity of mesothelioma cells to lysis by LAK and NK cells can be enhanced or induced by IFNγ [114], that the growth of human mesothelioma xenografts in nude mice is inhibited by IL-2 and IFNα [115], and that interferon can augment the sensitivity of mesothelioma cells to chemotherapeutic agents [62,113,116].

313

Encouraging progress has been made recently against limited malignant mesothelioma by using intrapleurally administered recombinant IFNγ (40 MU twice a week for two months) [117,118]. However, a subsequent study found that severe adverse reactions associated with the mode of administration hampered compliance [119]. A study using recombinant IFNβ$_{ser}$ (100 MU, five days per week for 6 weeks) [120] did not demonstrate any advantage for IFNβ over IFNγ, but it is possible that the intramuscular route used did not permit sufficient levels of interferon to develop in the plasma. A clinical trial of recombinant IFNα-2a (3–18 MU/day for 12 weeks) is under way in Australia [115]. So far, 4 out of 25 patients have responded positively, as evaluated by CT scanning (1CR, 3PR). The disease has been stabilized in 12 patients. A multicenter study is in progress in Scandinavia to assess the effects of methotrexate combined with recombinant IFNα (3 MU/day sc for nine days during each methotrexate cycle, then 3 MU TIW) and IFNγ (40 μg sc d3,7,11 during each methotrexate cycle, then 40 μg/week), following in vitro results that showed that the activity of methotrexate is greatest when combined with this interferon combination [121].

In view of the resistance of mesothelioma to other forms of treatment, continued investigations using interferon in combination with other therapies would seem to be justified.

Acknowledgments

The authors would like to thank Ms. Anna Ekman for preparing the tables and Graham Hand, M.A., for his invaluable editorial comments.

References

1. Baron S, Tyring SK, Fleischmann WR, Coppenhaver DH, Niesel DW, Klimpel GR, Stanton GJ, Hughes TK. 1991. The interferons — mechanisms of action and clinical applications. JAMA 266:1375–1383.
2. Rosenberg SA, Lotze MT, Yand JC, et al. 1989. Combination therapy with interleukin 2 and alpha interferon for the treatment of patients with advanced cancer. J Clin Oncol 7:1863–1874.
3. Redman BG, Flaherty L, Chou TH, et al. 1990. A phase I trial of recombinant interleukin 2 combined with recombinant interferon gamma in patients with cancer. J Clin Oncol 8:1269–1276.
4. Pestka S, Langer JA, Zoon KC, Samuel CE. 1987. Interferons and their actions. Ann Rev Biochem 56:727–777.
5. Wells V, Mallucci L. 1985. Expression of the 2–5 A system during the cell cycle. Exp Cell Res 159:27–36.
6. Contente S, Kenyon K, Rimoldi D, Friedman RM. 1990. Expression of gene rrg is associated with reversion of NIH 3T3 transformed by LTR-c-H-ras. Science 249:796–798.

314

7. Langdon SP, Rabiasz GJ, Anderson L, Ritchie AA, Fergusson RJ, Hay FG, Miller EP, Mullen P, Plumb J, Miller WR, Smyth JF. 1991. Characterisation and properties of a small cell lung cancer cell line and xenograft WX322 with marked sensitivity to alpha-interferon. Br J Cancer 63:909–915.

8. Tamm L, Jasny BR, Pfeffer LM. 1987. Antiproliferative action of interferons. In Mechanisms of Interferon Action, Vol. 2, M Pfeffer (ed.). CRC Press: Boca Raton, FL, pp. 25–58.

9. Bepler G, Carney DN, Nau MM, Gazdar AF, Minna JD. 1986. Additive and differential biological activity of α-interferon A, difluoromethylornithine and their combination on established human lung cancer cell lines. Cancer Res 46:3413–3419.

10. Sekar V, Atmar VJ, Joshi AR, Krim M, Kuehn G. 1983. Inhibition of ornithine decarboxylase in human fibroblast cells by type I and type II interferons. Biochem Biophys Res Commun 114:950–954.

11. Yasui H, Takai K, Yoshida R, Hayaishi O. 1986. Interferon enhances tryptophan metabolism by inducing pulmonary indoleamine 2,3-dioxygenase: its possible occurrence in cancer patients. Proc Natl Acad Sci USA 83:6622–6626.

12. Fleischmann WR Jr, Newton RC, Fleischmann CM, Colburn NH, Brysk MM. 1984. Discrimination between nonmalignant and malignant cells by combination of IFNγ and IFNα/β. J Biol Response Mod 3:397–405.

13. Billiau A. 1983. The pharmacokinetics and toxicology of interferon. In Interferons: From Molecular Biology to Clinical Application, DC Burke and AG Morris (eds.). Cambridge University Press: Cambridge, pp. 255–276.

14. Marley GM, Doyle LA, Ordóñez JV, Sisk A, Hussain A, Chiu Yen R-W. 1989. Potentiation of interferon induction of class I histocompatibility complex antigen expression by human tumor necrosis factor in small cell lung cancer cell lines. Cancer Res 49:6232–6236.

15. Schwartz BD. 1991. HLA molecules: sentinels of the immune response. Am J Respir Cell Mol Biol 5:211–212.

16. Funa K, Gazdar AF, Mattson K, Niiranen A, Koivuniemi A, Öberg K, Wilander E, Doyle A, Linnoila RI. 1986. Interferon-mediated in vivo induction of β_2-microglobulin on small-cell lung cancers and mid-gut carcinoids. Clin Immunol Immunopathol 41:159–164.

17. Crawford J, Ringenberg S, Propert K, Glenn L, Modeas C, Christenson V, Jaffe H, Green M. 1989. A dose response study of the biological activity of interferon-gamma (IFN-G) in patients with advanced non-small cell lung cancer (NSCLC). Proc ASCO 8:A867.

18. Jabbar SAB, Twentyman PR. Relationship between growth inhibition by cytokines (interferon and tumour necrosis factor) and receptor binding in human lung cancer cell lines.

19. Suarez-Pestano ER, Bjorklund GC, Bergh J, Larsson R, Nilsson K, Pereda CM. 1991. Development of a new interferon alpha-resistant cell line from small-cell lung carcinoma cell line H-82. J Tumor Marker Oncol 6(4):73.

20. Thomassen MJ, Wiedemann HP, Barna BP, Farmer M, Ahmad M. 1988. Induction of in vitro tumoricidal activity in alveolar macrophages and monocytes from patients with lung cancer. Cancer Res 48(14):3949–3953.

21. Murray HW, Scavuzzo D, Jacobs JL, Kaplan MH, Libby DM, Schindler J, Roberts RB. 1987. In vitro and in vivo activation of human mononuclear phagocytes by interferon-gamma. J Immunol 138:2457–2462.

22. Sechler JMG, Malech HL, White CJ, Gallin JI. 1988. Recombinant human interferon-gamma reconstitutes defective phagocyte function in patients with chronic granulomatous disease of childhood. Proc Natl Acad Sci 85:4874–4878.

23. Jaffe HA, Buhl R, Mastrangeli A, Holroyd KJ, Saltini C, Czerski D, Jaffe HS, Kramer S, Sherwin S, Crystal RG. 1991. Organ specific cytokine therapy. J Clin Invest 88:297–302.

24. Badger AM, Meunier PC, Weiss RA, Bugelski PJ. 1988. Modulation of rat broncho-alveolar lavage cell function by the intratracheal delivery of interferon-gamma. J Interferon Res 8:251–260.

315

25. Debs RJ, Fuchs HJ, Philip R, Montgomery AB, Brunette EN, Liggitt D, Patton JS, Shellito JE. 1988. Lung-specific delivery of cytokines induces sustained pulmonary and systemic immunomodulation in rats. J Immunol 140:3482–3488.

26. Kawatsu H, Hasegawa Y, Takagi E, Shimokata K. 1991. Human alveolar macrophages of anergic patients with lung cancer lack the responsiveness to recombinant interferon gamma. Chest 100:1277–1280.

27. Tsuruo T, Lida H, Tsukagoshi S, Olu T, Kishida T. 1982. Different susceptibilities of cultured mouse cell lines to mouse interferon. Gann 73:42–47.

28. Twentyman PR, Workman P, Wright KA, Bleehen NM. 1985. The effects of α and γ interferons on human lung cancer cells grown in vitro or as xenografts in nude mice. Br J Cancer 52:21–29.

29. Carney DN. 1991. Lung cancer biology. Eur J Cancer 27:366–369.

30. Lagadec PF, Saraya KA, Balkwill FR. 1991. Human small cell lung cancer cells are cytokine-resistant but NK/LAK sensitive. Int J Cancer 48(2):311–317.

31. Grönberg A, Ferm M, Tsai L, Kiessling R. 1989. Interferon is able to reduce tumor cell susceptibility to human lymphokine-activated killer (LAK) cells. Cell Immunol 118:10–21.

32. Gazdar AF, Kadoyama C, Venzon D, Park J-G, Tsai C-M, Linnoila RI, Mulshine JL, Ihde DC, Giaccone G. 1992. Association between histological type and neuroendocrine differentiation on drug sensitivity of lung cancer cell lines. J Natl Cancer Inst Monogr 13:191–196.

33. Munker M, Munker R, Saxton RE, Koeffler HP. 1987. Effect of recombinant monokines, lymphokines and other agents on clonal proliferation of human lung cancer cell lines. Cancer Res 47:4081–4085.

34. Jabbar SAB, Twentyman PR. 1990. The use of clonogenic assays in assessing the response of human lung cancer cell lines to alpha- and gamma-interferons alone or in combination with adriamycin. Int J Cancer 46:546–551.

35. Schiller JH, Groveman DS, Schmid SM, Willson JKV, Cummings KB, Borden EC. 1986. Synergistic antiproliferative effects of human recombinant α54- or β$_{ser}$-interferon with γ-interferon on human cell lines of various histogenesis. Cancer Res 46:483–488.

36. Wadler S, Schwartz EL. 1990. Antineoplastic activity of the combination of interferon and cytotoxic agents against experimental and human malignancies: a review. Cancer Res 50:3473–3486.

37. Carmichael J, Fergusson RJ, Wolf CR, Balkwill FR, Smyth JF. 1986. Augmentation of cytotoxicity of chemotherapy by human α-interferons in human non-small cell lung cancer xenografts. Cancer Res 46:4916–4920.

38. Cole SP, Campigotto BM, Johnson JG, Elliot BE. 1991. Differential growth inhibition and enhancement of major histocompatiability complex Class I antigen expression by interferons in a small cell lung cancer cell line and its doxorubicin-selected multidrug-resistant variant. Cancer Immunol Immunother 33:274–277.

39. Tanio Y, Watanabe M, Osaki T, Tachibana I, Kawase I, Kuritani T, Saito S, Masuno T, Kodama N, Furuse K, et al. 1992. High sensitivity to peripheral blood lymphocytes and low HLA Class I antigen expression of small cell lung cancer cell lines with diverse chemo-radiosensitivity. Jpn J Cancer Res 83(7):736–745.

40. Kardamakis D, Gillies NE, Soulhami RL, Bewerley PCL. 1989. Recombinant human interferon alpha-2b enhances the radiosensitivity of small cell lung cancer in vitro. Anticancer Res 9:1041–1044.

41. Dritschilo A, Mossman K, Gray M, Sreevalan T. 1982. Potentiation of radiation injury by interferon. Am J Clin Oncol 5:79–82.

42. Carney DN, Mitchell JB, Kinsella TT. 1983. In vitro radiation and chemotherapy sensitivity of established cell lines of human small cell lung cancer and its large cell morphological variants. Cancer Res 43:2806–2811.

43. Chang AYC, Keng PC. 1987. Potentiation of radiation cytotoxicity by recombinant interferons, a phenomenon associated with increased blockage at the G_2–M phase of the cell cycle. Cancer Res 47:4338–4341.

316

44. Lvovsky EA, Mossman KL, Levy HB, Dritschilo A. 1985. Response of mouse tumour to interferon inducer and radiation. Int J Radiat Oncol Biol Phys 11:1721–1726.
45. Tsai C-M, Ihde DC, Kadoyama C, Venzon D, Gazdar AF. 1990. Correlation of in vitro drug sensitivity testing of long-term small cell lung cancer cell lines with response and survival. Eur J Cancer 26(11/12):1148–1152.
46. Salmon SE. 1990. Chemosensitivity testing: another chapter. J Natl Cancer Inst 82(2): 82–83.
47. Färkkilä M, Niiranen A, Mattson K, Salmi T, Iivanainen M, Cantell K. 1986. Neurotoxicity of high- or low-dose natural IFN-α and of recombinant IFN-γ in patients with lung cancer. In The Biology of the Interferon System. Elsevier: Amsterdam.
48. Mattson K, Niiranen A, Pyrhönen S, Färkkilä M, Cantell K. 1991. Recombinant interferon gamma treatment in non-small cell lung cancer. Acta Oncol 30(5):607–610.
49. Known S, Stoopler M, Cunningham-Rundles S, Oettgen HF. 1980. Phase II trial of human leukocyte interferon in non-small cell lung cancer. Proc Am Assoc Cancer Res 21:179.
50. Stoopler MB, Krown SE, Gralla RJ, Cunningham-Rundles S, Stewart WE, Oettgen HF. 1980. Phase II trial of human leukocyte interferon in non-small cell lung cancer. In II World Conference on Lung Cancer, Abstracts. Copenhagen, p. 221.
51. Figlin RA, Sarna GP, Callaghan M. 1983. Alpha (human leukocyte)-interferon as treatment for non-small cell carcinoma of the lung: a phase II trial. J Biol Respir Modif 2:343–347.
52. Leavitt RD, Duffey P, Aisner J. 1984. A phase II study of recombinant leukocyte-A interferon in non-small cell carcinoma of the lung. Proc ASCO 3:52.
53. Grunberg SM, Kempf RA, Itri LM, Venturi CL, Boswell WD, Mitchell MS. 1985. Phase II study of recombinant alpha interferon in the treatment of advanced non-small cell lung carcinoma. Cancer Treat Rep 69:1031–1032.
54. Olesen BK, Ernst P, Nissen MH, Hansen HH. 1987. Recombinant interferon A (IFL-rA) therapy of small cell and squamous cell carcinoma of the lung: a Phase II study. Eur J Cancer Clin Oncol 23(7):987–989.
55. Niiranen A, Holsti LR, Cantell K, Mattson K. 1990. Natural interferon-alpha alone and in combination with conventional therapies in non-small cell lung cancer. Acta Oncol 29: 927–930.
56. van Zandwijk N, Jassem E, Dubbelman R, Braat MCP, Rumke P. 1990. Aerosol application of interferon-alpha in the treatment of bronchioloalveolar carcinoma. Eur J Cancer 26:738–740.
57. Kinnula V, Cantell K, Mattson K. 1990. Effect of inhaled natural interferon-alpha on diffuse bronchioloalveolar carcinoma. Eur J Cancer 26:740–741.
58. Jones DH, Bleehen NM, Slater AJ, George PJM, Walker JR, Dixon AK. 1983. Human lymphoblastoid interferon in the treatment of small cell lung cancer. Br J Cancer 47: 361–366.
59. Jackson D, Caponera M, Muss H, Ruduick S, Spurr C, Capizzi R. 1984. Interferon α_2 in advanced small cell carcinoma of the lung. Proc ASCO 3:226.
60. Mattson K, Holsti LR, Niiranen A, Kivisaari L, Iivanainen M, Sovijärvi A, Cantell K. 1985. Human leukocyte interferon as part of a combined treatment for previously untreated small cell lung cancer. J Biol Respir Modif 4:8–17.
61. Newman HFV, Bleehen NM, Galazka A, Scott E. 1987. Small cell lung carcinoma: a phase II evaluation of r-interferon-γ. Cancer 60:2938–2940.
62. Sklarin N, Chahinian AP, Feuer EJ, Lahman LA, Szrajer L, Holland JF. 1988. Augmentation of activity of cis-diamminedichloroplatinum (II) and mitocycin C by interferon in human malignant mesothelioma xenografts in nude mice. Cancer Res 48:64–67.
63. Walsh C, Speyer JL, Wernz J, Hochster H, Grossberg H, Chachoua A, Molinaro P, Meyers M, Blum RH. 1989. Phase I study of the combination of alpha-2 interferon and cisplatinum. J Biol Respir Modifiers 8(1):11–15.
64. Schiller JH, Storer B, Dreicer R, Rosenquist D, Frontiera M, Carbone PP. 1989.

Randomized phase II-III trial of combination beta and gamma interferons and etoposide and cisplatin in inoperable non-small cell lung cancer of the lung. J Natl Cancer Inst 81:1739–1743.

65. Rosso R et al. 1989.

66. Bowman A, Fergusson RJ, Allan SG, Stewart ME, Gregor A, Cornbleet MA, Greening AP, Crompton GK, Leonard RCF, Smyth JF. 1990. Potentiation of cisplatin by alpha-interferon in advanced non-small cell lung cancer (NSCLC): a phase II study. Ann Oncol 1:351–353.

67. Rosell R, Carles J, Ariza A, Moreno I, Ribelles N, Solano V, Pellicer I, Barnadas A, Abad A. 1991. A phase II study of days 1 and 8 cisplatin and recombinant alpha-2B interferon in advanced non-small cell lung cancer. Cancer 67:2448–2453.

68. Ardizzoni A, Rosso R, Salvati F, Scagliotti G, Soresi E, Ferrara G, Pennucci C, Baldini E, Cruciani AR, Antilli A, Tonachella R, Rinaldi M, Genovese G, Crippa M, Gatti E, Fortini C. 1991. Combination chemotherapy and interferon-α2b in the treatment of advanced non-small cell lung cancer. Am J Clin Oncol 14(2):120–123.

69. Kataja V. 1993. Combination of cisplatin (CDDP) and interferon alfa-2a in advanced non-small cell lung cancer (NSCLC); an open non-randomized multicentre study. Proc ASCO 12:350(A1177).

70. Giaccone G, Donadio M, Bonardi G, Silvestro L, Viano I, Cotevino G, Vinzio M, Genazzani E, Calciati A. 1989. Phase II study of alpha-interferon plus bleomycin in advanced non-small cell lung cancer. Anticancer Res 9:405–408.

71. Lind MJ, Gomm S, Simmonds AP, Ashcroft L, Kamthan A, Gurney G, Thatcher N. 1991. A phase II study of ifosfamide and a$_{2b}$-interferon in advanced non-small cell lung cancer. Cancer Chemother Pharmacol 28:142–144.

72. Jansen RLH, Slingerland R, Hoo Goey S, Franks CR, Bolhuis RLH, Stoter G. 1992. Interleukin-2 and interferon-α in the treatment of patients with advanced non-small-cell lung cancer. J Immunother 12:70–73.

73. Cellerino R, Tummarello D, Graziano F, Santo A, Pasini F, Isidori P, Pedeli A, Ferretti B, Pieroni V. 1993. Advanced non-small cell lung cancer (ANSCLC): phase II study with rIL-2 & α-IFN in patients responsive or stable to induction chemotherapy. Proc ASCO 12:348(A1169).

74. Jett JR, Su JQ, Maksymiuk AW. 1992. Phase III trial of recombinant interferon gamma (r IFN-γ) in complete responders (CR) with small cell lung cancer (SCC). Proc ASCO 11:267(A956).

75. Mattson K, Niiranen A, Pyrhönen S, Holsti LR, Kumpulainen E, Cantell K. 1992. Natural interferon alpha as maintenance therapy for small cell lung cancer. Eur J Cancer 28A (8/9):1387–1391.

76. Kohne-Wompner CH, Koschel G, Pawel JV, Wilke H, Vallee D, Bremer K, Schroder M, Kaukel E, Eberhard W, et al. 1992. Carboplatin, etoposide, vincristine chemotherapy plus radiotherapy in limited desease small-cell lung cancer followed by maintenance with interferon alpha-2B versus observation. Proc ASCO 11:A1027.

77. Kelly K, Bunn PA, Musuka N, Beasley K, Crowley J, Livingston R. 1993. The role of alpha interferon (rINFα2A) maintenance in patients with limited stage SCLC responding to concurrent chemoradiation: a southwest oncology study. Proc ASCO 12:330(A1099).

78. Glisson BS, Palmer JL, Shin DM, Wester M, Markowitz AB. 1993. Phase II trial of interferon alfa (IFN) + etoposide/cisplatin induction and IFN/MEGACE maintenance in extensive small cell lung cancer. Proc ASCO 12:354(A1194).

79. Mattson K, Maasilta P, Halme M, Niiranen A, Pyrhönen S, Riska K, Cantell K, Eklund J. 1993. Chemotherapy plus alpha-interferon in the treatment of small cell lung cancer. Am Rev Respir Dis 147(4):A748.

80. Nederman T, Benediktsson G. 1982. Effects of interferon on growth rate and radiation sensitivity of cultured, human glioma cells. Acta Radiol Oncol 21:231–234.

81. Gould M, Kakria R, Olson B, Borden E. 1984. Radiosensitization of human bronchogenic carcinoma cells by interferon beta. J Interferon Res 4(1):123–128.
82. Holsti LR, Mattson K, Niiranen A, Standertskiöld-Nordenstam C-G, Stenman S, Sovijärvi A, Cantell K. 1987. Enhancement of radiation effects by alpha interferon in the treatment of small cell carcinoma of the lung. Int J Radiat Oncol Biol Phys 13:1161–1166.
83. Real FX, Known SE, Nisce LZ, Oettgen HF. 1985. Unexpected toxicity from radiation therapy in two patients with Kaposi's sarcoma receiving interferon. J Biol Respir Modif 4:141–146.
84. Jermy A, Rees GJG, Rees RC. 1983. Lack of interferon induction by radiotherapy. Br J Radiol 56:274.
85. Maasilta P, Holsti LR, Halme M, Kivisaari L, Cantell K, Mattson K. 1992. Natural alpha-interferon in combination with hyperfractionated radiotherapy in the treatment of non-small cell lung cancer. Int J Radiat Oncol Biol Phys 23:863–868.
86. Torrisi J, Berg C, Bonnem E, Dritschilo A. 1986. The combined use of interferon and radiotherapy in cancer management. Semin Oncol 13(Suppl 2):78–83.
87. Torrisi J, Berg C, Harter K, Lvovsky E, Yeung K, Wooley P, Bonnem E, Dritschilo A. 1986. Phase I combined modality clinical trial of alpha-2 interferon and radiotherapy. Int J Radiat Oncol Biol Phys 12:1453–1456.
88. Cottler-Fox M, Torrisi J, Spitzer TR, Deeg HJ. 1990. Increased toxicity of total body irradiation in patients receiving interferon for leukaemia. Lancet 335:174.
89. Hagberg H, Blomkvist E, Ponten U, Persson L, Muhr C, Eriksson B, Öberg K, Olssn Y, Lilja A. 1990. Does alpha-interferon in conjugation with radiotherapy increase the risk of complications in the central nervous system? Ann Oncol 1:449.
90. Kinnula V, Mattson K, Cantell K. 1989. Pharmacokinetics and toxicity of inhaled human interferon alpha in patients with lung cancer. J Interferon Res 9:419–423.
91. Maasilta P, Halme M, Mattson K, Cantell K. 1991. Pharmacokinetics of inhaled recombinant and natural alpha interferon. Lancet 337:371.
92. Halme M, Maasilta P, Repo H, Ristola M, Taskinen E, Mattson K, Cantell K. 1994. Inhaled recombinant interferon gamma in humans: pharmocokinetics and effects on chemiluminescence responses of alveolar macrophages and peripheral blood neutrophils and monocytes. Int J Radiation Oncol Biol Phys. In Press.
93. Halmc M, Maasilta P, Mattson K, Cantell K. 1994. Pharmacokinetics and toxicity of inhaled human natural interferon-beta in patients with lung cancer. Respiration 61:105–107.
94. Esgro JJ, Whitworth P, Fidler IJ. 1990. Macrophages as effectors of tumor immunity. Immunol Allergy Clin North Am 10:705–729.
95. Bocci V, Carraro F, Naldini A, Borrelli E, Biagi G, Gotti G, Ciomarelli PP. 1990. Interferon levels in human pulmonary tumours are lower than plasma levels. J Biol Regul Homeostat Agents 4:153–156.
96. Bocci V, Pessina GP, Pacini A, Paulesu L, Muscettola M, Mogensen KE. 1984. Pulmonary catabolism of interferons: alveolar absorption of ^{124}I-labeled human interferon alpha is accompanied by partial loss of biological activity. Antiviral Res 4:211–220.
97. Halme M, Maasilta P, Repo H, Leirisalo-Repo M, Taskinen E, Mattson M, Cantell K. 1994. Subcutaneously administered recombinant interferon gamma in humans: pharmaco-kinetics and effects on chemiluminescence responses of alveolar macrophages, blood neutrophils and monocytes. Immunother 15:283–291.
98. Huland E, Huland H, Heinzer H. 1992. Interleukin-2 by inhalation: local therapy for metastatic renal cell carcinoma. J Urol 147:344–348.
99. Bocci V. 1992. Physicochemical and biological properties of interferons and their potential uses in drug delivery systems. Crit Rev Ther Drug Carrier Syst 9:91–133.
100. Beck LK, Kane MA, Bunn PA Jr. 1988. Innovative and future approaches to small cell lung cancer treatment. Semin Oncol 15:300–314.

319

101. Borden EC, Hawkins MJ. 1986. Biologic response modifiers as adjucants to other therapeutic modalities. Semin Oncol 13:144–152.
102. Itri LM, Campion M, Dennin RA, et al. 1987. Incidence and clinical significance of neutralizing antibodies in patients receiving recombinant IFN-α_{2a} by intramuscular injection. Cancer 59:668–674.
103. Von Wussow P, Freund M, Block B, et al. 1987. Clinical significance of anti-IFN-α antibody titers during interferon therapy. Lancet 2:635–636.
104. Öberg K, Alm G, Magnusson A, Lundqvist G, Theodorsson E, Wide L, Wilander E. 1989. Treatment of malignant carcinoid tumors with recombinant interferon alfa-2b: development of neutralizing interferon antibodies and possible loss of antitumor activity. J Natl Cancer Inst 81:531–535.
105. Feldman M, Londei M, Buchan G. 1987. Interferons and autoimmunity. In Interferon, Vol. 9, I Gresser (ed.). Academic Press: New York, pp. 73–90.
106. Von Wussow P, Pralle H, Hockkeppel H-K, Jakschies D, Sonnen S, Schmidt H, Müller-Rosenau D, Franke M, Haferlach T, Zwingers T, Rapp U, Delcher H. 1991. Effective natural interferon α therapy in recombinant interferon α-resistant patients with hairy cell leukaemia. Blood 78:38–43.
107. Smith JW, Longo DL, Urba WJ, Clark JW, Watson T, Beveridge J, Conlon KC, Sznol M, Creekmore SP, Alvord WG, Lawrence JB, Steis RG. 1991. Prolonged continuous treatment of hairy cell leukemia patients with recombinant interferon-α2a. Blood 78(7): 1664–1671.
108. Steinmann GG, Göd B, Rosenkaimer F, Adolf G, Bidlingmaier G, Frühbeis B, Lamche H, Lindner J, Patzelt E, Schmähling C, Schneider F-J. 1992. Low incidence of antibody formation due to long-term interferon-α_{2c} treatment of cancer patients. Clin Invest 70:136–141.
109. Pelin-Enlund K, Husgafvel-Pursiainen K, Tammilehto L, Klockars M, Jantunen K, Gerwin BL, Harris CC, Tuomi T, Vanhala E, Mattson K, Linnainmaa K. 1990. Asbestos-related malignant mesothelioma: growth, cytology, tumorigenicity and consistent chromosome findings in cell lines from five patients. Carcinogenesis 11(4):673–681.
110. Manning LS, Whitaker D, Murch AR, et al. 1991. Establishment and characterisation of five human malignant mesothelioma cell lines derived from pleural effusions. Int J Cancer 47:285–290.
111. Hand AMS, Husgafvel-Pursiainen K, Tammilehto L, Mattson K, Linnainmaa K. 1991. Malignant mesothelioma: the antiproliferative effects of cytokine combinations on three human mesothelioma cell lines. Cancer Lett 58:205–210.
112. Christmas TI, Manning LS, Davis MR, Robinson BWS, Garlepp MJ. 1991. HLA expression and malignant mesothelioma. Am J Respir Cell Mol Biol 5:213–220.
113. Hand AMS, Husgafvel-Pursiainen K, Pelin K, Vallas M, Suitiala T, Ekman A, Mattson M, Mattson K, Linnainmaa K. 1992. Interferon-α and -γ in combination with chemotherapeutic drugs: in vitro sensitivity studies in four human mesothelioma cell lines. Anti-Cancer Drugs 3:687–694.
114. Manning LS, Bowman RV, Darby SB, Robinson BS. 1989. Lysis of human malignant mesothelioma cells by natural killer and lymphokine-activated killer cells. Am Rev Respir Dis 139:1369–1374.
115. Robinson BWS, Bowman R, Christmas T, Musk AW, Manning LS. 1991. Immunotherapy for malignant mesothelioma: use of interleukin-2 and interferon alpha. In Interferons and Cytokines, HC Thomas, M Talpaz, and R Penny (eds.). Mediscript: London, 1991.
116. Chahinian AP, Norton L, Holland JF, et al. 1984. Experimental and clinical activity of mitocycin C and cis-diamminedichloroplatinum in malignant mesothelioma. Cancer Res 44:1688–1692.
117. Boutin C, Viallat JR, Astoul P. 1990. Treatment of mesothelioma with interferon gamma and interleukin-2. Rev Pneumol Clin 46(5):211–215.
118. Chicheportiche C, Laurent JC, Bethaj M, Rey F, Astoul P, Ponchetet P, et al. 1992.

Immuno-biological monitoring of patients with malignant pleural effusions treated with intrapleural interferon γ. Proc Am Assoc Cancer Res 33:246(A1476).

119. Douillard JY, Boutin C, Bignon J, Guerin JC, Van Derschueren R, Brandely M. 1992. Intrapleural recombinant human gamma interferon (rhγ IFN) in the treatment of malignant pleural mesothelioma. Proc ASCO 11:307(A1037).

120. Von Hoff DD, Metch B, Lucas JG, Balcerzak SP, Grunberg SM, Rivkin SE. 1990. Phase II evaluation of recombinant interferon-β (IFN-β_{ser}) in patients with diffuse mesothelioma: a Southwest Oncology Group study. J Interferon Res 10:531–534.

121. Hand AMS, Pelin K, Halme M, Mattson M, Ekman A, Linnainmaa K. Submitted. Interferons and methotrexate: in vitro sensitivity studies in 4 malignant mesothelioma cell lines.

15. New antineoplastic agents in lung cancer 1988–1993

Stefan C. Grant and Mark G. Kris

Introduction

Chemotherapy is the standard initial treatment for patients with small cell lung cancer (SCLC), and combination chemotherapy can prolong the lives of patients with non-small cell lung cancer (NSCLC) [1,2]. Despite these developments, most patients develop metastatic disease, and lung cancer remains the leading cause of death from cancer [3]. Over the past five years, a number of new agents with activity against lung cancer have been identified, offering the potential for improved control of this disease. A number of these drugs have novel mechanisms of action. Additionally, the understanding of the pharmacokinetics of 'older' agents has expanded, resulting in the more effective use of the available chemotherapeutic drugs. At the same time, we have also learned that many new agents have insufficient antitumor activity against lung cancer to warrant further development. Agents identified between 1988 and 1993 with potential usefulness in lung cancer patients are presented in table 1 and discussed in detail below.

Agents identified

Chloroquinoxaline sulfonamide

Chloroquinoxaline sulfonamide (CQS) is a sulfonamide specifically selected for development because of its substantial activity against lung tumors in the in vitro human tumor colony-forming assay [4]. In a phase I trial where dose levels ranged from 18 to 4870 mg/m^2, one major and six minor responses were observed in 52 NSCLC patients who had previously received chemotherapy [5]. The drug is currently being evaluated in a phase II trial in NSCLC patients, using a dosing schedule guided by pharmacokinetic modeling.

Heine H. Hansen, (ed), Hansen: Lung Cancer.
© *1994 Kluwer Academic Publishers. ISBN 0-7923-2835-3. All rights reserved.*

Table 1. Chemotherapeutic agents for the treatment of lung cancer identified 1988–1993

Non-small cell lung cancer (response rate ≥15%)	Small cell lung cancer (response rate ≥20%)
CPT-11	CPT-11
Edatrexate	Epirubicin
Etoposide (oral)	Etoposide (oral)
Fotomustine	Gemcitabine
Gemcitabine	Paclitaxel
Paclitaxel	Teniposide
Docetaxel	
Vinorelbine	

CPT-11

Camptothecin is a plant alkaloid derived from Camptotheca acuminata, a shrub found throughout Asia [6]. Although initial clinical trials were disappointing, it was subsequently discovered that an intact lactone ring, not present in the parent compound, is necessary for activity [7]. Thereafter a number of compounds were produced, either as semisynthetic derivatives or de novo, including 7-ethyl-10-(4-[1-piperidino]-1-piperidin) carbonyloxy-camptothecin (CPT-11) (figure 1). This agent is a water-soluble compound with an intact lactone ring. Other members of the class include topotecan and nine amino camptothecin.

These agents have a unique intranuclear target, the enzyme topoisomerase I, which is involved in the relaxation of supercoiled DNA [8]. Camptothecins permit the topoisomerase to uncoil, produce a single strand break in the DNA, and prevent the resealing of the break by the enzyme [7]. In preclinical animal studies, CPT-11 demonstrated antitumor activity against a number of tumors including the Lewis lung carcinoma [9,10].

Phase I trial. Seventeen patients with advanced NSCLC were studied in a phase I trial reported in 1991 [11]. CPT-11 was administered weekly at a dose of 50, 100, 125, and 150 mg/m^2, with at least three patients being entered at each dose level. The median age was 64 years, and 16 of the patients had an ECOG performance status of 1 or 2. Thirteen of the patients were men. Twelve patients had stage IV NSCLC, and the remainder had stage III disease. One patient had received prior chemotherapy. The dose-limiting toxicities were myelosuppression and diarrhea. Nausea and vomiting occurred in 53% of patients (24% grade 3 or 4), and 41% of patients experienced diarrhea, including four cases of grade 3 or 4 diarrhea, both of which occurred at a dose ≥125 mg/m^2. The major hematologic toxicity was leukopenia, with two patients at the 150 mgm^2 dose level experiencing grade

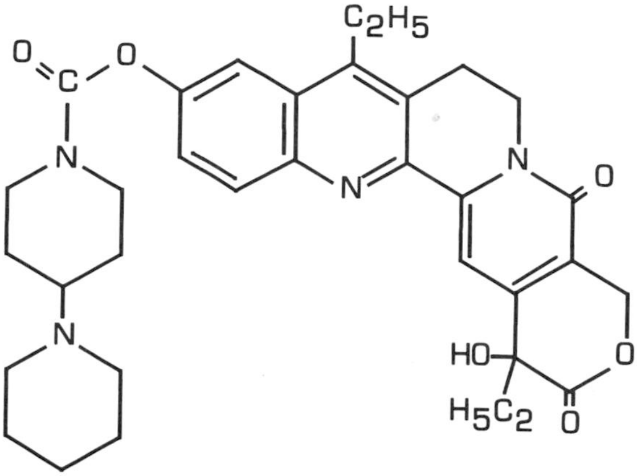

Figure 1. Structure of CPT-11.

4 leukopenia. Thrombocytopenia was reported to be milder, although grade 4 toxicity was observed in the two patients with grade 4 leukopenia. Other toxicities included anemia, alopecia (12%), abnormal serum tests of liver function, and renal insufficiency following dehydration from severe diarrhea. One patient experienced drug-induced pneumonitis that responded to treatment. Two partial responses were observed among 11 NSCLC patients assessable for response. The authors recommended $100 \, mg/m^2$ weekly as the phase II dose of CPT-11.

Phase II trials in NSCLC. Fukuoka et al. [12] studied CPT-11 in 73 patients with inoperable NSCLC who had not received prior therapy. Patient characteristics are summarized in table 2. Standard criteria [13] were used to evaluate both response and toxicity. CPT-11 was administered weekly as a 90-minute infusion after a prick skin test. The starting dose was $100 \, mg/m^2$. Treatment was delayed for leukopenia, with dose attenuations being incorporated. Treatment was discontinued for any grade 4 toxicity. Seventy-two patients were assessable for both response and toxicity, with a median follow-up of 17 months. Twenty-three patients (32%) achieved a partial response (95% confidence intervals: 20%–44%). Response rates were similar in patients with locoregional and stage IV disease (31% and 33%). The median duration of response was 15 weeks (range, 7 to 31 weeks), with no difference being observed between patients with locoregional and stage IV disease. The median duration of survival was 42 weeks for all patients and 40 weeks for patients with stage IV disease. The toxicities observed were similar to those seen in the phase I trial and are summarized in table 2. The dose-limiting toxicities were leukopenia and diarrhea. Other major side-effects were nausea and vomiting, diarrhea, anemia, and alopecia. Mild thrombocytopenia, constipation, low-grade fever, mucositis and skin rash,

Table 2. Summary of phase II trials of CPT-11

CPT-11	NSCLC [12]	SCLC [14]	[15]
Total number of patients	73	15	41
(adequate for response)	(72)	(14)	(35)
Male: Female	53:20	12:3	33:8
PS (ECOG)			
0, 1	53	6	28
2	19	9	13
Stage	I, II = 3	LD = 5	LD = 12
	III = 30	ED = 10	ED = 29
	IV = 40	—	—
Prior chemotherapy	0	15	27
Response rate	32%	47%	33%
(95% confidence intervals)	(20% to 44%)	(21% to 72%)	—

and elevations in serum liver enzymes were observed. Six patients developed pulmonary toxicity. Two had grade 4 toxicity (3%) with one death.

Phase II trials in SCLC. Sixteen patients with refractory (1) or relapsed (15) SCLC were studied by Masuda et al. [14]. Patient characteristics are summarized in table 2. Treatment schedule, dose, and dose attenuation were similar to the trial in patients with NSCLC reported by Fukuoka [12], as were the criteria for assessing response and toxicity. Of 15 patients assessable for response, seven (47%) achieved a partial response (95% confidence limits, 21%–72%), with a median duration of response of 58 days (range: 28 to 156 days). The median survival for all eligible patients was 187 days. Toxicities were similar to those seen in other trials, with leukopenia being dose limiting. Grade 3 and 4 pulmonary toxicity was observed in two patients and was fatal in one.

Another trial reported by the same authors [15] studied CPT-11 at the same dose and schedule in both previously untreated and treated SCLC patients. Patient characteristics were similar (table 2). Among 27 previously treated patients, there were two complete responses and seven partial responses (33% major response rate). Four partial responses were observed in eight previously untreated patients. The overall major response rate was 37%. The median time to response was 28 days (range: 12 to 57 days), and median duration of response was 50 days (range, 28 to 116 days). The median survival for all patients was 246 days.

Combination chemotherapy trials. The phase II trials of CPT-11 established the activity of this unique agent in patients with lung cancer. Using an MTT (cytotoxicity) in vitro assay, Takada et al. [14] evaluated the antitumor activity of CPT-11 in combination with agents commonly used in the treatment of lung cancer. SN-38, an active metabolite of CPT-11, was combined with doxorubicin, vindesine, etoposide, cisplatin, and mitomycin. Based on the results of this study, the combination of CPT-11 and cisplatin was selected and evaluated against human lung cancer xenografts in nude mice. A synergistic effect was reported in two of three tumor cell lines studied. The authors proposed clinical trials to evaluate CPT-11 in combination with cisplatin or etoposide.

A phase I trial combined cisplatin at a dose of $80\,mg/m^2$ given every four weeks, with CPT-11 given on days, 1, 8, and 15 of a 28-day cycle [16]. The initial dose of CPT-11 was $30\,mg/m^2$, with increments of $10\,mg/m^2$ until dose-limiting toxicity was reached. Twenty-three previously untreated patients (10 women) with stage IIIB (4) or IV (19) non-small cell lung cancer were studied, and all were assessable for response and toxicity. The median age was 64 years (range: 38–75). The maximum tolerated dose of CPT-11 was $70\,mg/m^2$, with leukopenia and diarrhea being the dose-limiting toxicities. Of the 23 patients, 13 partial responses (57%) were observed. It was concluded that the combination of cisplatin and CPT-11 was highly active in NSCLC, and further studies are warranted. The authors proposed a dose of $60\,mg/m^2$ of CPT-11 for subsequent studies in combination with cisplatin. This combination is currently being studied in SCLC.

Docetaxel (Taxotere®)

Docetaxel (figure 2) is produced from a noncytotoxic precursor, 10-deacetyl baccatin III, extracted from the needles of the European yew, Taxus baccata. Docetaxel's mechanism of action is similar to that of paclitaxel; however, it appears to be 2.5 to 5 times more potent in certain cell lines [17]. In preclinical studies, it has demonstrated antitumor activity against tumor cell lines in vitro and in vivo, including a paclitaxel resistant cell line, J7.TAX-50, and Lewis lung [18]. For phase I trials, the agent was solubilized in 50% polysorbate 80 and 50% dehydrated alcohol.

Phase I trials. Phase I studies have evaluated docetaxel administered every three weeks as a 24-hour infusion [17], a six-hour infusion [19], or a one-hour infusion [20]. Docetaxel has been given, without premedication, over one hour for five days every three weeks [21], and as a one-hour infusion weekly [22]. The major limiting toxicity was neutropenia, with the nadirs occurring by day 7 and resolving by day 14. Peripheral neuropathies were seen, particularly in patients who had previously received either vincristine or cisplatin. Other adverse rations were alopecia, mucositis, skin rash, and thrombocytopenia, which were generally mild. Infusion-related hypersensitivity reactions were seen, but their incidence appears lower than that

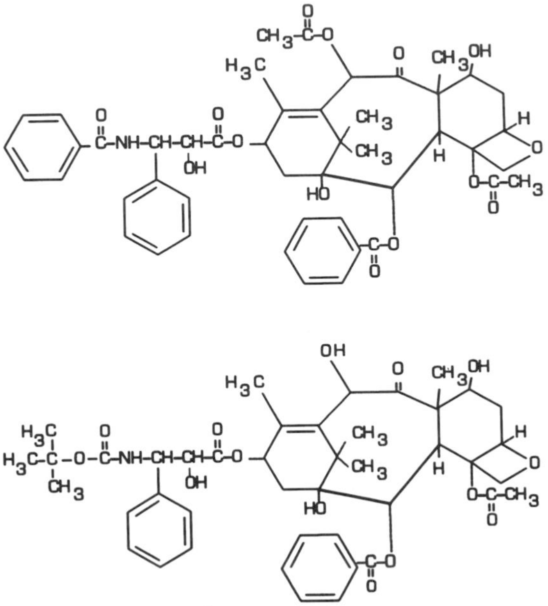

Figure 2. Structure of paclitaxel (top) and docetaxel (bottom).

observed with paclitaxel, even though docetaxel was administered as a short infusion without premedication.

Phase II trials in NSCLC. Three phase II studies, in both previously treated and untreated patients with NSCLC, are underway and have been reported in abstract form. Docetaxel was administered at a dose of $100\,mg/m^2$ intravenously every three weeks [23–25]. Patient characteristics are shown in table 3. Responses were observed both in previously untreated patients and

Table 3. Phase II trials of docetaxel in NSCLC

Docetaxel	[23]	[24]	[25]
Patients entered (adequate for response)	31 (20)	43 (24)	22 (18)
Male:Female	17:14	35:8	14:8
Performance status	NR	NR	60%–90%
Stage	NR	NR	IIIB/IV
Prior chemotherapy	15	0	0
Response rate (95% confidence interval)	30% (12%–54%)	33% (16%–55%)	28% (10%–54%)

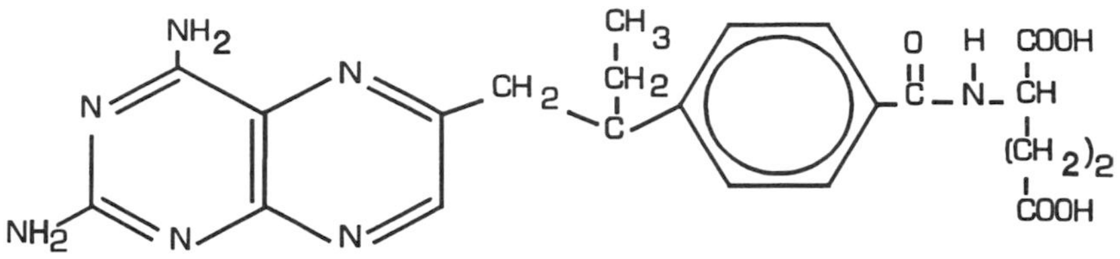

Figure 3. Structure of edatrexate.

in patients who had received cisplatin chemotherapy. Although all three trials include patients in whom it was too early to evaluate response, response rates of 28% to 33% have been reported. Additional singe-agent trials and the testing of docetaxel in combination with cisplatin are planned.

Edatrexate

Edatrexate (10-ethyl-10-deazaaminopterin, 10EdAM, EDX) (figure 3) is an antifolate antimetabolite. Compared to 10-deazaaminopterin and methotrexate, edatrexate has an increased differential in membrane transport between normal tissues and tumor cells as well as a preferential increase in the polyglutamylation and intracellular accumulation of cytotoxic polyglutamates in tumor cells [26–28]. Edatrexate is metabolized in the liver and excreted in bile. In mouse studies, activity superior to methotrexate as well as the parent compound 10-deazaaminopterin was demonstrated [27, 29–31]. Phase I trials evaluated dosage levels from 5–120 mg/m^2 I.V. given weekly, with or without a rest period, in adults with advanced solid tumors [32]. The most common and dose-limiting toxicity in each trial was mucositis. Although the median leukocyte nadir was within the normal range, 15% of all patient courses were complicated by 2+ leukopenia, and 15% of patient courses were complicated by 2+ or greater thromobocytopenia. A macular rash on the trunk and extremities was noted in 12 patients (19%) and occurred more commonly in patients receiving edatrexate on the weekly schedule. Partial remissions were observed in patients with NSCLC and breast cancer.

Phase II trials in NSCLC. In 1988, Shum et al. reported a major response rate of 32% (95% confidence interval: 15%–55%) in a phase II study of 20 patients with stage III or IV NSCLC who had not previously received chemotherapy [33]. The median response duration was 15.4 months (range 5.5 to 41 months), and the median survival was 8.0 months. Toxicities were qualitatively similar but generally milder than those in the phase I trials.

The second phase II study of edatrexate in 31 NSCLC patients was reported by Lee et al. [34]. The initial edatrexate dose was 80 mg/m^2 weekly. Three partial remissions (10%) as well as nine minor responses (30%) were documented. Adverse effects were generally mild and similar to those noted in previous studies. The median survival for all 31 patients was 10.8 months.

A third phase II study of edatrexate given at a dose of 80 mg/m^2 weekly to 49 untreated NSCLC patients was conducted at University College Hospital, London [35]. The median WHO performance status was 0 (range 0–2). Employing standard WHO response criteria, partial responses were seen in 6 of 45 assessable patients (13%; 95% confidence intervals, 6%–26%). Again a high minor response rate was observed, occurring in 20%. The median duration of response was 10 weeks, and toxicities were similar to those observed in prior trials.

Combination chemotherapy trials in NSCLC. Sirotnak et al. studied edatrexate in combination with other cytotoxic agents and observed a synergistic effect [36,37]. Based on this, Kris et al. [38] explored a combination of edatrexate, mitomycin, and vinblastine in patients with stage III or IV NSCLC. In this study, a major objective response rate of 58% (95% confidence intervals: 47%–67%) was observed. The median response duration was 9.5 months, and the median survival was 13.6 months. With a median follow up of 13.3 months (range 3–23 months), the one-year survival was 54%. With the exception of an increased incidence of leukopenia, the toxicities seen in this study were similar in type and severity to those seen in the single-agent phase II trials, demonstrating that edatrexate can be given safely at its phase II dose with the combination of vinblastine and mitomycin. This regimen is currently being evaluated in a randomized multicenter phase III trial comparing it to the combination of mitomycin and vinblastine alone.

Again based on the data of Sirotnak demonstrating antitumor synergy, Lee et al. studied edatrexate in combination with cisplatin and cyclophosphamide [39,40]. Thirty-two previously untreated patients with stage IIIB (four patients) or stage IV (28 patients) NSCLC were treated. All had a Zubrod's performance status of at least 2, and 22 of the patients were men. The first 16 patients received edatrexate 80 mg/m^2 intravenously on days 1 and 8; cyclophosphamide 800 mg/m^2 on day 1; and cisplatin 80 mg/m^2 on day 1, repeated every three weeks. Doses were attenuated according to toxicities. In the second 16 patients, staring doses were reduced by 12.5% because of the toxicities experienced by the first group. Seven of 15 evaluable patients (47%) in the first group and 4 of 15 (27%) of the second group had major tumor responses, with an overall response rate of 37%. Toxicities seen in this study were similar to those seen in early studies, but with more severe myelosuppression. Four patients treated with leucovorin had alleviation of their stomatitis.

Phase II trials in SCLC. The North Central Cancer Treatment Group evaluated edatrexate in SCLC [41]. Eleven untreated and 19 previously treated patients received 80 mg/m^2 edatraxate weekly. No responses were observed, and toxicities were similar to those observed in prior trials.

Epirubicin

Epirubicin (4'-epidoxorubicin) is a stereoisomer of doxorubicin. In preclinical studies, equitoxic doses of epirubicin produced equivalent antitumor activity to doxorubicin, with less cardiotoxicity being observed in rabbits [42–44]. In phase I trials, the major toxicity was myelosuppression [45].

Phase II trials in NSCLC. Joss et al. conducted a phase II trial of epirubicin in 98 patients with NSCLC [46], of which 75 were evaluable for response. Initially administered at a dose of $90\,mg/m^2$ every three weeks, epirubicin doses were attenuated or escalated in individual patients according to their nadir blood counts. All patients were ambulatory, and half had experienced no or minimal weight loss. Seventy-three patients had not received prior chemotherapy. Partial responses were observed in only four patients (major response rate, 5%; 95% confidence limits, 0.2%–10%). A second trial evaluated doses from 70 to $85\,mg/m^2$ and reported a 12% response rate [47]. A subsequent phase I–II trial [45] evaluated doses of $15\,mg/m^2$ to $60\,mg/m^2$ given daily for three days repeated every three weeks. After treating 35 patients, the maximum tolerated dose (MTD) was defined as $55\,mg/m^2$ daily for three days, and an additional 30 patients were treated at a daily dose of $50\,mg/m^2$. Once again, the major toxicity was myelosuppression. No complete responses were seen. An overall response rate of 19% (95% confidence limits, 10% to 31%) was reported. Martoni et al. administered epirubicin at doses from 120 to $165\,mg/m^2$ and reported a 29% response rate [48]. The improved response rates observed at higher doses suggests that this agent may be useful in NSCLC.

Phase II trials in SCLC. Three trials have demonstrated the activity of epirubicin in SCLC. The Clinical Trials Group of the National Cancer Institute of Canada treated 40 previously untreated patients with extensive stage disease [49]. The starting dose was $100\,mg/m^2$ (eight patients) or $120\,mg/m^2$ administered intravenously every three weeks. Three complete and 17 partial responses (50%) were observed. The major toxicity was myelosuppression. Alopecia, nausea and vomiting, and declines in cardiac ejection fractions were also observed.

A second study evaluated a dose of $120\,mg/m^2$ given every three to four weeks, in a similar patient population [50]. Of 80 patients entered, 71 were evaluable for response. An overall response rate of 48% was reported, with four complete and 30 partial responses. Toxicities were similar to those observed previously.

Macchiarini administered epirubicin every three weeks at a dose of $100\,mg/m^2$ for the first cycle and $140\,mg/m^2$ in subsequent cycles [51]. Nineteen patients were entered, of which 18 were eligible. Eleven patients had limited-stage disease. The overall response rate was 33% (two complete responses, four partial responses; 95% confidence limits, 14%–52%).

331

Etoposide: prolonged oral administration

Etoposide (VP-16) is a phase-specific drug, acting during late S phase or early G2 phase of the cell cycle, and has been shown, in preclinical studies, to be schedule dependent [52–54]. It is currently used as a first-line agent in SCLC, and is commonly administered to patients with NSCLC. The initial studies of intravenous etoposide reported response rates of 50% for SCLC [55], with response rates of 7% for NSCLC [56]. In 1989, Slevin et al. demonstrated the schedule dependence of etoposide in SCLC [52]. Thirty-nine previously untreated patients with extensive-stage SCLC were randomized to receive either $500 \, mg/m^2$ as a continuous intravenous infusion over 24 hours or $100 \, mg/m^2$ given over two hours daily for five days, both repeated every 21 days. In the group of patients receiving the single dose of chemotherapy, a partial response of 10% (2/20) was observed. In contrast, amongst those patients receiving the five-day treatment, an 84% partial response rate (17/19) and a 5% complete response rate was seen. Further, the median survival of this group was 10 months, compared to 6.3 months for those patients receiving etoposide as a single dose. When etoposide became available as an oral capsule, it became feasible to administer the agent over even longer periods. A series of studies have been conducted that have evaluated the activity of oral etoposide in both SCLC and NSCLC.

Phase II trials in NSCLC. Three studies evaluated the administration of etoposide capsules over three weeks in NSCLC [53,54,57]. The results are summarized in table 4. In each trial, a dose of $50 \, mg/m^2$ etoposide was given daily for 21 days of a four-week cycle. Because the drug is only available as a 50-mg capsule, doses were averaged over two or three days to achieve the desired dose. Most patients had not received chemotherapy prior to entry into the trials. Response rates of 4% [57], 20% (26% in untreated patients) [54], and 23% [53] were observed. Nonhematologic toxicities were generally

Table 4. Single-agent phase II trials of oral etoposide given on a chronic schedule in patients with NSCLC

Etoposide — chronic, oral schedule	[57]	[53]	[54]
Patients entered	46	25	25
(adequate for response)	(43)	(22)	(25)
Male : Female	36:7	12:13	20:5
Performance status		2 = 0;	
ECOG (KPS)	(50–100)	17 = 1; 6 = 2	Median = 2
Prior chemotherapy	0	2	6
Response rate	5%	23%	20%
(95% confidence interval)	(1%–16%)	(10%–43%)	(4%–36%)

mild, although alopecia occurred in 46% to 100% of patients. Nausea was also common, but was usually mild (grade 1 or 2).

Phase II trials in SCLC. The activity of etoposide against SCLC also appears to be enhanced by prolonged administration. Twenty elderly or unfit patients received 50 mg twice daily for 14 days of a 21-day cycle for a maximum of six cycles [58]. The median age was 70 years, and the median Karnofsky performance status was 60%. Fifteen patients had extensive stage disease. In this group of patients, an 85% major response rate was observed (95% confidence limits, 62%–97%), with two patients achieving a complete response and 15 a partial response. The major toxicity was myelosuppression.

Prolonged oral administration of etoposide has also demonstrated activity against refractory or relapsed SCLC [59]. Twenty-two patients who had previously received chemotherapy were treated with 50 mg/m^2/day for 21 days of a 28-day cycle. Eleven patients had received cyclophosphamide and doxorubicin, with either vincristine (CAV) or etoposide (CAE) or both (CAVE). Four of these patients had subsequently been treated with cisplatin and intravenous etoposide (EP). An additional nine patients had received EP as initial therapy, while two patients had been treated with high-dose cyclophosphamide etoposide and cisplatin. Only four patients had not received etoposide previously. The overall response rate was 46%, with 64% of patients who had not received chemotherapy for at least 90 days having a major response. Among the patients who had received treatment within 90 days of entering the study, only 13% responded. Once again, the most important side effect was myelosuppression, with six episodes of fever and neutropenia.

In all reported trials, the major toxicity has been myelosuppression. The most appropriate regimen for prolonged oral administration remains unresolved. One trial compared etoposide 50 mg daily for 21 days of a 28-day cycle to 50 mg twice daily for 14 days of a 21-day cycle. [60] A major response rate of 80% was observed in 40 patients who received the twice-daily regimen, compared to 59% in 27 patients treated with 50 mg once daily for 21 days. Patients in both groups received equivalent amounts of etoposide. Despite the difference in response rates, median times of remission and survival were similar.

Combination chemotherapy trials. Oral etoposide in combination with cisplatin has been evaluated in both SCLC and NSCLC. Twenty-two patients with extensive stage SCLC were treated with cisplatin 100 mg/m^2 very 28 days, together with etoposide 50 mg/m^2/day for 21 days, for a total of four cycles [61]. The overall response rate was 82% (95% confidence interval, 62%–93%), with two complete (9%) and 16 partial responses (73%). The median duration of response was 7.0 months, with a median survival of 10 months. Myelosuppression was the most frequent adverse reaction. Although the observed results were no better than those reported with either single-agent oral etoposide or with cisplatin plus intravenous etoposide, the authors suggest that improved results may be seen if the etoposide dose is administered twice daily.

Twenty-three patients with stage III (seven patients) or IV (16 patients) non-small cell lung cancer were treated with cisplatin, $80\,mg/m^2$ every 28 days, plus oral etoposide, $50\,mg/m^2$/day for 21 days of a 28-day cycle [62]. Seven of 23 patients (30%; 95% confidence interval, 12%–49%) achieved a partial response, lasting for 5+ to 18+ weeks. The most frequent toxicity was myelosuppression with 47% of patients experiencing leukopenia, 9% thrombocytopenia, and 31% grade 3 or 4 anemia. Again, these results were comparable to those observed in prior trials with similar doses of cisplatin and three to five intravenous doses of etoposide.

Fotemustine

Phase II trials in NSCLC. The nitrosurea fotemustine was administered to patients with NSCLC at a dose of $100\,mg/m^2$ on days 1 and 3, then $100\,mg/m^2$ on day 43, and repeated every three weeks [63]. Sixty-two patients were evaluable for response, 57% of patients had received chemotherapy, and 67% of patients had stage IV disease. The overall response rate was 16% (95% confidence intervals, 7%–25%), with a 14-week median duration of response. Six partial responses were observed in 29 patients who had not received chemotherapy prior to entry into the study (23% response rate). The dose-limiting toxicity was thrombocytopenia, with 7% of patients experiencing grade 4 toxicities.

Combination chemotherapy trials. In a subsequent trial, fotemustine was combined with cisplatin and given to patients with NSCLC [64]. The first six patients received fotemustine $100\,mg/m^2$ on days 1 and 8, and cisplatin $120\,mg/m^2$ on day 1. Patients were evaluated after six weeks, and those without disease progression were treated with fotemustine $100\,mg/m^2$ and cisplatin $100\,mg/m^2$ repeated every three weeks. Three responses were observed. The only observed toxicity was cisplatin-induced nausea and vomiting. Subsequent patients also received cisplatin $100\,mg/m^2$ on day 22. Twenty-four patients received this regimen, of which 16 were evaluable at the time of the report. Seven patients had previously received chemotherapy. Four partial responses were observed in the 16 patients. Leukopenia, thrombocytopenia, and nausea and vomiting were the major adverse reactions.

Gemcitabine

Gemcitabine (2′,2′-difluorodeoxycytidine, dFdCyd) is a pyrimidine antimetabolite that differs from cytarabine at the 2′ position of the carbohydrate

334

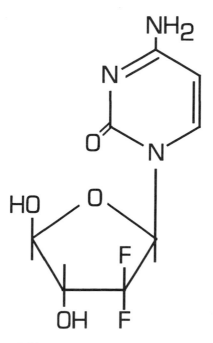

Figure 4. Structure of gemcitabine.

moiety (figure 4). It was initially developed as an antiviral agent, but pre-clinical studies found it to be markedly more potent than other difluoro-pyrimidines as an antitumor agent in vitro. Shown to be cell-cycle specific, blocking cells at the S and late G_1 phase, it is retained in human tumor cells for long periods [65]. Experiments with implanted mouse tumors, as well as human tumor xenografts including the LX-1 lung carcinoma, demonstrated antitumor activity [65,66].

Phase I trials. A phase I trial evaluated doses ranging from 10 to 1000 mg/m² weekly for three out of every four weeks [66]. A total of 50 previously treated patients, including six patients with NSCLC, were studied, and the maximum tolerated dose was defined as 790 mg/m². The dose-limiting toxicity was myelosuppression. Thrombocytopenia was the most common toxicity, although anemia and granulocytopenia were also observed. Other toxicities were generally mild and included nausea and vomiting, anorexia, and malaise. Transient fevers were observed after administration of the first dose in 43% of patients, and 5 of 22 patients treated with a dose of at least 525 mg/m² developed a generalized rash, which responded to topical steroids and reduction in the dose of gemcitabine. Pharmacokinetic evaluation showed gemcitabine to have a terminal half-life of 14 hours, with most of the agent being metabolized and then excreted in the urine. Two objective responses were observed in 28 patients assessable for response. A partial response lasting two months was observed in a patient with adenocarcinoma of the lung who was treated at a dose of 525 mg/m^2.

Phase II trials in NSCLC and SCLC. A number of phase II trials have evaluated gemcitabine, using a variety of doses and schedules [67–70]. Patient characteristics, and results are shown in table 5. Gemcitabine has demonstrated major objective response rates ranging from 17%–26% in NSCLC patients and 37% in a group of 14 individuals with SCLC who had previously received chemotherapy [70]. Myelosuppression was the most important adverse effect in all trials.

Paclitaxel (Taxol®)

Paclitaxel (figure 2) is the prototype of a new class of agents, the taxanes. Isolated from the bark of the Pacific yew tree, Taxus brevifolia, it demonstrated activity against B16 melanoma and human mammary tumor xenografts in preclinical screening [71]. The agent affects the equilibrium between microtubules and their basic subunits, tubulin dimers. Paclitaxel induces excessive polymerization of tubulin, stabilizes microtubules, and prevents their disassembly [72–74]. In tissue culture, paclitaxel inhibits cell replication during the G$_2$ or M phase of the cell cycle [73]. Some indicate that paclitaxel affects cells during interphase by interfering with other cell functions involving microtubules, such as intracellular transport, signal transduction, and motility [75,76]. Paclitaxel is a complex molecule and is insoluble in aqueous solution. It requires formulation in ethanol and polyoxyethylated castor oil (Cremophor EL). It is unclear whether hypersensitivity reactions observed with paclitaxel are due to the drug itself, to its cremophor vehicle, or both.

Phase I trials. Initial studies evaluated paclitaxel when given by single infusions, ranging from 3 hours to 24 hours [77–80]. Partial responses were observed in patients with NSCLC [78], adenocarcinoma of unknown primary [78], and melanoma [79]. Doses as high as 275 mg/m^2 were administered over 24 hours [79]. The dose-limiting toxicity was neutropenia, which did not appear to be schedule dependent in these trials. The onset of neutropenia is usually around day 8, with recovery by days 15 to 21. Myelosuppression does not appear to cumulative, and thrombocytopenia and anemia are seldom significant. Paclitaxel induces a peripheral neuropathy that is cumulative. The neuropathy is characterized by numbness, parasthesias, and burning in a glove-and-stocking distribution. Examination often reveals sensory loss for vibration and proprioception as well as fine touch and temperature [81]. Involvement of motor and autonomic nerves can also occur, especially in patients with preexisting neuropathies. Transient myalgias and arthralgias have been seen and cardiac rhythm disturbances can

336

Table 5. Phase II trials evaluating gemcitabine

Gemcitabine	Non-small cell lung cancer			Small cell lung cancer [70]
	[67]	[68]	[69]	
Gemcitabine dose	800 mg/m² weekly for 3 of 4 weeks	90 mg/m² twice weekly	1000 mg/m² IV weekly for 3 of 4 weeks	1000 mg/m² IV weekly for 3 of 4 weeks
Patient number (adequate for response)	56 (47)	23 (16)	43 (17)	14 (8)
Male:Female	38:21	11:12	NR	NR
Performance status	PS 0 = 23 PS 1 = 23 PS 2 = 13	PS 0 = 8 PS 1 = 13 PS 2 = 2	PS 0 = 2 PS 1 = 41 —	PS 0,1 = 14 — —
Stage				
IIIA	17	1	NR	—
IIIB	20	3	NR	—
IV	21	19	NR	—
Prior chemotherapy	0	0	NR	14
Response rate (95% confidence limits)	26% (14%–40%)	19% (4%–46%)	17% (4%–43%)	37% (9%–76%)

occur. Transient asymptomatic bradycardia, reported in up to 29% of patients, is not an indication for discontinuing therapy. Alopecia is almost universal at doses greater than $135 \, \text{mg/m}^2$.

Hypersensivity reactions during paclitaxel infusions were an early dose-limiting toxicity. Symptoms include hypotension, dyspnea, bronchospasm, pruritus, urticaria, and flushing. Other reactions such as abdominal and extremity pain, angioedema, and diaphoresis also occur, usually within a few minutes of initiating the infusion. The incidence of these hypersensivity reactions is decreased by the prophylactic administration of dexamethasone, diphenhydramine, and cimetidine, and has been recommended by the NCI and phase I investigators (table 6) [80,82–84].

Phase II trials in NSCLC. Two phase II trials have evaluated paclitaxel given as a 24-hour infusion every three weeks to patients with advanced NSCLC (table 7) [85,86]. The starting dose of paclitaxel was $200 \, \text{mg/m}^2$ in the M.D. Anderson Cancer Center study, while a dose of $250 \, \text{mg/m}^2$ was administered in the Eastern Cooperative Oncology Group (ECOG). All patients received the premedication shown in table 5. One complete response and five partial responses were observed in 24 assessable patients in the M.D. Anderson study, for a major response rate of 24% (95% confidence intervals, 8%–41%). The median duration of response was 6.8 months, and the median survival was 10 months. The ECOG trial reported five partial responses in 24 assessable patients (21%; 95% confidence intervals, 7%–42%). The median response duration was 6.4 months, and the median survival was 8 months. Adverse effects were similar in both trials. Grade 3 or 4 leukopenia occurred in 83% of patients in the ECOG study. Thrombocytopenia and anemia were mild or absent. Other toxicities were similar to those observed in the phase I trials.

Phase II trial in SCLC. A phase II study of paclitaxel is being conducted in previously untreated patients with extensive-stage SCLC. The results of this ECOG trial are unavailable; however, activity against this disease has been demonstrated (D.S. Ettinger, personal communication).

Combination chemotherapy trials. The combination of paclitaxel and cisplatin has been evaluated in a phase I trial, in untreated or minimally treated patients with a variety of solid tumors [84]. Doses of cisplatin: palcitaxel ranged from $50 \, \text{mg/m}^2 : 110 \, \text{mg/m}^2$ to $75 \, \text{mg/m}^2 : 200 \, \text{mg/m}^2$. The drugs were each given every three weeks, and either cisplatin or paclitaxel was administrated first in successive cohorts of patients. The paclitaxel was given as a 24-hour infusion, and premedication was routinely given (see table 6). A total of 182 courses were administered to 44 patients at six dose levels. The dose-limiting toxicity was neutropenia, with over three quarters of patients having grade 3 or 4 toxicity. More severe neutropenia was observed when cisplatin was administered before paclitaxel. Although only

Table 6. Pretreatment regimen for paclitaxel [82]

Dexamethasone	20 mg PO/IV 14 hours and 7 hours, then 20 mg IV 30 minutes before paclitaxel
Diphenhydramine	50 mg IV 30 minutes before paclitaxel
H_2-antagonist	300 mg IV cimetidine, 50 mg IV ranitidine, or 20 mg famotidine 30 minutes before paclitaxel

Table 7. Phase II trials of paclitaxel in non-small cell lung cancer

Paclitaxel	[86]	[85]
Patients entered	27	25
(adequate for response)	(25)	(24)
Male : Female	14 : 11	17 : 7
Performance status (%)		
ECOG 0	3 (12%)	9 (38%)
ECOG 1	13 (52%)	15 (62%)
ECOG 2	9 (36%)	—
Stage		
IIIA	1 (4%)	—
IIIB	2 (8%)	—
IV	22 (88%)	24 (100%)
Prior chemotherapy	0	0
Response rate	24%	21%
(95% confidence interval)	(9%–45%)	(7%–42%)

27% of patients had symptomatic or objective neurotoxicity, it did appear to be both dose related and cumulative. Cardiac arrhythmias, including both bradycardias and ventricular tachycardias, were observed with paclitaxel infusions. Alopecia occurred in all patients. Thirteen patients with NSCLC were entered into this trial. Partial responses were observed in two patients, and one patient had a pathologically confirmed complete response (major response rate 23%).

Teniposide (VM-26)

Teniposide is a plant product with a toxicity profile similar to that observed with etoposide, with myelosuppression being most prominent.

Phase II trials in NSCLC. Most studies evaluating this agent in NSCLC patients have reported overall negative results [87–89]. One trial evaluated doses from 120 mg/m² to 180 mg/m² on days 1, 3, and 5 every three weeks [90] in 42 patients, of whom 34 had not received prior chemotherapy. Seven partial responses were observed, six in previously untreated patients. The overall response rate was 17% (95% confidence limits, 6%–28%), suggesting that this agent may be useful at higher doses.

Phase II trials in SCLC. Teniposide is an active agent in patients with SCLC. It has been studied in eight phase II trials entering 201 patients. The overall response rate was 37%, with individual response rates ranging from 0% to 91% [55]. One randomized trial comparing etoposide to teniposide has been reported [91]. Ninety-four patients, 70 years of age or older, were randomly assigned to receive either etoposide (70–803mg/m^2) or teniposide (70 or 90 mg/m^2) intravenously for five days every three weeks. The overall response rates were 65% for etoposide and 71% for teniposide, with complete response rates of 24% and 23%, respectively. Although the median survival was 8.5 months for etoposide-treated patients and 11.3 months for those who received teniposide, this difference was not statistically significant. While teniposide has been shown to be an active agent in SCLC patients, two decades of research have failed to establish its role in the management of this disease. Whether teniposide provides any advantage over etoposide (or other agents, for that matter) remains questionable. The available data suggest what it is, at best, equivalent to intravenous etoposide.

Vinorelbine

Vinorelbine is a vinca alkaloid that has shown anticancer activity against mouse tumors, human tumor xenografts including NSCLC xenografts, and a human bronchial squamous cell tumor in vitro. In these experiments, the activity of vinorelbine was greater than that of the related vinca alkaloids, vincristine, and vinblastine. Compared to the other vinca alkaloids, vinorelbine has a long terminal half-life and a large volume of distribution, reflecting marked tissue uptake. Tissue uptake is particularly prominent in lung tissue [92]. Phase I trials evaluated intravenous vinorelbine given weekly. In heavily pretreated patients the maximum tolerated dose ranged from 27.5 to 43 mg/m^2 [93,94]. The dose-limiting toxicity was neutropenia. Peripheral neuropathy was seen.

Phase II trials in NSCLC. A phase II study entered 83 patients with inoperable NSCLC [92]. Pretreatment patient characteristics and results are shown in table 8. The agent was administered intravenously weekly at a dose of 30 mg/m^2. An objective response rate of 33% (95% confidence limits, 20%–40%) was observed in the 70 assessable patients. For all 78 eligible patients, the response rate was 29%. The median response duration was 8.5 months, with a median survival of 8.3 months. Myelosuppression was the most important toxicity, with grade 3 or 4 neutropenia occurring in 13% of cycles. Other significant adverse reactions included stomatitis, nausea and vomiting, diarrhea, and alopecia. Constipation (grade 3 or 4,

340

Table 8. Phase II trials of vinorelbine, single agent and in combination with cisplatin

Vinorelbine (VNB)	Single-agent VNB		Cisplatin+VNB [96]
	[92]	[95]	
Patient number	83	80	32
(adequate for response)	(78)	(48)	(30)
Male:Female	75:3	28:20	27:5
Performance status	ECOG 0 = 11	NR	Median KPS 80%
	ECOG 1 = 39	NR	Range 70%–100%
	ECOG 2 = 28	NR	
Stage			
I–II	10%	—	—
IIIA	21%	4	2
IIIB	17%	−8	11
IV	52%	36	19
Response rate	33%	29%	23%
(95% confidence limits)	(20%–40%)	(17%–44%)	

8% of patients), peripheral neuropathies (grade 3, 12%), and transient jaw pain occurred.

In a second trial, reported in abstract form, 80 patients were entered [95]. Forty-eight were evaluable at the time of review. Patient criteria are also shown in table 8. Fourteen of 48 patients (29%; 95% confidence interval, 17%–44%) achieved a partial response. The median duration of response was 7.5+ weeks. Toxicity was similar to that seen in other trials.

Phase II trials in SCLC. The EORTC has conducted a phase II trial evaluating vinorelbine in previously treated SCLC patients [19]. Twenty-five eligible patients who had received one prior chemotherapy regimen and who had been off treatment for at least three months received a dose of $30 \, \text{mg/m}^2$ intravenously weekly. Fifteen patients had also received radiotherapy. The median performance status was 1. A partial response was observed in four patients for a response rate of 16% (95% confidence interval, 4%–36%). Toxicities were similar to those observed in prior trials.

Combination chemotherapy trials. A phase I–II trial combined vinorelbine with cisplatin in patients with NSCLC [96]. Cisplatin was administered at a dose of $120 \, \text{mg/m}^2$ on day 1, day 29, and then every six weeks. Vinorelbine was administered weekly at three dose levels, namely, 20, 25, and $30 \, \text{mg/m}^2$. Patient characteristics are shown in table 8. No objective responses were observed in the patients treated at the $20 \, \text{mg/m}^2$ dose level. Of the 21 assessable patients treated with either 25 or $30 \, \text{mg/m}^2$, seven patients achieved a partial response (33%; 95% confidence interval, 13–53%). The

341

median response duration was 7.5+ months, and the median survival was 11 months. The dose-limiting toxicity was neutropenia, with over half the patients experiencing grade 3 or 4 toxicity. Other toxicities were similar.

Zeniplatin

Zeniplatin is a third-generation platinum compound that, in human tumor xenografts, has a spectrum of antitumor activity different from that of cisplatin [97]. A phase II trial was undertaken in 30 chemotherapy-naive patients with advanced NSCLC, of which 26 patients had stage IV disease [97]. A dose of $145\,mg/m^2$ was administered every three weeks. The median performance status was 1. Twenty-eight patients were assessable for response. Six patients had a partial response (response rate 21%; 95% confidence interval, 9%–39%). Nausea and leukopenia were the major adverse reactions. Because of toxicity observed in trials conducted in patients with other primary sites of cancer, this agent has been withdrawn from clinical use.

Conclusions

Over the past five years, a number of chemotherapeutic agents with substantial antitumor activity against lung cancer have become available. Several of these are members of new classes of drugs. It is possible that the inclusion of these agents in combination chemotherapy regimens may make substantial inroads in the treatment of this disease. The clinical trials in the next five years will determine if this indeed is the case.

References

1. Rapp E, Pater JL, Willan A, et al. 1988. Chemotherapy can prolong survival in patients with advanced non-small cell lung cancer: Report of a Canadian multicenter randomized trial. J Clin Oncol 6:633–641.
2. Dillman R, Seagren S, Propert K, et al. 1990. A randomized trial of induction chemotherapy plus high-dose radiation versus radiation alone in stage III non-small cell lung cancer. N Engl J Med 323:940–945.
3. Boring C, Squires T, Tong T. 1993. Cancer statistics, 1993. CA C ancer J Clin 43(1):7–26.
4. Rigas JR, Kris MG, Tong W, et al. 1991. Phase I trial of chloroquinoxaline sulfonamide (CQS): A unique agent with activity in NSCLC stem cell assay (abstract). Lung Cancer 7(Suppl):108.
5. Carey R, Comis R, Anbar D, et al. 1983. Cancer and leukemia group B phase II non-small cell lung carcinoma trial: axiridinylbenzoquinone (AZQ). Cancer Treat Rep 67(1):95–96.
6. Chabner BA. 1992. Camptothecins (editorial). J Clin Oncol 10(1):3–4.
7. Hertzberg RP, Holden KG, Hecht SM, et al. 1987. Characterization of structural features of camptothecin essential for topoisomerase I interaction and for induction of protein-linked DNA breaks in cells (abstract). Proc Am Assoc Cancer Res 28:7.

342

8. Maxwell A, Gellert M. 1986. Mechanistic aspects of DNA topoisomerases. Adv Protein Chem 38:69–107.

9. Kunimoto T, Nitta K, Tanaka T, et al. 1987. Antitumor activity of 7-ethyl-10-[4-(1-piperidion)-1-piperidion [arbonyloxy-camptothecin, anovelwater-soluble derivative of camptothecin, against murine tumors. Cancer Res 47:5944–5947.

10. Matsuzaki T, Yokokura T, Mutai M. 1988. Inhibition of spontaneous and experimental metastasis by a new derivative of camptothecin, CPT-11, in mice. Cancer Chemother Pharmacol 21:308–312.

11. Negoro S, Masahiro F, Masuda N, et al. 1991. Phase I study of weekly intravenous infusions of CPT-11, a new derivative of camptothecin, in the treatment of advanced non-small cell lung cancer. J Natl Cancer Inst 83(16):1164–1168.

12. Fukuoka M, Niitani H, Suzuki A, et al. 1992. A Phase II study of CPT-11, a new derivative of camptothecin, for previously untreated non-small-cell lung cancer. J Clin Oncol 10:16–20.

13. WHO Handbook for Reporting Results of Cancer Treatment. 1979. World Health Organization: Geneva.

14. Takada M, Fukuoka M, Kudoh S, et al. 1992. Synergistic effects of CPT-11 and cisplatin or etoposide on human lung cancer cell lines and xenografts in nude mice (abstract). Proc Am Assoc Cancer Res 33:226.

15. Negoro S, Fukuoka M, Niitani H, et al. 1991. Phase II study of CPT-11, new camptothecin derivative, in small cell lung cancer (SCLC). Proc Am Soc Clin Oncol 10:241.

16. Fukuoka M, Takada M, Nakagawa K, et al. 1992. CPT-11 dose in combination with cisplatin for advanced non-small cell lung cancer (abstract). Proc Am Soc Clin Oncol 11:293.

17. Bissett D, Setanoians A, Cassidy J, et al. 1993. Phase I and pharmacokinetic study of taxotere (RP 56976) administered as a 24-hour infusion (abstract). Cancer Res 53:523–527.

18. Bissery M, Guernard D, Gueritte-Voegelin F, et al. 1991. Experimental antitumor activity of taxotere (RP 56976, NSC 628503), a taxol analogue. Cancer Res 51:4845–4852.

19. Jassem J, Karnicka-Miodkowska H, van Pottelsberghe C, et al. 1992. EORTC phase II study of navelbine (NVB) in previously treated patients (PT) with small cell lung carcinoma (SCLC). Proc Am Soc Clin Oncol 11:309.

20. Extra J, Rousseau F, Bruno R, et al. 1993. Phase I and pharmacokinetic study of taxotere (RP 56976; NSC 628503) given as a short intravenous infusion (abstract). Cancer Res 53:1037–1042.

21. Pazdur R, Newman RA, Newman BM, et al. 1992. Phase I trial of taxotere: Five-day schedule. J Natl Cancer Society 84(23):1781–1788.

22. Vandenberg T, Pritchard KI, Eisenhauer E. 1992. Phase II study of weekly 10-EDAM (Edatrexate) as first line chemotherapy for metastatic breast cancer: A National Cancer Institute of Canada Clinical Trials Group study (abstract). Proc Am Soc Clin Oncol 11:51.

23. Burris H, Eckardt J, Fields S, et al. 1993. Phase II trials of taxotere in patients with non-small cell lung cancer (abstract). Proc Am Soc Clin Oncol 12:335.

24. Cerny T, Wanders J, Kaplan S, et al. 1993. Taxotere is an active drug in non small cell lung (NSCLC) cancer: A phase II trial of the early clinical trials group (ECTG) (abstract). Proc Am Soc Clin Oncol 12:331.

25. Rigas JR, Francis PA, Kris MG, et al. 1993. Phase II trial of taxotere in non-small lung cancer (NSCLC) (abstract). Proc Am Soc Clin Oncol 12:336.

26. Rumberger BG, Barrueco JR, Sirotnak FM. 1990. Differing specificities for 4-aminofolate analogues of folylpolyglutamyl synthetase from tumors and proliferative intestinal epithelium of the mouse with significance for selective antitumor action. Cancer Res 50:4639–4643.

27. Sirotnak FM, DeGraw JI, Moccio DM, et al. 1984. New folate analogues of the 10-deaza-aminopterin series; basis for structural design and biochemical and pharmacologic properties. Cancer Chemother Pharmacol 12:18–25.

28. Samuels LL, M MD, M SF. 1985. Similar differential for total polyglutamylation and

cytotoxicity among various folate analogs in human and murine tumor cells in vitro. Cancer Res 45:1488-1495.

29. Schmid FA, Sirotnak FM, Otter GM. 1985. New folate analogs of the 10-deaza-aminopterin series. Markedly increased activity of the 10-ethyl analogue compared to the parent compound and methotrexate against some human tumor xenografts in nude mice. Cancer Treat Rep 69:551–553.

30. Braakhuis BJM, van Dongen GAMS, Bagnay MBS, et al. 1989. Preclinical chemotherapy on human head and neck cancer xenografts grown in athymic nude mice. Chemother Head Neck Cancer Xenogr (November/December):511–515.

31. Brown DH, Braakhuis BJM, Van Dongen GAMS, et al. 1989. Activity of the folate analog 10-ethyl, 10-deaza-aminopterin (10-EdAM) against human head and neck cancer xenografts. Anticancer Res 9:1549–1552.

32. Kris M, Kinahan J, Gralla R, et al. 1988. Phase I trial and clinical pharmacological evaluation of 10-ethyl-10-deazaaminopterin in adult patients with advanced cancer. Cancer Res 48:5573–5579.

33. Shum K, Kris M, Gralla R, et al. 1988. Phase II study of 10-ethyl-10-deaza-aminopterin in patients with stage III and IV non-small cell lung cancer. J Clin Oncol 6(3):446–450.

34. Lee JS, Libshitz HI, Murphy WK, et al. 1990. Phase II study of 10-ethyl-10-deaza-aminopterin (10-EdAM; CGP 30 694) for stage IIIb or IV non-small cell lung cancer. Invest New Drugs 8:299–304.

35. Souhami R, Hartley J, Allen R, et al. 1991. 10-EDAM (10-Ethyl-10-Deazaaminopterin) in untreated advanced non small cell lung cancer (SCLC) (abstract). Lung Cancer 7(Suppl): 134.

36. Schmid FA, Sirotnak FM, Otter GM, et al. 1987. Combination chemotherapy with a new folate analog: Activity of 10-ethyl-deaza-aminopterin compared to methotrexate with 5-fluorouracil and alkylating agents against advanced metastatic disease in murine tumor models. Cancer Treat Rep 71:727–732.

37. Sirotnak FM, Schmid FA, I DJ. 1989. Intracavitary therapy of murine ovarian cancer with cis-Diamminedichloroplatinum (II) and 10-ethyl-10-deazaaminopterin incorporating systemic leucovorin protection (abstract). Cancer Res 49:2890–2893.

38. Kris MG, Gralla RJ, Potanovich LM, et al. 1990. Assessment of pretreatment symptoms and improvement after EDAM+mitomycin+vinblastine in patients with inoperable non-small cell lung cancer (abstract). Proc Am Soc Clin Oncol 9:229.

39. Lee JS, Libshitz HI, Murphy WK, et al. 1990. Phase II trial of 10-ethyl-10-deaza-aminopterin (10-edam) with cytoxan (CTX) and cisplatin (CDDP) for stage IIIB/IV non-small cell lung cancer (NSCLC) (abstract). Proc Am Soc Clin Oncol 9:241.

40. Lee JS, Libshitz H, Fossella F, et al. 1992. Brief communication. Improved therapeutic index by leucovorin of edatrexate, cyclophosphamide, and cisplatin regimen for non-small cell lung cancer. J Natl Cancer Inst 84:1039–1040.

41. Wiesenfeld M, Su J, Jett J. 1992. Phase II study of edatrexate (10–EDAM) in patients with small cell carcinoma (SCC) of the lung (abstract). Proc Am Soc Clin Oncol 11:311.

42. Casazza A, DiMarco A, Bertazzoli C. 1978. Antitumor activity, toxicity, and pharmacological properties of 4'-epiadriamycin. In Current Chemotherapy, W Siegenthaler and R Luthy (eds.). American Society of Microbiology; Washington, DC, pp. 1257–1260.

43. Casazza A. 1979. Experimental evaluation of anthracycline analogues. Cancer Treat Rep 63:835–844.

44. Zbinden G, Brandle E. 1975. Toxicologic screening of daunorubicin (NSC-82151) and their derivatives in rats. Cancer Chemother Rep 59:707–715.

45. Feld R, Wierzbicki R, Walde PLD, et al. 1992. Phase I–II study of high-dose epirubicin in advanced non-small-cell lung cancer. J Clin Oncol 10(2):297–303.

46. Joss R, Hansen H, Hansen M, et al. 1984. Phase II trial of epirubicin in advanced squamous, adenocarcinoma and large cell carcinoma of the lung. Eur J Cancer Oncol 20:495–499.

47. Kalman L, Kris M, Gralla R, et al. 1983. Phase II trial of 4′-epi-doxorubicin in patients with non-small cell lung cancer. Cancer Treat Rep 67(6):591–592.
48. Martoni A, Melotti B, Guaraldi M, et al. 1990. Activity of high dose epirubicin (HD EPI) in non small cell lung cancer (NSCLC). Proc Am Soc Clin Oncol 9:237.
49. Blackstein M, Eisenhauer EA, Wierzbicki R, et al. 1990. Epirubicin in extensive small-cell lung cancer: A phase II study in previously untreated patients: A National Cancer Institute of Canada Clinical Trials Group study. J Clin Oncol 8:385–389.
50. Eckhardt S, Kolaric K, Vukas D, et al. 1990. Phase II study of 4′-epi-doxorubicin in patients with untreated, extensive small cell lung cancer. Med Oncol Tumor Pharmacother 7(1):19–23.
51. Macchiarini P, Danesi R, Mariotti R, et al. 1990. Phase II study of high-dose epirubicin in untreated patients with small-cell lung cancer. Am J Clin Oncol 13(4):302–307.
52. Slevin ML, Clark PI, Joel SP, et al. 1989. A randomized trial to evaluate the effect of schedule on the activity of etoposide in small-cell lung cancer. J Clin Oncol 7:1333–1340.
53. Waits TM, Johnson DH, Hainsworth JD, et al. 1992. Prolonged administration of oral etoposide in non-small-cell lung cancer: A phase II trial. J Clin Oncol 10(2):292–296.
54. Estape J, Palombo H, Sanchez-Lloret J, et al. 1992. Chronic oral etoposide in non-small cell lung carcinoma. Eur J Cancer 28A(4/5):835–837.
55. Grant SC, Gralla RJ, Kris MG, et al. 1992. Single agent chemotherapy trials in small-cell lung cancer, 1970–1990. The case for studies in previously treated patients. J Clin Oncol 10(3):484–498.
56. Itri LM, Gralla RJ. 1982. A review of etoposide in patients with non-small cell lung cancer (NSCLC). Cancer Treat Rev 9:115–118.
57. Saxman S, Loehrer Sr. PJ, Logie K, et al. 1991. Phase II trial of daily oral etoposide in patients with advanced non-small cell lung cancer (abstract). Invest New Drugs 9:253–256.
58. Clark P, Cottier B, Joel S, et al. 1990. Prolonged administration of single-agent oral etoposide in patients with untreated small cell lung cancer (SCLC). Proc Am Soc Clin Oncol 9:226.
59. Johnson DH, Greco FA, Strupp J, et al. 1990. Prolonged administration of oral etoposide in patients with relapsed or refractory small-cell lung cancer: A phase II trial. J Clin Oncol 8(10):1613–1617.
60. Clark P, Cottier B, Joel S, et al. 1991. Two prolonged schedules of single-agent oral etoposide of differing duration and dose in patients with untreated small cell lung cancer (SCLC) (abstract). Proc Am Soc Clin Oncol 10:268.
61. Murphy PB, Hainsworth JD, Greco FA, et al. 1992. A phase II trial of cisplatin and prolonged administration of oral etoposide in extensive-stage small cell lung cancer. Cancer 69:370–375.
62. Fukuda M, Nakano S, Fukuoka M, et al. 1991. Chronic daily administration of oral etoposide and cisplatin for advanced non-small cell lung cancer (NSCLC) (abstract). Lung Cancer 7(Suppl):118.
63. Monnier A, Pujol JL, Cerinna ML, et al. 1991. Fotemustine: French multicenter phase II study in 67 patients with advanced non small cell lung carcinoma (NSCLC) (abstract). Lung Cancer 7(Suppl):119.
64. Riviere A, Le Cesne A, Benoliel C, et al. 1991. Phase II pilot study of fotemustine–cisplatin combination in 24 patients with advanced non small cell lung carcinoma (abstract). Lung Cancer 7(Suppl):119.
65. Hertel L, Boder G, Kroin J, et al. 1990. Evaluation of the antitumor activity of gemcitabine (2′,2′-difluoro-2′-deoxycytidine). Cancer Res 50:4417–4422.
66. Abbruzzese J, Grunewald R, Weeks E, et al. 1991. A phase I clinical, plasma, and cellular pharmacology study of gemcitabine. J Clin Oncol 90(3):491–498.
67. Lund B, Anderson H, Walling J, et al. 1991. Phase II study of gemcitabine in non small cell lung cancer (NSCLC) (abstract). Lung Cancer 7(Suppl):121.
68. Lund B, Ryberg M, Anderson H, et al. 1992. A phase II study of gemcitabine in non-small

cell lung cancer (NSCLC) using a twice weekly schedule (abstract). Proc Am Assoc Cancer Res 33:226.

69. Abratt R, Bezwoda W, Falkson G, et al. 1992. Efficacy and safety of gemcitabine in non-small cell lung cancer–Phase II study results (abstract). Proc Am Soc Clin Oncol 11:311.

70. Eisenhauer E, Cormier Y, Gregg R, et al. 1992. Gemcitabine is active in patients (PTS) with previously untreated extensive small cell lung cancer (SCLC) — A phase II study of the National Cancer Institute of Canada Clinical Trial Group (NCIC CTG) (abstract). Proc Am Soc Clin Oncol 11:309.

71. Rowinsky E, McGuire W. 1992. Taxol: Present status and future prospects. Contemp Oncol (March):29–36.

72. Schiff PB, Fant J, Horwitz SB. 1979. Promotion of microtubule assembly in vitro by taxol. Nature 277:665–667.

73. Schiff PB, Horwitz SB. 1980. Taxol stabilizes microtubules in mouse fibroblast cells. Proc Natl Acad Sci USA 77:1561–1565.

74. Parness J, Horwitz SB. 1981. Taxol binds to polymerized microtubules in vitro. J Cell Biol 91:479.

75. Fuchs DA, Johnson RK. 1978. Cytologic evidence that taxol, an antineoplastic agent from Taxus brevifolia, acts as a mitotic spindle poison. Cancer Treat Rep 62:1219.

76. Rowinsky EK, Donehower RC, Jones RJ. 1988. Microtubule changes and cytotoxicity in leukemic cells treated with taxol. Cancer Res 48:4093–4100.

77. Kris M, O'Connell J, Gralla R, et al. 1986. Phase I trial of taxol given as a 3-hour infusion every 21 days. Cancer Treat Rep 70(5):605–607.

78. Brown T, Havlin G, Weiss G, et al. 1991. A phase I trial of taxol given by a 6-hour intravenous infusion. J Clin Oncol 9(7):1261–1267.

79. Wiernik P, Schwartz E, Einzig A, et al. 1987. Phase I trial of taxol given as a 24-hour infusion every 21 days: Responses observed in metastatic melanoma. J Clin Oncol 5(8):1232–1239.

80. Rowinsky E, Burke P, Karp J, et al. 1989. Phase I and pharmacodynamic study of taxol in refractory acute leukemias. Cancer Res 49:4640–4647.

81. Rowinsky EK, Cazenave LA, Donehower RC. 1990. Taxol: A novel investigational antimicrotubule agent. J Natl Cancer Inst 82(15):1247–1259.

82. Weiss R, Donehower R, Wiernik P, et al. 1990. Hypersensitivity reactions from taxol. Am J Clin Oncol 8:1263–1268.

83. Donehower RC, Rowinsky EK, Grochow LB, et al. 1987. Phase I trial of taxol in patients with advanced cancer. Cancer Treat Rep 71:1171–1177.

84. Rowinsky E, Gilbert M, McGuire W, et al. 1991. Sequences of taxol and cisplatin: A phase I and pharmacologic study. J Clin Oncol 9(9):1692–1703.

85. Chang AY, Kim K, Glick J, et al. 1993. Phase II study of taxol, merbarone, and piroxantrone in stage IV non-small-cell lung cancer: The Eastern Cooperative Oncology Group results. J Natl Cancer Inst 85(5):388–394.

86. Murphy WK, Fossella FV, Winn RJ, et al. 1993. Phase II study of taxol in patients with untreated advanced non-small-cell lung cancer. J Natl Cancer Inst 85(5):384–388.

87. Spremulli E, Schulz JJ, Speckhart VJ, et al. 1980. Phase II study of VM-26 in adult malignancies. Cancer Treat Rep 64(1):147–149.

88. Samson MK, Baker LH, Talley RW, et al. 1978. VM-26: A clinical study in advanced carcinoma of the lung and ovary. Eur J Cancer 14:1395–1399.

89. Creech RH, Mehta CR, Cohen M, et al. 1981. Results of a phase II protocol for evaluation of new chemotherapeutic regimens in patients with inoperable non-small cell lung carcinoma. Cancer Treat Rep 65(5–6):431–438.

90. Giaccone G, Donadio M, Ferrati P, et al. 1987. Teniposide in the treatment on non-small cell lung carcinoma. Cancer Treat Rep 71(1):83–85.

91. Bork E, Ersbøll J, Dombernowsky P, et al. 1991. Teniposide and etoposide in previously untreated small-cell lung cancer: A randomized study. J Clin Oncol 9:1627–1631.

92. Depierre A, Lemaire E, Dabouis G, et al. 1991. A phase II study of navelbine (Vinorelbine) in the treatment of non-small-cell lung cancer. Am J Clin Oncol 14(2):115–119.

93. Besenval M, Delgado M, Demarez JP, et al. 1989. Safety and tolerance of navelbine in phase I–II clinical studies. Semin Oncol 16(2)(Suppl 4):37–40.

94. Mathe G, Reizenstein P. 1985. Phase I pharmacologic study of a new vinca alkaloid: Navelbine. Cancer Lett 27:285–293.

95. Kubotal K, Furusel K, Niitani H: 1991. A late phase II study of navelbine (vinorelbine), a new vinca alkaloid derivative, in non small cell lung cancer (abstract). Lung Cancer 7(Suppl):117.

96. Berthaud P, Le Chevalier T, Ruffie P, et al. 1992. Phase I–II study of vinorelbine (Navelbine.113) plus cisplatin in advanced non-small cell lung cancer. Eur J Cancer 28A(11):1863–1865.

97. Jones AL, Davies C, Smith IE. 1991. Phase II study of zeniplatin, an active new agent in advanced non-small cell lung cancer (NSCLC) (abstract). Lung Cancer 7(Suppl):125.

16. Pulmonary blastomas

Michael N. Koss

Introduction

Pulmonary blastomas are malignant tumors characterized by glands and/or mesenchyme that microscopically resemble the glycogen-rich tubules or embryonic stroma seen in fetal lung of 10–16 weeks gestation (the pseudoglandular stage of lung development) [1].

Initially, blastomas were considered to be biphasic neoplasms composed of both malignant epithelium and stroma [2–5]. However, in 1982, Kradin and associates [8] described an epithelial variant that has been given names such as well-differentiated fetal adenocarcinoma (WDFA) [6], pulmonary adenocarcinoma of fetal type, well-differentiated adenocarcinoma simulating fetal lung tubules [7], pulmonary endodermal tumor resembling fetal lung [8,10] and pulmonary blastoma, epithelial variant [11]. For reasons to be mentioned below, it appears that epithelial blastomas are histogenetically linked to biphasic blastomas.

In 1988, Manivel and associates [9] studied a group of childhood blastomas and noticed that they consisted solely of embryonic malignant stroma. Glands were present in some of the tumors, but they were benign in appearance and considered to be entrapped epithelium rather than neoplastic. These neoplasms might be considered blastomas because of the embryonic appearance of the stroma, but they appear to be distinctly separate clinically, pathologically, and histogenetically from the biphasic and epithelial blastomas of adults. They are considered in a separate section below.

Clinical features

Pulmonary blastomas are rare, probably representing only 0.25% to 0.5% of primary pulmonary malignancies [5,13].

While more research concerning biphasic tumors than epithelial blastomas has been published, this probably reflects the late recognition of the epithelial variant. In fact, in one large series, the two tumors were encountered equally as frequently, and men and women were nearly equally affected [6].

Heine H. Hansen, (ed), Hansen: Lung Cancer.
© 1994 Kluwer Academic Publishers. ISBN 0-7923-2835-3. All rights reserved.

Table 1. Differential diagnostic features of three different types of pulmonary blastomas [6,9]

Feature	Epithelial blastomas	Biphasic blastomas	Pleuropulmonary blastomas
Clinical			
% Pts <10 years old	0	8	91
Smoker	Often	Often	No
Mediastinal tumor only	Never	Never	Often
Average size (cm)	4.5	10.1	NA
Asymptomatic	Often	Occasional	Rare
Prognosis	Good	Poor	Poor
Pathological			
Malignant epithelium/malignant stroma	+/−	+/+	−/+
Morules	86%	43%	−
Chromogranin-positivity	Frequent	Frequent	−

+ = present; − = absent.

Curiously, despite their embryonic microscopic appearance, neither biphasic nor epithelial blastomas occur often in children [6] (table 1). Not only are they tumors of adults, but most (approximately 80%) of the patients are smokers, suggesting that the same environmental agents that are etiological factors in lung cancer play a role in these tumors, despite their fetal appearance [6,12].

Fever, cough, chest pain, and hemoptysis are the usual symptoms, but 25% to 40% of patients are asymptomatic [5,6,12]. Patients with epithelial blastomas show symptoms less often than those with biphasic tumors. This is likely due to the smaller size of epithelial tumors, which also tend to grow more slowly than their biphasic counterparts (table 1) [6].

Chest x-ray films typically show a solitary intrapulmonary mass, usually away from the hilum (figure 1).When bronchoscopic or needle biopsies are attempted, they produce a correct or suggestive diagnosis in only one third of cases. Both the histologic resemblance to other tumors (such as carcinoid tumor) and small sample size may be causative factors.

Pathologic findings

Pulmonary blastomas are large (range, 1–28 cm; median, 6 cm), well-demarcated, unencapsulated peripheral pulmonary masses (figure 2) [6]. They are typically solitary; occasionally, a dominant mass with satellite lesions can occur. Epithelial tumors are significantly smaller than biphasic blastomas (table 1). The tumors are not usually intrabronchial, but we have encountered tumors with an endobronchial component. The cut surface is bulging with a fish-flesh surface; it is typically variegated in color, with

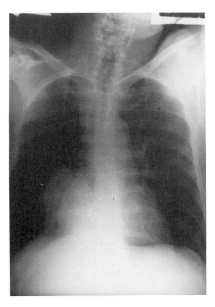

Figure 1. Chest x-ray in a patient with pulmonary blastoma of adults. The tumor in this case presented as a mass in the posterior segment of the lower lobe, right lung.

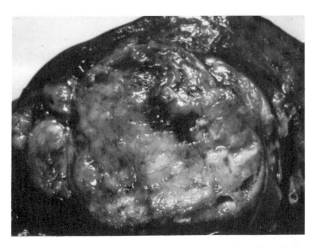

Figure 2. Gross appearance of pulmonary blastoma of adults. The tumor presented as a circumscribed, bulging fleshy mass in lung with areas of cavitation (center).

admixtures of white, tan, or brown. The tumors frequently show foci of cystic breakdown (figure 2).

Microscopically, *epithelial blastomas* are composed of complex branching tubules lined by nonciliated columnar cells with clear or lightly eosinophilic cytoplasm (figure 3). The nuclei of the glandular cells are relatively uniform,

351

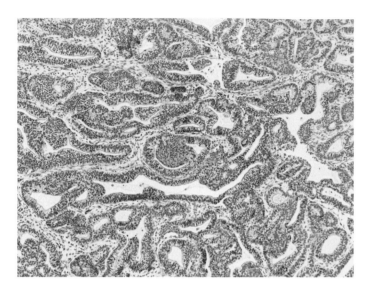

Figure 3. Microscopic appearance of pulmonary blastoma, epithelial variant (well-differentiated fetal adenocarcinoma). The tumor shows a complex pattern of branching glands embedded in a scant benign spindle cell stroma.

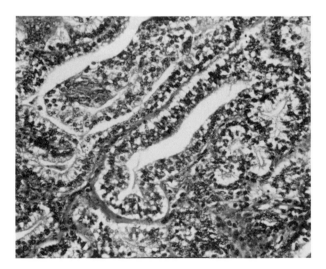

Figure 4. Microscopic appearance of pulmonary blastoma, epithelial variant (well-differentiated fetal adenocarcinoma). The glandular lining cells show numerous subnuclear clear vacuoles, producing a resemblance to endometrium.

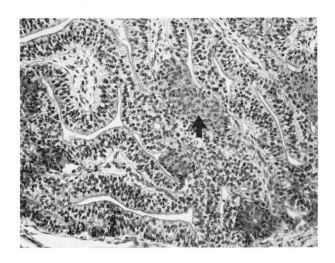

Figure 5. Microscopic appearance of pulmonary blastoma, epithelial variant (well-differentiated fetal adenocarcinoma). The closely packed, branching glands are lined by columnar cells with clear cytoplasm. A solid nest of cells (morule) with optically clear nuclei is present (arrow).

oval or round, with little hyperchromasia. Subnuclear and supranuclear cytoplasmic vacuoles are characteristically present, producing a distinctly endometrioid appearance (figure 4). The clear cytoplasm of these neoplastic glands is due to abundant glycogen, which is at least partially dissolved during processing of the tissues.

A variety of glandular patterns can be seen, ranging from cribriform arrays to cords, ribbons, or solid epithelial nests that sometimes show a basal palisade [6]. In the case of biphasic tumors, the solid epithelial nests may fade into the malignant stroma. Occasionally, squamous pearls can be present [5,11,13].

The bases of the glands show solid nests of cells with ample eosinophilic cytoplasm, so-called morules, in 43% of biphasic tumors and 86%–100% of cases of epithelial tumors (figure 5) [6,12]. These nests consist of solid balls of cells with ample eosinophilic cytoplasm and, on occasion, optically clear nuclei. The combination of glands and morules can produce a resemblance to adenoacanthoma of the uterus.

Small amounts of mucin may be present within glands, but intracellular mucin is unusual. Argyrophilic granules can sometimes be found within scattered morules and less frequently within columnar glandular cells.

Both mitoses and necrosis can be seen in the epithelial component of blastomas. The former, at least, does not appear to be of prognostic importance.

In addition to the malignant glands described above, epithelial blastomas show a scant, benign stroma of spindled myofibroblastic cells (figures 3–5) [6–8,10,12].

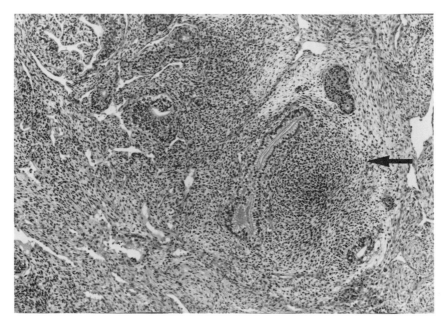

Figure 6. Pulmonary blastoma of adults, biphasic variant. There are scattered malignant glands lined by clear cells and a malignant stroma of embryonic or 'blastematous' appearance. Note the stromal compaction around a gland (arrow).

By electron microscopy, the neoplastic glands have a distinct basal lamina, apical junctional complexes, glycogen-free spaces, and microvilli on the apical surface of lining cells.

Biphasic blastomas show malignant glands and a malignant stroma of embryonic or 'blastematous' appearance that shows a tendency to condense around the glands (figure 6). The stromal cells lie in a myxoid stroma and are most often small, oval and spindled, but they may sometimes show striking pleomorphism (figure 7). About 25% of cases show immature striated muscle or cartilage (figure 8). Osseous differentiation is found in about 5% of tumors [5,6]. Short fascicles of 'fetal-type' smooth muscle have been described in a number of cases [11].

As noted above, epithelial and biphasic tumors are histogenetically linked. Support for this idea comes from the finding that composite tumors occur, that is, neoplasms consisting of areas of epithelial blastoma with separate foci showing a biphasic pattern. We have also encountered rare cases that show a combination of yolk sac tumor and either epithelial or biphasic blastoma [14].

Focal neuroendocrine differentiation is frequent in these tumors. Both chromogranin and neuron-specific enolase are seen, especially in morules, in 64% to 72% of cases [6]. Other neuroendocrine markers can also be found. These include calcitonin and gastrin-releasing peptide, bombesin, leucine

354

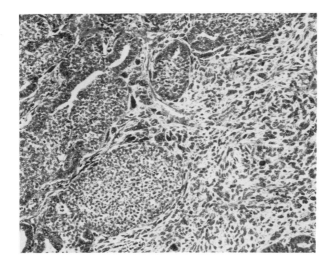

Figure 7. Pulmonary blastoma of adults, biphasic variant. A pleomorphic spindle cell sarcoma is present adjacent to epithelial nests and small glands.

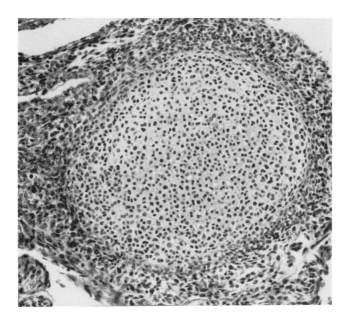

Figure 8. Pulmonary blastoma of adults, biphasic variant, showing an island of immature cartilage. Cartilage or striated muscle can occur in up to 25% of cases.

355

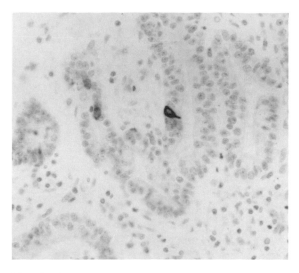

Figure 9. Immunohistochemical staining for calcitonin in pulmonary blastoma of adults. A single glandular lining cell is decorated by the antibody in this field. This figure well illustrates the sparse staining for hormonal markers typical of these tumors.

and methionine enkephalin, somatostatin, and serotonin (figure 9) [6,7,10, 12]. Morules and glands also stain with antibody to N-CAM [16]. Electron microscopy supports the presence of neuroendocrine differentiation. In particular, there are scattered cells within glands and morules that show typical dense-core granules [12]. The histological appearance and staining of the morules for neuroendocrine markers have suggested to some that these are analogues of neuroepithelial bodies [17].

While a high percentage of cases show immunoreactivity for neuro-endocrine markers, the number of hormonally reactive cells in any one case is relatively small (figure 9). This finding is useful to distinguish these tumors from carcinoids, which they superficially resemble at the light-microscopic level.

Other immunoreactants can also be seen in the epithelial component of blastomas. The glandular cells not only react for cytokeratin, carcino-embryonic antigen, alpha-fetoprotein, and epithelial membrane antigen but also for Clara cell antigen and surfactant apoprotein [11,12,16]. In this regard, it should be recalled that fetal lung shows development of Clara cells and of type 2 pneumocytes at 13 weeks and 22 weeks of gestation, res-pectively, so that the tumor immunohistochemically mimics the developing fetal lung [11,16]. Finally, the glandular component of the tumors expresses sialosylated Lewis X antigen, suggesting an endodermal origin for the epithelium [16].

Some authors have found particularly strong immunoreactivity for sur-factant apoprotein in morules [12]. This finding has been correlated by electron microscopy with the presence of morules merging into cells containing lamellar inclusions to suggest that morules represent developing alveolar buds, rather than neurepithelial bodies [12]. Ultrastructurally, the optically clear nuclei seen in morules consist of intranuclear aggregates of fine filaments or fibrils measuring 7–10 nm in diameter [12].

The malignant stromal cells of biphasic blastomas contain vimentin, musclespecific actin and, on occasion, desmin. Myoglobin and S-100 protein are found when, respectively, malignant striated muscle and cartilage are present.

Ultrastructurally, the spindle 'stromal' cells surrounding the glands have typical myofibroblastic features, including well-developed rough endoplasmic reticulum, peripheral cytoplasmic filaments forming dense bodies, pinocytotic vesicles, and an investing basal lamina.

The diagnosis of pulmonary blastoma has on occasion been made using fine-needle aspiration [18]. Cytological studies show round to oval uniform epithelial cells that are characteristically smaller than those seen in typical adenocarcinoma of the lung [19]. The nuclei show an even chromatin distribution with inconspicuous nucleoli. Biphasic tumors also show a concurrent population of short spindle cells with hyperchromatic cells.

Treatment and prognosis

Surgical excision is the primary treatment of adult-type pulmonary blastomas. Combination chemotherapy may be of palliative benefits when there is metastasis, but there are no rigorous studies of its efficacy [6].

Biphasic blastomas recur in 40% to 50% of cases, most commonly in thorax, but distant metastases also occur in a variety of extrathoracic organs.

Patients with biphasic blastomas have as poor a survival as those with common lung carcinomas [5,6]. While there are individual reports of long-term tumor-free survival [20], two thirds of patients with biphasic tumors die within two years of diagnosis, 16% survive five years, and only 8% survive 10 years [6]. Prognosis is partly dependent on stage of the tumor, with stage 1 'blastomas' having a five-year survival of about 25% [6].

The separation of epithelial and biphasic blastomas is important because the clinical behavior and prognosis of WDFA is different. For example, epithelial blastomas recur in about 30% of cases, but they do so most frequently in lung, rather than in distant sites. Invasion of the chest wall and metastasis to hilar, periaortic, and mediastinal lymph nodes and brain also occur in fatal cases.

The overall prognosis of epithelial blastomas is strikingly better than that of biphasic tumors. Tumor-associated mortality is only 10% to 14% (median follow-up, 95 months). This reduced mortality is likely due to a lower level of biological aggressiveness, as well as the tendency of these blastomas to recur in lung where they can be easily resected [6,12].

Factors that predict poor outcome for pulmonary blastomas are listed in

Feature	Epithelial	Biphasic
Clinical[a]		
Thoracic adenopathy (x-ray)	Yes	No
Metastases (presentation)	Yes	Yes
Tumor recurrence	Yes	Yes
Gross pathologic[a]		
Gross tumor size (≥ 5 cm)	No	Yes
Histologic[a,b]		
Nuclear pleomorphism	?Yes	No
Lymphatic invasion	Yes	NA
Multifocal necrosis	Yes	NA
Restricted neuroendocrine differentiation	Yes	NA

[a] Koss et al. [6].
[b] Nakatani et al. [12].
NA = Data not available.

table 2. Nakatani and associates [9] have suggested that cytologic atypia, necrosis, and restricted neuroendocrine expression suggest a poor prognosis for epithelial tumors, but these features seem more in keeping with clear cell adenocarcinoma of the adult type than with epithelial blastoma.

Cystic and pleuropulmonary blastomas of childhood

Childhood blastomas differ both clinically and pathologically from those of adults. Clinically, they are more varied in location, occurring as solitary pleural masses as well as intrapulmonary tumors. Grossly, they exist in a spectrum of cystic to solid tumors. Thin-walled cystic tumors can occur that characteristically show an underlying cambium layer of rhabdomyosarcomatous mesenchyme. These tumors, which we term cystic blastomas, were previously classified under a variety of names, including pulmonary sarcoma arising in mesenchymal cystic hamartoma, embryonal sarcoma, and pulmonary rhabdomyosarcoma arising in congenital cystic adenomatoid malformation or bronchogenic cyst [9,21–23].

The term *pleuropulmonary blastoma* has been used to describe solid tumors that consist of a malignant embryonic-appearing mesenchyme with either no epithelial component or with a benign, entrapped epithelium [9]. It seems likely that most or all of the previously reported 'biphasic' blastomas of children fall into this tumor category [9,24].

Clinical features

Predominantly cystic lesions occur within the lungs of children who are usually 1 to 4 years old. The patients may be asymptomatic or they may have cough, fever, shortness of breath, or on occasion severe dyspnea due to pneumothorax [21].

Pleuropulmonary blastomas are largely solid, multilobulated masses that occur in the mediastinum and pleura as often as they are found in lung. The patients range from 30 months to 12 years of age, but we have now encountered microscopically similar pulmonary tumors in adults. The patients typically have nonproductive cough, fever, or chest pain [9,25–27].

Pathologic features

Cystic tumors are intrapulmonary single or multiloculated lesions that involve one or more lobes and that show thick nodular walls. Pleuropulmonary blastomas are predominantly solid masses that measure 8–23 cm in diameter, weighing up to 1100 grams. As implied above, these solid tumors may also show a cystic component, producing a spectrum from largely cystic to totally solid tumors.

Histologically, cystic tumors are lined by benign alveolar or ciliated columnar epithelial cells. Beneath the epithelium, there is a 'cambium' layer of primitive oval and spindled rhabdomyoblasts in a fibrovascular stroma (figure 10).

Pleuropulmonary blastomas consist of oval or stellate stromal cells in a myxoid stroma, but frequently there are large, pleomorphic mesenchymal cells with numerous mitoses [9,25]. The stroma often shows alternating bands of compact and loose cells (figures 11 and 12). Foci of cells with eosinophilic cytoplasm suggestive of rhabdomyosarcoma are common, and

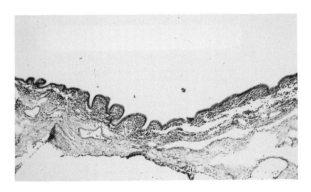

Figure 10. Cystic blastoma of childhood. The thin-walled, epithelial-lined cyst shows an underlying layer of compact cells (cambium layer).

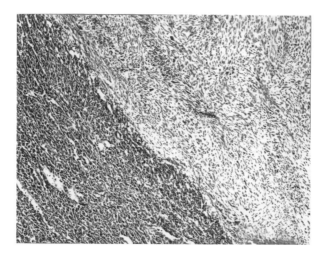

Figure 11. Pleuropulmonary blastoma of childhood. Alternating zones of compact cells and spindle cells in a myxoid stroma are present.

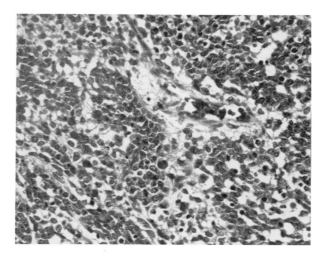

Figure 12. Pleuropulmonary blastoma of childhood. High-magnification microscopic view to show compact aggregates of primitive, oval cells in a myxoid stroma.

spindle cells resembling fascicles of smooth muscle can occasionally be seen. Foci of malignant cartilage and fat may also be present.

As noted above, cysts or small glandular spaces can be present in pleuropulmonary blastomas. They are usually lined by histologically benign epithelial cells that are probably entrapped bronchiolar, alveolar, or mesothelial cells.

The stromal cells and especially the pleomorphic giant cells are decorated

360

with antibodies to vimentin, alpha-1-antitrypsin, and alpha-1-antichymo-trypsin. Rhabdomyosarcomatous cells contain desmin and myoglobin, while chondroid elements stain for S-100 protein. The benign entrapped epithelial components stain for epithelial membrane antigen and cytokeratin [9,25,26].

Treatment and prognosis

Relatively few cases of these rare tumors have been reported with long-term follow-up, so only provisional comments can be made about treatment, survival, and prognostic factors [27]. Primary treatment for childhood cases is surgical resection, but adjuvant combination chemotherapy and radio-therapy has also been employed [27]. Recurrences are also treated with the same regimen. Gallium-67 scintigraphy can be used to document complete removal of the tumors and recurrence [28].

Fatal cases of pleuropulmonary blastoma show massive local recurrence, particularly in the mediastinum. There may be bilateral pulmonary metastases or spread to brain, spinal cord, skull, and skeletal muscle. Histologically, the metastases consist of malignant mesenchyme without an epithelial component.

Patients with intrapulmonary thin-walled cystic lesions may also have tumor recurrence and metastases, but they are more likely to have surgically resectable neoplasms than those with pleuropulmonary blastomas. Long-term survival occurs in 25% to 50% of children with solid lesions and in over 50% of those with thin-walled cystic lesions. Overall disease-free survival is 40% [27].

References

1. Sobin LH, Yesner R. 1981. International histological classification of tumors, No 1. Histological typing of lung tumors. WHO: Geneva, p. 30.
2. Barnett NR, Barnard W. 1945. Some unusual thoracic tumors. Br J Surg 32:447–457.
3. Barnard WG 1952. Embryoma of the lung. Thorax 7:229–301.
4. Spencer H. 1961. Pulmonary blastomas. J Pathol Bacteriol 82:161–165.
5. Francis D, Jacobsen M. 1983. Pulmonary blastoma. Curr Top Pathol 73:265.
6. Koss M, Hochholzer L, O'Leary T. 1991. Pulmonary blastomas. Cancer 67:2368–2381.
7. Kodama T, Shimosato Y, Watanabe S, Koide T, Naruke T, Shimose J. 1984. Six cases of well differentiated adenocarcinoma simulating fetal lung tissues in pseudoglandular stage: comparison with pulmonary blastoma. Am J Surg Pathol 8:725–744.
8. Kradin RL, Young RH, Dickersin GIC, Kirkham SE, Mark EJ. 1982. Pulmonary blastoma with argyrophil cells lacking sarcomatous features (pulmonary endodermal tumor resembling fetal lung). Am J Surg Pathol 6:165–172.
9. Manivel JC, Priest JR, Watterson J, Steiner M, Woods W, Wick M, Dehner L. 1988. Pleuropulmonary blastoma. The so-called pulmonary blastoma of childhood. Cancer 62: 1516–1526.
10. Manning JT Jr, Ordonez NJ, Rosenberg HS, Walker WE. 1985. Pulmonary endodermal tumor resembling fetal lung. Arch Pathol Lab Med 109:48–50.

11. Yousem SA, Wick MR, Randhawa P, Manivel JC. 1990. Pulmonary blastoma. An immunohistochemical analysis with comparison with fetal lung in its pseudoglandular stage. Am J Clin Pathol 93:167–175.
12. Nakatani Y, Dickersin GR, Mark EJ. 1990. Pulmonary endodermal tumor resembling fetal lung: a clinicopathologic study of five cases with immunohistochemical and ultrastructural characterization. Hum Pathol 21:1097–1107.
13. Jacobsen M, Francis, D. 1980. Pulmonary blastoma. Acta Pathol Microbiol Scand: 151–160.
14. Siegel RJ, Bueso-Ramos C, Cohen C, Koss M. 1991. Pulmonary blastoma with germ cell (yolk sac) differentiation: report of two cases. Mod Pathol 4:566–570.
15. Muller-Hermelink HK, Kaiserling E. 1986. Pulmonary adenocarcinoma of fetal type: alternating differentiation argues in favor of a common endodermal stem cell. Virch Arch (Pathol Anat) 409:195–210.
16. Inoue H, Kasai K, Shinada J, Yoshimura H, Kameya T. 1992. Pulmonary blastoma. Comparison between its epithelial components and fetal bronchial epithelium. Acta Pathol Jpn 42:884–892.
17. Chefjec G, Cosnow I, Gould NS, Husain AN, Gould VE. 1990. Pulmonary blastoma with neuroendocrine differentiation in cell morules resembling neuroepithelial bodies. Histopathology 17:353–358.
18. Cosgrove MM, Chandrasoma PT, Martin SE. 1991. Diagnosis of pulmonary blastoma by fine-needle aspiration biopsy: cytologic and immunocytochemical findings. Diagn Cytopathol 7:83–87.
19. Yokoyama S, Hayashida Y, Nagahama J, Kashima K, Nakayama I, Tanaka K, Hadama T, Mizuki M. 1992. Pulmonary blastoma: A case report. Acta Cytol 36:293–298.
20. Gibbons JRP, McKeown F, Field TW. 1981. Pulmonary blastoma with hilar lymph node metastases: survival for 24 years. Cancer 47:152–155.
21. Hedlund GL, Bisset GS, Bove KE. 1989. Malignant neoplasms arising in cystic hamartomas of the lung in childhood. Radiology 173:77–79.
22. Becroft DMO, Jagusch MF. 1987. Pulmonary sarcoma arising in mesenchymal cystic hamartomas (abstract). Pediatr Pathol 7:478.
23. Krous HF, Sexauer CL. 1981. Embryonal rhabdomyosarcoma arising within a congenital bronchogenic cyst in a child. J Pediatr Surg 16:506–508.
24. Ashworth TG 1983. Pulmonary blastoma, a true congenital neoplasm. Histopathology 7:585–594.
25. Cohen M, Emms M, Kaschula ROC. 1991. Childhood pulmonary blastoma: a pleuropulmonary variant of the adult-type pulmonary blastoma. Pediatr Pathol 11:737–749.
26. Dehner LP. 1992. Tumors and tumor-like lesions of the lung and chest wall in childhood: clinical and pathologic review. In Pediatric Pathology, JT Stocker and LP Dehner (eds.). Lippincott: Philadelphia, 232.
27. Calabria R, Srikanth MS, Chamberlin K, Bloch J, Atkinson JB. 1993. Management of pulmonary blastoma in children. Am Surg 59:192–196.
28. Howman-Giles R, Dalla Pozza L, Uren R. 1993. Ga-67 scintigraphy in pulmonary blastoma in a child. Clin Nucl Med 18:120–122.

17. Psychosocial issues in lung cancer patients

Jürg Bernhard and Patricia A. Ganz

Introduction

Lung cancer is a major cause of death in industrialized countries. In contrast to other cancers (e.g., breast), there have been few studies of quality of life, coping, behavioral interventions, and other psychosocial issues in patients with lung cancer. There are several possible explanations to consider. Metastatic disease is frequently present at the time of lung cancer diagnosis, and the limited survival time of these patients diminishes the opportunity for psychosocial investigations. Similarly, psychosocial interventions for patients with cancer are more likely to be applied in patients with longer survival times. In addition, the poor performance status and rapid disease progression in many lung cancer patients inhibits studies that require patient attentiveness and cognitive effort. Lastly, until recently, lung cancer has primarily affected men, and male patients may be more reluctant to participate in psychosocial research in which their emotional concerns are discussed.

Few lung cancer patients arc candidates for curative therapy, and therefore treatment for most patients is palliative rather than curative, i.e., treatment is directed towards symptom relief, with generally only modest improvement in survival time with chemotherapy. In this situation, patients and their families must confront and adjust to many fundamental changes in everyday life. In addition, family members play an important role in the physical and emotional care of the lung cancer patient. More research is needed on the psychosocial concerns in lung cancer to facilitate the development of supportive interventions for the patient, family, and social network, as well as to monitor more effectively the risks and benefits of treatment.

In this review (based on our comprehensive discussions in [1,2]), we focus primarily on papers that deal specifically with lung cancer patients, tracing the historical development of this field and exploring current trends (table 1). However, many studies have examined heterogeneous populations of cancer patients. Although we acknowledge that lung cancer is not one disease with uniform treatment strategies (e.g., the differing role of surgery in non-small cell and small cell carcinoma), the psychosocial literature has

Heine H. Hansen, (ed), Hansen: Lung Cancer.
© *1994 Kluwer Academic Publishers. ISBN 0-7923-2835-3. All rights reserved.*

Table 1. Historical development of psychosocial issues in lung cancer

Period	Shift of emphasis
1950s–1960s	Personality traits as direct psychosocial risk factors
1960s–1970s	Smoking behavior as indirect psychosocial risk factors; prevention programs
1970s–1980s	General psychosocial impact of the disease and its treatment
1980s–1990s	'Quality of life' as a new endpoint in clinical trials Multidisciplinary interventions

rarely distinguished between the different histologies or stages. Future investigations may evaluate the psychosocial response to lung cancer and its treatments more appropriately according to medical and biologic factors [3].

Psychosocial factors in relation to the incidence of and mortality from lung cancer

The question of whether or not psychosocial factors influence the incidence and/or mortality in lung cancer patients has been investigated extensively. There are two proposed mechanisms through which psychosocial factors may influence the multi-factorial process resulting in the development of lung cancer. First, certain complex behaviors may lead to increased carcinogen exposure. There is increasing evidence that smoking behavior is acquired and influenced by psychological factors such as control of arousal and mood, as well as social norms and values, e.g., peer pressure, and that pharmacological, psychological, and social factors play an important role in the continuation of smoking [4]. These behaviors are therefore considered indirect psychosocial factors, as opposed to direct psychosocial factors, such as loss of a job or partner. Grief during bereavement may lead to changes in the immune or endocrine systems via psychological processes.

Indirect psychosocial factors

Lung cancer is the major malignancy for which indirect psychosocial factors have been shown to play a dominant role in etiology. Many aspects of smoking behavior have been studied, including age at starting, number and kind of cigarettes smoked, and inhaling pattern. Reviews of the association between smoking behavior and cancer have consistently concluded that 80% to 90% of lung cancer and about 30% of all cancer deaths are caused by smoking [5–7]. The risk of lung cancer in nonsmokers has increased by 25% to 35% due to passive smoking (breathing of others' tobacco smoke). In Scandinavia, the United Kingdom, and North America, the incidence of male lung cancer is rising only in older men, whereas in Mediterranean

364

Europe, where smoking is a more recently acquired habit, the incidence is still increasing in men of all ages [8]. A rising incidence and mortality from lung cancer has been observed in women in most Western countries [8–10]. In the U.S., by the late 1980s, lung cancer caused more deaths than breast cancer among women. Lung cancer mortality rates in women are increasing faster than for any other cancer type.

Consequently, the behavioral and social dimensions of smoking have been studied, and prevention strategies have been developed, mainly related to education (e.g., encouraging medical personnel to take leadership roles) and legislation (e.g., banning of tobacco advertising, limiting smoking in public places) [11–13].

There are some other indirect psychosocial risk factors that play a role in the development of lung cancer. An inverse relationship between lung cancer incidence and socioeconomic status has been observed in several studies [14]. Smoking habits contribute partly to these differences. Occupational risk factors are also strongly linked with lower social class (e.g., radon exposure in miners). Epidemiological studies have identified about 40 chemicals, groups of chemicals, or complex mixtures that are associated with the development of cancer; 12 of them have the lung as a target organ [15]. Environmental carcinogenesis may also play a role in the observed socioeconomic differences in lung cancer incidence. Lung cancer tends to be more common in urban than rural areas in virtually all parts of the world [14], although air pollution is estimated to have a minimal influence compared to cigarette smoking [10].

Direct psychosocial factors

Two main hypotheses have been suggested related to direct psychosocial risk factors: 1) there is a 'cancer personality,' i.e., certain personality traits predispose to cancer; and 2) severe personal losses lead to disorders of physical function via psychological changes. Most investigations in lung cancer have explored the first hypothesis, i.e., comparing personality traits in lung cancer patients to healthy controls or patients with other chronic diseases. A comprehensive review of this work does not show any specific psychosocial pattern for lung cancer [1]. Since lung cancer may have a latent period of several years, psychological data collected a few months before diagnosis may not in fact reflect the premorbid personality of the individual, but rather the morbidity of disease, or a complex interaction of both.

A few truly prospective studies suggest that direct psychosocial factors such as depression influence subsequent risk of lung cancer and other malignancies [16]. However, recent epidemiological studies call into question the causal connection between depressive symptoms and cancer morbidity and mortality [17,18]. The hypothesis related to personal loss has not specifically been formulated with regard to lung cancer. The risk of death after the loss of a marriage partner has been discussed, especially for men

365

[19]. These data do not support loss as a specific risk factor for death from cancer in the surviving partner. Rather, the increased morbidity and mortality in the bereaved individual reflects vulnerability to multiple diseases.

Smoking and personality factors have also been studied as combined risk factors for lung cancer. However, more systematic work would be necessary to elucidate the postulated synergistic interactions between personality, stress, smoking, and genetic predisposition [20].

In summary, risk factors for lung cancer should be considered from more than a purely biomedical perspective, including risk behavior and socioeconomic conditions. Prevention of lung cancer and other smoking-related neoplasms can primarily be accomplished by developing strategies that address the psychological and social behaviors associated with smoking.

Psychosocial issues related to the disease and its treatment

To distinguish disease from treatment-related problems experienced by lung cancer patients is a somewhat arbitrary process, since some problems may be manifestations of both the disease and/or its treatment. Similarly, separation of the physical symptoms from the psychologic effects of the lung cancer experience can be difficult. For clarity, this section is organized according to the topics given in table 2. Specific recommendations for supportive care in lung cancer [21] and for psychiatric symptom management in cancer patients [22] have recently been presented, and are not discussed here.

Adjustment to diagnosis and course of disease

There is often a lag time of several weeks between the initial symptoms and the final diagnosis of lung cancer in both industrialized [23] and developing countries [24]. This delay may partly be explained by the patient's fear,

Table 2. Psychosocial issues related to lung cancer and its treatment

Adjustment to diagnosis and course of disease
Physical symptoms and functional status
Pain
Dyspnea
Nausea, vomiting, and appetite disorders
Cognitive changes and organic mental disorders
Paraneoplastic syndromes
Fatigue
Sleep disturbance
Psychologic distress
Social interaction
Sexual dysfunction

especially in smokers, and because the initial symptoms may mimic other conditions. Pessimism and a fatalistic outlook about the availability of any effective treatment can also contribute to delay [25].

The initial psychological response to a diagnosis of lung cancer may be anticipatory depression, even before diagnosis is established [26], disbelief, and shock, followed by recognition of the existential crisis, with anxious searching for the best treatment available [25]. Development of a trusting relationship between the patient and physician during this early phase is crucial for the patient's adjustment and compliance with treatment. Each change in the often rapid course of disease or treatment affects the patient as well as his or her family. Giving timely information to the patient and the family regarding the specific clinical issues will assist and encourage them in their adjustment, for example, during periods with significant treatment-related toxicity or in preparation for terminal care (e.g., decision between home care and institutional care).

A large variation in psychological adjustment can be observed both within a patient over time, as well as between patients, that is closely related to the underlying biological processes. In general, there is a positive relationship between quality of life and good physical functioning, and better quality of life with more limited disease in lung cancer patients [27]. Other medical problems (frequently related to smoking) such as cardiovascular disease can complicate the disease course.

Of particular interest is a patient's smoking history. Many patients do not seem to acknowledge the close relationship between their smoking behavior and the development of their lung cancer [28]. The neglect of this relationship may be aimed at restoring their self-esteem rather than denying the seriousness of the disease [29]. A personal sense of failure ('Why me?') may occur within an individual patient with or without smoking history. Good health is associated with personal responsibility, whereas having a serious disease such as lung cancer often is associated with a sense of failure. Even when an individual patient has no known etiologic risk factors, the patient and significant others may consider him or her responsible in some way for the disease; similarly, nonsmoking patients may feel they are the victim of passive smoking. Causal attributions appear to play an important role in the patient's as well the spouse's adjustment and should therefore be addressed by the primary care giver.

Smoking behavior may still be a relevant issue for lung cancer patients. Recently, it was reported that smoking cessation significantly reduces the risk of second primary cancer in long-term cancer-free survivors of small cell lung cancer [30]. There is little information about the rate of smoking cessation in lung cancer patients [31]. Smoking habits were studied in 52 patients who had survived more than five years after surgery for lung cancer [32]. Ninety-six percent of the patients were smokers before their operation, 56% stopped smoking preoperatively, and no patients smoked in the immediate postoperative period; however, 48% became regular smokers again, usually within a year of the operation. For the individual lung cancer patient, smoking cessation may be important for relief of dyspnea and cough. Whereas some patients feel that being able to quit smoking is a helpful step in their coping process, others prefer to continue to smoke. For these patients, quitting smoking results in an additional stress. Clinically, the approach to the lung cancer patient must be individualized. More systematic information with regard to smoking behavior and smoking cessation, as well as the related psychosocial and biomedical adjustment, would be useful in clinical practice.

Physical symptoms and functional status

There are a wide range of serious physical symptoms in lung cancer that affect the patients' everyday lives [33]. These symptoms are not always specific for this disease (e.g., dyspnea and cough), and are shared with other respiratory diseases. However, some physical symptoms are more specific for lung cancer as opposed to other pulmonary conditions (e.g., pain from pleural or chest wall involvement, weight loss, and anorexia) and lead to more serious physical and functional consequences for the lung cancer patient.

The physical symptoms of lung cancer have a serious impact on the individual's functional or performance status as defined by the ability to do certain physical activities, especially related to mobility, work, and self-care. The first systematic assessment of this key concept was introduced by Karnofsky and Burchenal in 1949 [34]. They developed a single-item scale rated by physicians, as an additional descriptive measure for chemotherapy trials. The scale has been found to be a major predictor of prognosis and survival in lung cancer patients [35] and has become a standard stratification variable in clinical trials, mostly assessed by short forms (4- or 5-point grading scales [36–38]) adapted from the original 10-point scale. This type of instrument has been criticized for being a crude measure with only modest interrater reliability [39–44], and modifications have been proposed [41]. Nevertheless, the patient's functional ability has important biologic as well as psychosocial consequences in clinical research and practice. For example, a patient may stress how important it is to live as before and to be able to work again after primary treatment.

Treatments for lung cancer often burden the patient with additional physical symptoms [33]. Most investigations have been focused on chemotherapy side effects. Limited information is available about the psychosocial impact of lung cancer surgery, probably due in part to the fact that surgery is usually performed with curative intent. Surgically treated lung cancer patients have been followed with physician-rated performance status that gives only a rough picture of the patients' physical well-being and neglects their subjective experience. Similarly, there have been only limited evaluations of the psychosocial effects of radiotherapy in lung cancer. Both treatment modalities warrant more extensive study of their psychosocial effects.

Pain

Despite the importance of pain in palliative care, only a few descriptive studies deal with pain in lung cancer specifically. In 164 patients with early lung cancer, pain was present in 40%, and a relationship was described between the location of the neoplasm, the location of the pain, and the characteristics of the sensory changes [45]. From several reviews, it can be concluded that pain is experienced in 30% to 40% of lung cancer patients with early disease and 60% to 90% with advanced disease. In ambulatory lung cancer patients with excellent performance status, 39% reported 'persistent or frequent' pain [46]. In about half of these patients, pain interfered substantially with their functioning and quality of life.

Suffering from pain is one of the major concerns of lung cancer patients. In contrast to other types of cancer, patients with lung cancer may experience pain early in the disease from the chest lesion or from metastatic sites in bone. Poor pain control can exacerbate fears about dying. Appropriate treatment, as well as information about pain and pain management, is important for patient's adjustment to the disease and facilitates a trusting physician–patient relationship. Chronic pain is frequently associated with psychological symptoms (e.g., sleep disorders, reduction in appetite) and with clinical signs and symptoms that may mimic a depressive disorder [47]. Chronic pain is also a burden to the patient's family, who may have feelings of helplessness and anxiety [48] and need special support.

The intervention strategy for controlling pain depends on the specific cause(s) of pain in the individual cancer patient. A multidisciplinary approach may be required in the management of cancer pain, including adequate analgesia, neurosurgical and anesthetic interventions, and psychiatric assistance. In spite of the frequency of pain in patients with advanced lung cancer, there have been few systematic evaluations of multidisciplinary pain interventions, and this presents a challenge for future research.

Dyspnea

Dyspnea is a common symptom in lung cancer patients throughout the entire course of the disease. It can be caused by the tumor, its treatment, medical complications of the debilitated state, or underlying lung or cardiac disease. Dyspnea in lung cancer is often associated with severe fatigue, impaired cognitive function and poor appetite, all of which can promote the patient's social withdrawal [49,50]. In a study of 1754 terminally ill cancer patients, 70% had dyspnea, and 28% rated their symptom severity as 'moderate or worse' during their last six weeks of life [51]. In addition to lung or pleural involvement by the tumor, the presence of underlying lung or cardiac disease and low Karnofsky performance status were significantly associated with dyspnea, whereas age and sex did not show a relationship.

In the case of increased dyspnea, the patient's attention is focused on controlling breathing. As with pain, the patient may perceive this symptom as an indication of advancing tumor growth and thereby experience considerable anxiety. The perception of increasing dyspnea and the related feelings of anxiety or panic may lead to a vicious cycle of decreased oxygen consumption and anxiety of suffocation. Skilled professional intervention is necessary to modify the patient's response to these physical symptoms, the related emotions, and the social environment. Ad hoc interventions are used by most clinicians in dealing with this problem, and some supportive techniques by nurses have been described (e.g., nasal administration of oxygen, instruction in breathing [52]). More systematic investigation of a multidisciplinary management of dyspnea, e.g., possibly the development of specific behavioral strategies, could aid clinical practice.

Nausea, vomiting, and appetite disorders

Nausea and vomiting are among the most important concerns of patients who are to receive chemotherapy. In a review of the frequency of nausea and vomiting in clinical trials of combination chemotherapy in inoperable non-small cell lung cancer, acute nausea and vomiting were commonly reported in 70% to 80% of the patients receiving cisplatin [53]. While there has been considerable improvement in antiemetic therapy during the past few years, nausea and vomiting are still a problem. Although not commonly reported in the clinical trial literature, subacute and delayed nausea and vomiting are also seen in lung cancer patients receiving chemotherapy, and this has received some attention from clinicians and researchers [54]. Frequently, patients experience nausea and vomiting for up to a week after platinum-based chemotherapy, resulting in weight loss, dehydration, and a decline in performance status for some individuals. Persistent nausea and vomiting may be caused by other factors, such as brain metastases and hypercalcemia.

Nausea or vomiting can occur with either chemotherapy or radiotherapy. In a study of non-small cell lung cancer, patients were randomized to receive either radiation therapy or four cycles of combination chemotherapy including cisplatin [53]. Of the chemotherapy patients, 80% reported nausea and 69% had vomiting two weeks after the start of treatment; five weeks after the last cycle, 61% still reported nausea and 44% had spells of vomiting. Of the radiotherapy patients, 43% reported nausea and 11% vomiting two weeks after start of treatment, whereas only 14% reported nausea and 5% vomiting 14 weeks after start of treatment.

370

Conditioned responses to chemotherapy treatment are prevalent in cancer patients and can occur before treatment, generally labeled as 'anticipatory nausea and vomiting' (e.g., vomiting approaching the hospital), as well as during or after treatment. The prevalence of conditioned nausea and vomiting ranges from 18% to 57% in over 20 studies [55]. The presence and severity of conditioned as well as treatment-induced nausea and vomiting varies widely between patients, and the factors underlying individual differences are not yet clear. Anticipatory nausea, vomiting, and related symptoms are probably due largely to maladaptive learning; this learning generally follows a respondent conditioning paradigm [55]. Individual variables, especially anxiety, are associated with the development of the conditioned responses.

Sophisticated measures of the frequency and intensity of nausea and vomiting have been developed for the evaluation of antiemetic regimens; however, these measures do not routinely evaluate the affective consequences of nausea and vomiting. In addition, many of the antiemetic medications have side effects of their own (e.g., extrapyramidal symptoms, excessive sedation). Behavioral interventions, especially relaxation techniques (hypnosis, progressive muscle relaxation) have been developed and studied in a variety of cancers. Symptom relief has been reported in controlled trials, mainly focused on anticipatory reactions due to chemotherapy [56]. There is increasing evidence that nonspecific interventions, such as distraction by video games [57] or relaxing by listening to music, can effectively control the side effects of chemotherapy. However, this kind of intervention has not been tested extensively in controlled lung cancer trials.

A related problem is learned food aversion in patients receiving chemotherapy. This response is usually established when food ingestion has been temporally paired with chemotherapy administration and its associated nausea and vomiting, and can occur even after a single course of chemotherapy. Any type of food may be targeted, and highly preferred items eaten every day are often most problematic. In a comparison of lung and breast cancer patients, pretreatment reductions in appetite were found in 57% of the lung cancer patients as compared with 19% of the breast cancer patients [58]. Aversions were formed to food ingested anywhere from 24 hours before to more than 24 hours after treatment, and these had a median duration of less than one month. An emetic episode was not a necessary condition.

Nausea, vomiting, and appetite disorders may have an important impact on the patient's well-being. Prevention and management strategies for these problems should be studied further. In addition to the effective use of antiemetics, behavioral interventions should be used to reduce or prevent anticipatory nausea and vomiting, food aversions, or increased anxiety and physiological arousal.

A wide range of changes in psychological well-being have been reported in lung cancer patients, from daily fluctuations in a 'normal' range to psychiatric disorders such as major depression or organic anxiety disorder. Some clinical reports refer to the potential underlying interactions between biological and psychosocial processes, e.g., manic spmptoms in a patient with small cell lung cancer, apparently caused by ectopic ACTH production [68], a paraneoplastic syndrome.

Several authors who have studied the process of adjustment in cancer of the lung and other sites concluded that most patients cope fairly well with their disease. However, special attention has to be given to a high-risk group for poor psychosocial adaptation. In a screening trial for psychological morbidity, 274 patients with advanced small-cell lung cancer completed the Hospital Anxiety and Depression Scale (HADS) [69]. Thirty-six percent of patients met the criteria for morbidity, with equal proportions of 'depression' 'anxiety', and mixed 'depression–anxiety'; 22% were estimated as 'borderline' cases [70].

Patients may anticipate a lung cancer diagnosis and be distressed before the diagnosis. In patients attending a chest clinic, symptoms of major depression were observed in 16% of 134 lung cancer patients before the establishment of their diagnosis [26]. This prevalence of depression was higher than that found in patients with non-malignant chest conditions or healthy controls. Past psychiatric history and presence of metastases were most significantly correlated with depression. At a subsequent evaluation of the lung cancer patients (2–3 months later), a minority (16%) of the subset (50 patients) with inoperable lung cancer had major depression. Patients not receiving a specific treatment were more likely to be depressed or dissatisfied [71].

In lung cancer, it is especially difficult to discriminate between underlying biological and psychological factors causing depression. Depressive symptoms are frequently observed in patients with organic mental syndromes. In addition, the somatic symptoms of depression, e.g., extreme fatigue and sleep disorders, can be confused with constitutional symptoms from the tumor or its treatment. Altered mood or behavior may be simply labeled as reactive or appropriate to a lung cancer diagnosis, and the possibility of a severe and treatable depression or organic mood disorder may not be considered without a psychiatric consultant.

In clinical experience, chemotherapy and radiotherapy can play a helpful role in the ability of some patients to adjust psychologically to their diagnosis. First, tumor response to treatment can improve physical performance and alleviate symptoms; the extent of disease-related symptoms has been shown to correlate highly with subjective well-being in several small cell and non-small cell lung cancer trials. In addition, treatment is usually associated with hope, which helps some patients deal with the course of the disease and cope with their anxiety. In a group of patients with different types of cancer, treatment status was the most important variable for prediction of anxiety [48]. Patients receiving palliative care displayed significantly higher anxiety scores than did patients under active treatment or follow-up care.

In 454 patients with small cell lung cancer, the relationship of psychological distress to medical and demographic factors was examined [72]. A significant relationship was found between the patients' performance status, extent of disease, and psychological distress as measured by the Profile of Mood States (POMS [73]), a patient-rated standardized measure of mood. Marital status, age, and education did not predict psychological distress. Physical impairment showed an approximately linear relationship to increasing levels of psychological distress, suggesting that performance status and extent of disease may be used to identify those patients who are potentially at high risk for psychological distress. However, these physical factors alone accounted for a very limited amount of the variability in mood disturbance (10%–15%).

Other factors such as past psychiatric history, social support, and coping behavior can be important, too. In addition, personality factors may contribute substantially to the patient's adjustment. As earlier research in this field indicates, there may be subgroups of lung cancer patients, as in any other chronic disease, who do not express their needs and emotions [1]. Clinicians must consider the patient's experience with past illness and life events to better evaluate the individual patient's adjustment to disease and treatment.

Social interaction

In clinical experience and empirical work [74], mostly in studies related to psychosocial risk factors [1], lung cancer patients show a tendency toward social withdrawal. This behavior has also been shown toward family members in cases where patients are reluctant to discuss their fears. Symptoms of the disease, especially impaired functional status, dyspnea, and pain, impose limitations on the patients' social life. Furthermore, many patients seem to dislike being dependent on others. It is very likely that social withdrawal is a direct consequence of the disease.

Like every serious or fatal disease, lung cancer affects the patient's family and social environment. Few data are available in this area. Differing supportive care interventions may be helpful for the patient and spouse or next of kin. These options are critically important in lung cancer patients, since the spouse is often the primary caregiver and experiences disruption and changes in her or his own life.

Sexual dysfunction

This area has been restricted to case reports and clinical impressions, for example, that almost all patients were able to resume normal sexual activity after lung surgery [75]. A comparison of lung cancer patients in different clinical phases shows increasing sexual impairment with progression of disease, comparable to colorectal cancer patients [27].

Developing new endpoints for clinical trials in lung cancer

When cancer treatments are curative, the short- and long-term side effects are usually outweighed by prolongation of disease-free survival and overall survival. When treatment is mainly palliative, such as for metastatic non-small cell lung cancer, with only modest prolongation in survival anticipated, then the cost–benefit relationship between increased survival and treatment-related toxicity will vary from individual to individual. Ideally, the treatment toxicity should always be minimized, but even under the best of circumstances it may be difficult for the clinician to estimate treatment benefit prospectively. Therefore, the patient's *subjective experience* is an important concept that is increasingly being used to estimate treatment benefit.

Quality of Life has thereby become a widely used catch phrase and key word in clinical papers covering nearly all psychosocial aspects of cancer and has been studied with different research strategies. However, a broad consensus in the literature defines quality of life as a multidimensional construct, including the central dimensions of physical, psychological, and social well-being. These include functional status (performance of self-care activities, mobility, physical activities, and role activities such as work or household responsibilities); disease and treatment-related symptoms (specific symptoms from the disease, such as pain or dyspnea, or from treatment toxicity, such as nausea or hair loss); psychological functioning (anxiety or depression that may be secondary to the disease or its treatment); and social functioning (disruptions in normal social activities). Additional considerations include spiritual or existential concerns, sexual functioning and body image, and satisfaction with health care. Of course, this definition is not final. More specific concepts may be defined with regard to a given setting, e.g., a phase III trial in early non-small cell lung cancer.

Clinical decision making

Quality of life assessment, i.e., the trade-off between 'quantity' and 'quality' of survival, can be illustrated in its simplest form at the level of clinical decision making for an individual patient. Multiple factors contribute to treatment decisions, such as the histology of the cancer, the stage of disease,

376

the functional status of the patient, and the specific pattern of metastases. Besides these fairly objective features of the illness, non-medical factors have also been shown to influence decisions. In a review of 1808 hospital charts of patients with non-small cell lung cancer, treatment was found to vary according to social and economic factors [76]. Patients were more likely to be treated with surgery if they were married, had private medical insurance, or resided farther from the cancer treatment center. Among patients not undergoing surgery, those with private insurance were more likely to receive either radiation or chemotherapy. The relationship between the type of treatment and socioeconomic factors was not based on apparent differences in tumor stage or functional status. The socioeconomic factors did not show an influence on survival. However, taking into account this kind of interaction in prospective investigations could at least partly clarify the impact of socioeconomic factors on survival.

Both physicians and patients may have their personal treatment preferences. Pulmonary physicians have been examined by presenting several case vignettes and asking them how they would choose to be managed if they themselves developed non-small cell lung cancer [77]. Their answers were remarkably similar, in view of their diverse backgrounds, and corresponded to treatment recommendations in standard textbooks. Interestingly, an exception was observed in the vignettes of patients with locally advanced and distant metastatic disease, where the physicians preferred no chemotherapy.

The preferences of cancer patients with regard to receiving information have been studied extensively, and it has been found that most patients prefer to have information about their diagnosis and prognosis. The vast majority (92%) of a mixed cancer sample wanted to receive all the information about their disease, good or bad [78]. However, almost one third of these patients preferred to leave decisions about their medical care and treatment to their doctor. Interestingly, this subgroup was composed primarily of older male patients who were married and had a lower performance status. Of all the diagnostic groups, lung cancer patients were more likely to prefer leaving therapeutic decisions to the physician. For some patients, it may be too burdensome to actively participate in the treatment decision.

Patients may be quite averse to accepting the risks of surgery, including the possibility of immediate death, as has been found in a small sample of 14 patients with 'operable' lung cancer [79]. Using a sophisticated measure of efficacy for each potential therapy, it was found that the patient's attitude toward treatment had a major effect on the choice of treatment, besides the presentation of survival data.

The risk–benefit ratio in lung cancer treatment has also been discussed in relationship to participation in clinical trials. The value of clinical trials for the community is evident, as a necessary step in developing and optimizing effective treatments; however, for the individual patient, the decision to participate is much more complex. The treatment experience in advanced non-small cell lung cancer as reported in the Eastern Cooperative Oncology Group (ECOG) trials has been reviewed [80]. The whole group of 2714 patients had a median survival of 4.2 months, and only 15% showed objective tumor response. Of the whole group, 39% experienced at least one episode of 'severe or worse' toxicity from therapy. The more intensive chemotherapy protocols showed some improvement in median survival and response rates, but at the expense of greater toxicity. It has been concluded that subgroups of patients unlikely to benefit from trial participation should be identified, and patient preferences should be incorporated in the final decision.

In summary, clinical decision making in lung cancer is often a subtle task for the patient as well the clinician, based on biomedical and psychosocial criteria. More systematic information from clinical trials in regard to quality of life considerations is therefore necessary.

Methodological issues in quality of life assessment

Implementing assessments of the patients' subjective experience into clinical trials requires new methods and procedures if these assessments are to be added to the traditional 'hard' biomedical outcome measures. In lung cancer, where overall treatment benefits have been modest and only a paucity of information is available about the specific psychosocial needs of patients, there has been considerable interest in the development of quality of life assessment tools. For example, the questionnaire by the European Organization for Research on the Treatment of Cancer (EORTC) was developed in lung cancer patients [81].

Since ratings by an external observer usually reflect the observer's point of view rather than the patient's subjective experience, there has been a broad agreement that quality of life endpoints should include patient report [82], preferably combined with physician-rated measures. Physician-rated performance status has been the major reference scale in lung cancer, but has been criticized for several reasons (see above). Performance status represents an important physical but rather limited aspect of quality of life not accurately reflecting the patient's subjective experience. In general, physicians have been found to underestimate patients' symptoms [83]. A similar criticism has been made for physician-rated toxicity.

In estimating the risk/benefit of a treatment, clinicians are interested in the relative impact of disease versus treatment-related symptoms on patients' quality of life. As discussed above, some of the clinically most relevant aspects, such as fatigue and functional status, can be due to both the disease and/or treatment. From this perspective, assessing specific disease and treatment-related symptoms is complementary to more global measures, and studying the association of specific disease and treatment-related symptoms over time and in relation to the biomedical variables can give insight into various interactions. This approach can be helpful in defining risk factors for psychosocial adjustment and in developing intervention strategies. For example, in small cell lung cancer patients (limited and extensive disease) receiving six cycles of combination chemotherapy, patient-rated symptoms of the tumor were closely related to most aspects of their well-being; the initial prognostic factors (performance status, extent of disease, prior weight loss) had a dominant impact on patients' well-being, tumor-related symptoms, and toxicity over the whole induction phase [84]. Such a 'modular' concept including disease-specific aspects of quality of life has been adopted by the EORTC approach [81]. Another lung cancer instrument, the Lung Cancer Symptom Scale (LCSS [85]), combining a brief patient and observer rating was specifically designed to address the issues of palliation and symptom control in evaluating patients receiving new chemotherapy regimens; it was recently applied in a large multicenter trial.

Some of the first studies with patient-rated questionnaires in lung cancer patients have shown that feasibility issues have been underestimated [86–88]. The traditional methods for data collection and data management developed in the 1960s for multicenter clinical trials need to be modified for quality of life assessment. Staff and patients must make additional efforts in order to get an acceptable compliance rate and data quality. In lung cancer, this requirement may be more of a problem than with other cancer sites, because these patients frequently have impaired cognitive and functional status, are receiving aggressive treatment, and are of advanced age. In addition, poorly educated patients may have difficulties understanding comprehensive questionnaires [86]. Lack of compliance can lead to serious biases, for example, that data are available only from those patients with relatively good quality of life or from those who are satisfied with their physician and treatment. However, an estimate of the representativeness of a subsample with psychosocial data with regard to biomedical and demographic variables of the whole sample has usually been the exception than the rule. Implementation of quality of life assessment in the clinical trial setting is still in a developmental phase, and ways of improving compliance have been proposed [88]. Interviewing patients by telephone has been suggested as an alternative approach [89].

Responsiveness to the course of disease is one of the key criteria for a valid quality of life measure. It has repeatedly been demonstrated in lung cancer, both with comprehensive measures, such as the Cancer Rehabilitation Evaluation System (CARES [90,27]) or the Sickness Impact Profile (SIP [91,92]), as well as with short indicators, such as linear-analogue self-assessment scales (LASA [93]), that patient-rated variables can sensitively discriminate between different phases of disease. In addition, patient-rated quality of life at baseline, as shown with the Functional Living Index–Cancer [94] and other measures, has been found to predict biomedical outcome after controlling for the conventional prognostic factors in both small and non-small cell lung cancer patients in different stages [95–97].

This finding is a strong argument that patient-rated quality of life variables validly reflect the course of disease. The fact that these variables may be used in lung cancer as a prognostic factor as well as a treatment endpoint offers new applications in clinical research and practice. However, it also points to the potential underlying interactions between disease, treatment, and the patient's coping process, and this interaction has been underestimated in interpreting quality of life data as a treatment endpoint.

It has been more difficult to achieve an accurate evaluation of responsiveness to toxicity and other differences among different treatment regimens. The basic assumption that different chemotherapy regimens can have a different impact on psychological well-being, despite the absence of a significant difference in tumor response, was already demonstrated in the first randomized lung cancer trial to use a patient-rated well-being measure [98]. However, patients are often assessed at clinical visits several weeks after the intervention, which is too large an interval to reliably assess acute toxicity. To gain more information about the course of treatment, the British Medical Research Council (MRC) Lung Cancer Working Party has developed a daily diary card filled in by patients at home [99]. This approach is sensitive to short-term treatment effects [100] and treatment-related differences [101], and may therefore provide information on longitudinal patterns of a few quality of life variables. However, compliance problems have been reported, and further methodological investigations are necessary with regard to analysis of longitudinal data and psychometric properties (e.g., the effect of ongoing serial assessments on patients' self-report).

The choice of the assessment tool, as well as the timing and frequency of data collection, depends on the endpoints and design of the trial. Divergent findings, especially with regard to the impact of chemotherapy, are partly due to different assessment approaches, focusing on different aspects of quality of life or on different time frames (e.g., acute versus subacute or long-term toxicity). In addition, methodological problems such as confounding biomedical or psychosocial factors play a role (e.g., supportive care). Generally, quality of life endpoints should be studied in controlled investigations with an established methodology, just as response rate and survival are in conventional clinical trials.

Interpreting quality of life data presupposes not just clinical experience but also basic information about a measure's psychometric properties. Well-being scales, developed for the general population or psychiatric patients, rarely discriminate cancer patients from healthy controls. For example, female small cell lung cancer patients reported substantially more mood distress than males in a well-validated standard scale (POMS [73]) [72]; a comparable difference in mood distress has been reported between healthy females and males. However, the scores of the entire sample of lung cancer patients were not dissimilar to the mean values in healthy individuals. Also, with regard to frequency or intensity of specific symptoms, lung and other cancer patients have reported in many studies remarkably 'good' values [84],

380

suggesting a better adjustment in a majority of patients than generally assumed. Various contributing methodological and psychological factors have been discussed, for example, that patients reframe their norms in adjusting to their disease (e.g., modified criteria for 'good' physical well-being after response to primary chemotherapy).

Given the current state of this research, quality of life data have to be interpreted with special caution. More information is needed about the influence of other disease- and treatment-related factors, such as the setting of data collection (e.g., inpatient versus outpatient), the timing relative to the intervention, or specific supportive interventions (e.g., antiemetic treatment). Methodological investigations are crucial in implementing quality of life endpoints in clinical trials, including systematic evaluation and comparison of quality of life measures in all phases of disease and treatment. In addition, short indicators need to be developed that are applicable to patients with poor performance status where a more comprehensive assessment is not feasible.

Use of quality of life endpoints in lung cancer trials

During the 1980s, the limitations of the traditional endpoints in cancer clinical trials have been extensively discussed. Lung cancer was one of the first tumors for which quality of life variables were proposed as additional outcome measures. However, there are still relatively few clinical trials published with quality of life endpoints in lung cancer.

In most of the studies, 'quality of life' assessment has been restricted to physician-rated performance status or to nonexperimental investigations. Pioneering work in this field was done in patients treated with lung surgery, three decades after the concept of performance status was introduced. Patients were assessed with the Vitagram, a rough model integrating performance status and the course of the disease [102]. Follow-up data in patients cured by resection suggested a high quality of life [103]. In contrast, in those patients who subsequently died from residual disease, surgery did not show a palliative effect in comparison with nonsurgically treated patients.

The social consequences of brain and liver relapse were retrospectively compared in 370 small cell lung cancer patients [104]. Patients with relapse in the brain had more deterioration in performance status (Karnofsky) and spent a greater proportion of their remaining life in the hospital than did patients with initial relapse in the liver. These kinds of quality-of-life-oriented data emphasize the importance of additional outcome measures for treatment policy and should be considered in the discussion of prophylactic cranial irradiation.

A related aspect in policy development and quality of life is the cost of treatment. An economic evaluation was undertaken in a three-arm randomized comparison of two different cisplatin-based combination chemo-therapies versus best supportive care in advanced non-small cell lung cancer [105]. A modest survival benefit was associated with both chemotherapy regimens compared to supportive care alone. The patients receiving sup-portive care spent more time in the hospital and received more palliative radiation treatments than those receiving chemotherapy, leading to in-creased costs; the majority of costs in each treatment arm were related to hospitalization. However, the key question, namely, whether a lower hos-pitalization rate reflects an improved quality of life, cannot be answered without a prospective evaluation of patients' subjective experience.

Few controlled trials have been reported with patient-rated quality of life variables. In 95 non-small cell lung cancer patients with limited disease, chest radiotherapy was randomly compared with chemotherapy (cisplatin, etoposide). No difference in overall survival was found; however, other studies have shown a survival advantage in patients treated with chemo-therapy. Patient-rated general symptoms and psychosocial well-being at the start of treatment were the best predictive factors for patients' survival [95]. Two weeks after the start of treatment, patients receiving chemotherapy showed a significantly greater decline in psychosocial well-being, presumably due to toxicity. However, a general improvement was observed during the following 14 weeks, and no differences were detected between the two treatment groups [106]. In contrast to the disease-related symptoms, sym-ptoms of toxicity were not significantly correlated with well-being, pointing to the dominant impact of the course of disease on patients' emotional adjustment in this population [107].

In a multicenter trial, 300 patients with untreated limited and extensive-stage small-cell lung cancer and no progressive disease after the first cycle of chemotherapy were randomized to receive combination chemotherapy (cy-clophosphamide, vincristine, etoposide) either regularly 'planned' or given 'as required' [101]. 'Planned' treatment was given every three weeks; 'as required' treatment was given for tumor-related symptoms and for radio-logical progression of disease. Both groups were given a maximum of eight cycles. Patients receiving treatment as required received on average half as much chemotherapy as those receiving planned treatment, but did not show a significantly shorter survival. However, unexpectedly, in a subsample of 62 patients, all treated at one center, who had systematic quality of life assess-ment, patients who received treatment as required scored more severe symptoms in daily diary cards than patients receiving planned treatment. This finding may be explained by the fact that tumor-related symptoms are alleviated by chemotherapy, even if at the expense of toxicity. Similar results have been reported in metastatic breast cancer [108]. In addition, chemotherapy as an active intervention is associated with the potential for cure, and may support a subgroup of patients in coping with their disease.

Another potential application of quality of life endpoints is suggested by a study of the effects of home nursing care in progressive lung cancer [109].

One hundred sixty-six patients were randomly assigned to one of three programs: a specialized oncology home care program, a standard home care program, or an office care program. Patients were interviewed two months after diagnosis and at six-week intervals for six months. No differences in pain, mood disturbance, and current concerns were found among the three groups, but the two home care groups had significantly less symptom distress and greater social independence (six weeks longer) than the office care group.

We are aware of only one specific, controlled lung cancer trial in which quality of life endpoints were used to evaluate a psychosocial intervention program. The effect of psychotherapy for the spouses of newly diagnosed lung cancer patients was tested in a randomized study [110]. Over the six months of the intervention program, no differential changes were found in emotional, social, or physical function for either the patients or their principal supporters according to the experimental status. Methodological problems — sensitivity of instruments, patient selection, and conflicts between research goals and clinical goals — may explain these negative findings and are of considerable interest for designing similar evaluations of multidisciplinary interventions in lung cancer.

In summary, quality of life is a major endpoint in the treatment of the lung cancer patient and can best be approached in a multidisciplinary setting. However, more systematic data are necessary, especially with regard to surgery and radiotherapy. Furthermore, it can be anticipated that the pattern of patients' quality of life during the course of the disease and treatment is predicted not only by biomedical variables but also by psychosocial factors, such as coping behavior and social support, allowing for more specific subgroup comparisons. Improving patients' quality of life requires a selective but systematic inclusion of psychosocial data in clinical research and practice.

Discussion and recommendations

Lung cancer and AIDS will likely be the most common nonacute, life-threatening diseases in the early part of the coming century. These diseases have some epidemiological similarities, and both are predominantly preventable [9]. Neither disease was known at the beginning of this century, and now both are rapidly increasing worldwide, with the most prominent increases occurring in industrialized countries during the last decade. Based on tobacco consumption data, a decline in U.S. male lung cancer mortality of approximately 25% has been predicted by 2005 [111]. However, lung cancer mortality will increase in most European countries and Japan until 2000. As smoking becomes part of the culture of developing nations, lung cancer will continue to increase in incidence. The lung cancer epidemic in the next century will mostly occur in Asia [111].

Table 3. Recommendations for multidisciplinary investigations in lung cancer

---

Smoking prevention and cessation in healthy individuals
- effective implementation of behavioral strategies within the clinical routine

Supportive care and psychosocial interventions
- systematic data base on psychosocial issues related to the disease and its treatment
- defining subgroups of patients with poor psychosocial adjustment
- development and evaluation of multidisciplinary interventions

Quality of life endpoints within clinical trials
- evaluation of the available instruments in lung cancer patients in all phases of disease and treatment
- specific methodological investigations about the impact of other disease- and treatment-related factors on patients' self-report (e.g., setting of data collection)
- development of short indicators for patients with poor performance status
- longitudinal description of quality of life patterns over the course of disease and treatment; biological and psychosocial predictors

---

The importance of prevention strategies for lung cancer emphasizes the need for alliance between health professionals, behavioral scientists, and politicians. Smokers of all ages should be encouraged to quit, because cessation at any age has been shown to decrease lung cancer risk relative to that of current smokers, with much greater benefits for those quitting at younger ages [112]. Health practitioners can play a key role in the implementation of smoking prevention in the individual patient, although they may feel pessimistic about the effectiveness of their efforts [113]. For example, an education program substantially changed the way physicians counseled smokers [114], and the availability of simple but specific mechanisms (chart reminders, nicotine gum) helped primary care physicians increase their success rates in helping patients quit smoking [115]. For successful long-term abstinence, the person who is quitting or has quit smoking will require an individualized, ongoing, and intense support program, as well as a reinforcing social environment [116].

What can be done for the quality of life of lung cancer patients? In addition to the existential threat of a lung cancer diagnosis, there are many everyday problems and concrete needs that the patient and family will experience. For the patient and his or her family, providing information will assist and encourage them in their adjustment. However, more specific information than is currently available is essential for patient care, planning intervention programs, and optimally utilizing resources, as summarized in table 3.

Behavioral and other types of psychosocial interventions have been proposed as an adjunct to oncological treatment for use within the clinical routine. There are several areas where a multidisciplinary management approach can or could increase the quality of care in lung cancer patients, i.e., smoking cessation; prevention and management of anticipatory nausea and vomiting, as well as learned food aversions; sleep disorders; development of techniques to encourage self-care of dyspnea; and more complete relief of pain. However, multidisciplinary supportive interventions have to be systematically evaluated in comparison with the standard biomedical approaches.

In contrast to some of the other areas discussed, quality of life research in lung cancer has been investigated more extensively. To determine the relative benefit of a given treatment in terms of the patients' subjective experience is a challenge, and will probably remain a challenge for future lung cancer treatments. Lung cancer clinical trials may continue to provide the experimental testing ground for new methodologies in quality of life research. In this evolving field, collaboration between clinicians and social scientists must be promoted further.

In conclusion, this review identifies a number of areas that need further investigation. However, it also shows progress in recent years, mainly with regard to quality of life considerations, emphasizing the importance for integrating psychosocial issues into the routine medical care of lung cancer patients.

Acknowledgments

The authors wish to thank Drs. Christoph Hürny, Prudence Francis, James Rigas, Mark Kris, Nathan Cherny, and Paul Jacobsen for many stimulating conversations about the issues discussed in this review. Dr. Bernhard's contribution to this work was supported by the Swiss Cancer League, the Cancer League of Canton Glarus, Switzerland, and the Huggenberger-Bischoff Foundation of Cancer Research, Zurich, Switzerland.

References

1. Bernhard J, Ganz PA. 1991. Psychosocial issues in lung cancer patients (part 1). Chest 99:216–223.
2. Bernhard J, Ganz PA. 1991. Psychosocial issues in lung cancer patients (part 2). Chest 99:480–485.
3. Holland JC. 1992. Psycho-oncology: Overview, obstacles and opportunities. Psycho-Oncol 1:1–13.
4. Wetterer A, Troschke J. 1986. Smoker Motivation. A Review of Contemporary Literature. Springer: Berlin.
5. U.S. Department of Health and Human Services. 1982. The health consequences of smoking. Cancer: A Report of the Surgeon General. U.S. Department of Health and Human Services (DHHS Publication No. PHS 82-50179).
6. Royal College of Physicians. 1983. Health or Smoking? Pitman: London. Publishing.
7. World Health Organization. 1986. Tobacco or health. Report by the Director-General. Geneva: World Health Organization (EB77/1986/REC/1).
8. Parkin DM. 1989. Trends in lung cancer incidence worldwide. Chest 96:S5–S8.
9. Stanley K, Stjernswärd J. 1989. Lung cancer — a worldwide health problem. Chest 96:1S–5S.
10. Samet JM. 1993. The epidemiology of lung cancer. Chest 103:20S–29S.

11. Stjernswärd J, Stanley K, Eddy D, et al. 1986. National cancer control programs and setting priorities. Cancer Detect Prev 9:113–124.
12. Cullen JW. 1986. International control of smoking and the U.S. experience. Chest 89: 206S–218S.
13. Flay BR, Ockene JK, Tager IB. 1992. Smoking: Epidemiology, cessation, and prevention. Chest 102:277S–301S.
14. Fraumeni JF, Blot WJ. 1982. Lung and pleura. In Cancer Epidemiology and Prevention, D Schottenfeld and JF Fraumeni (eds.). WB Saunders: Philadelphia, 564–582.
15. Saracci R. 1988. Environmental carcinogenesis of lung cancer. LUCAE (Suppl. Fifth World Conference on Lung Cancer) 4:P17.
16. Persky VW, Kempthorne-Rawson J, Shekelle RB. 1987. Personality and risk of cancer: 20-year follow-up of the Western Electric Study. Psychosom Med 49:435–449.
17. Fox BH. 1989. Depressive symptoms and cancer. JAMA 262:1231.
18. Zonderman AB, Costa PT, McCrae RR. 1989. Depression as a risk for cancer morbidity and mortality in a nationally representative sample. JAMA 262:1191–1195.
19. Rogers MP, Reich P. 1988. On the health consequences of bereavement. N Engl J Med 319:510–512.
20. Eysenck HJ, Everitt B. 1991. Personality, stress, smoking, and genetic predisposition as synergistic risk factors for cancer and coronary heart disease. Integr Physiol Behav Sci 26:309–322.
21. Gradishar WJ, Magid D, Bitran JD. 1990. Supportive care of the lung cancer patient. Hematol Oncol Clin North Am 4:1183–1199.
22. Breitbart W, Holland JC, eds. 1993. Psychiatric Aspects of Symptom Management in Cancer Patients. American Psychiatric Press: Washington, DC.
23. G.I.V.I.O. (Interdisciplinary Group for Cancer Evaluation) 1989. Diagnosis and first-line treatment of patients with lung cancer in Italian general hospitals. Tumori 75:163–167.
24. Rahim MA, Sarma SK. 1984. Pulmonary and extrapulmonary manifestations in delayed diagnosis of lung cancer in Bangladesh. Cancer Det Prev 7:31–35.
25. Holland JC. 1989. Lung cancer. In Handbook of Psychooncology: Psychological Care of the Patient with Cancer, JC Holland and JH Rowland (eds.). Oxford University Press: New York, pp. 180–187.
26. Hughes JE. 1985. Depressive illness and lung cancer. I. Depression before diagnosis. Eur J Surg Oncol 11:15–20.
27. Ganz PA, Schag CAC, Lee JJ, Sim MS. 1992. The CARES: a generic measure of health-related quality of life for patients with cancer. Qual Life Res 1:19–29.
28. Mumma C, McCorkle R. 1982. Causal attribution and life-threatening disease. Int J Psych Med 12:311–319.
29. Levine J, Zigler E. 1975. Denial and self-image in stroke, lung cancer, and heart disease patients. J Consult Clin Psychol 43:751–757.
30. Richardson G, Tucker MA, Venzon DJ, et al. 1993. Proc Am Soc Clin Oncol 12:1080 (abstract).
31. Knudsen N, Schulman S, van der Hoek J, Fowler R. 1985. Insights on how to quit smoking: A survey of patients with lung cancer. Cancer Nurs 8:145–150.
32. Davidson G, Duffy M. 1982. Smoking habits of long-term survivors of surgery for lung cancer. Thorax 37:331–333.
33. Minna JD, Pass H, Glatstein E, Ihde DC. 1989. Cancer of the lung. In Cancer: Principles and Practice of Oncology, VT Devita, S Hellman, and SA Rosenberg (eds.). JB Lippincott: Philadelphia, pp. 591–705.
34. Karnofsky DA, Burchenal JH. 1949. The clinical evaluation of chemo-therapeutic agents in cancer. In Evaluation of Chemotherapeutic Agents, CM MacLeod (ed.). Columbia University Press: New York, pp. 191–205.
35. Stanley KE. 1980. Prognostic factors for survival in patients with inoperable lung cancer. J Natl Cancer Inst 65:25–32.

36. Zubrod CG, Schneiderman M, Frei E, et al. 1960. Appraisal of methods for the study of chemo-therapy of cancer in man: Comparative therapeutic trial of nitrogen mustard and triethylene thiophosphoramide. J Chron Dis 11:7–33.

37. Eastern Cooperative Oncology Group 1983. Functional assessment scale. In Clinical Oncology: A Functional Approach, P Rubin (ed.). American Cancer Society: New York, p. 91.

38. World Health Organization 1979. WHO Handbook for Reporting Results of Cancer Treatment. World Health Organization: Geneva.

39. Hutchinson TA, Boyd NF, Feinstein AR 1979. Scientific problems in clinical scales, as demonstrated in the Karnofsky index of performance status. J Chron Dis 32:661–666.

40. Yates JW, Chalmer B, Mckegney FP. 1980. Evaluation of patients with advanced cancer using the Karnofsky performance status. Cancer 45:2220–2224.

41. Schag CC, Heinrich RL, Ganz PA. 1984. Karnofsky performance status revisited: Reliability, validity and guidelines. J Clin Oncol 2:187–193.

42. Grieco A, Long CJ. 1984. Investigation of the Karnofsky performance status as a measure of quality of life. Health Psychol 3:129–142.

43. Mor V, Laliberte L, Morris JN, Wiemann M. 1984. The Karnofsky performance status scale. An examination of its reliability and validity in a research setting. Cancer 53: 2002–2007.

44. Klein Poelhuis EH, Hart AA, Burgers JM, Hermus RJ, Bruning PF. 1987. Assessment of quality of life: Scoring performance status in cancer patients. In The Quality of Life of Cancer Patients, NK Aaronson and J Beckmann (eds.). Monograph Series of the European Organization for Research and Treatment of Cancer, Vol. 17. Raven Press: New York, pp. 93–95.

45. Marino C, Zoppi M, Morelli F, et al. 1986. Pain in early cancer of the lungs. Pain 27:57–62.

46. Portenoy RK, Miransky J, Thaler HT, et al. 1992. Pain in ambulatory patients with lung or colon cancer. Cancer 70:1616–1624.

47. Foley KM. 1985. The treatment of cancer pain. N Engl J Med 313:84–95.

48. Cassileth BR, Lusk EJ, Strouse TB, et al. 1985. A psychological analysis of cancer patients and their next-of-kin. Cancer 55:72–76.

49. Brown ML, Carrieri V, Janson-Bjerklic S, Dodd MJ. 1986. Lung cancer and dyspnea: The patient's perception. ONF 13:19–23.

50. Ryan LS. 1987. Lung cancer: Psychosocial implications. Semin Oncol Nurs 3:222–227.

51. Reuben DB, Mor V. 1986. Dyspnea in terminally ill cancer patients. Chest 89:234–236.

52. Foote M, Sexton DL, Pawlik L. 1986. Dyspnea: A distressing sensation in lung cancer. ONF 13:25–31.

53. Kaasa S, Mastekaasa A, Thorud E. 1988. Toxicity, physical function and everyday activity reported by patients with inoperable non-small cell lung cancer in a randomized trial (chemotherapy versus radiotherapy). Acta Oncol 27:343–349.

54. Kris MG, Gralla RJ, Tyson LB, et al. 1989. Controlling delayed vomiting: Double-blind, randomized trial comparing placebo, Dexamethasone alone, and Metaclopramide plus Dexamethasone in patients receiving Cisplatin. J Clin Oncol 7:108–114.

55. Burish TG, Carey P. 1986. Conditioned aversive responses in cancer chemotherapy patients: Theoretical and developmental analysis. J Consult Clin Psychol 54:593–600.

56. Jacobsen PB, Redd WH. 1992. Behavioral aspects of oncology. In Behavioral Medicine: International Perspectives, DG Byrne and GR Gaddy (eds.). Ablex: Norwood, pp. 293–315.

57. Redd WH, Jacobsen PB, Die-Trill M, et al. 1987. Cognitive/attentional distraction in the control of conditioned nausea in pediatric cancer patients receiving chemotherapy. J Consul Clin Psychol 55:391–395.

58. Mattes RD, Arnold C, Boraas M. 1987. Learned food aversions among cancer chemotherapy patients. Incidence, nature, and clinical implications. Cancer 60:2576–2580.

59. Silberfarb PM, Philibert D, Levine PM. 1980. Psychosocial aspects of neoplastic disease: II. Affective and cognitive effects of chemotherapy in cancer patients. Am J Psychiatry 137:597–601.

60. Kaasa S, Olsnes BT, Mastekaasa A. 1988. Neuropsychological evaluation of patients with inoperable non-small cell lung cancer treated with combination chemotherapy or radiotherapy. Acta Oncol 27:241–246.

61. Licciardello JTW, Cersosimo RJ, Karp DD, et al. 1985. Disturbing central nervous system complications following combination chemotherapy and prophylactic whole-brain irradiation in patients with small cell lung cancer. Cancer Treat Rep 69:1429–1430.

62. Johnson BE, Becker B, Goff WB, et al. 1985. Neurologic, neuropsychologic and computed cranial tomography scan abnormalites in 2 to 10-year survivors of small cell lung cancer. J Clin Oncol 3:1659–1667.

63. Laukkanen E, Klonoff H, Allan B, et al. 1988. The role of prophylactic brain irradiation in limited stage small cell lung cancer: Clinical, neuropsychologic, and CT sequelae. Int J Radiat Oncol Biol Phys 14:1109–1117.

64. Hürny C, Bernhard J, Joss R, et al. 1993. 'Fatigue and malaise' as a quality of life indicator in small cell lung cancer patients. Support Care Cancer 1:316–320.

65. Aaronson NK, Bullinger M, Ahmedzai S. 1988. A modular approach to quality-of-life assessment in cancer clinical trials. Recent Results Cancer Res 111:231–249.

66. Breitbart W. 1987. Suicide in cancer patients. Oncology 1:49–54.

67. Hu DS, Silberfarb PM. 1991. Management of sleep problems in cancer patients. Oncology 5:23–27.

68. Collins C, Oakley-Browne M. 1988. Mania associated with small cell carcinoma of the lung. Aust NZ J Psychiatry 22:207–209.

69. Zigmond AS, Snaith RP. 1983. The hospital anxiety and depression scale. Acta Psychiatrica Scand 67:361–370.

70. Hopwood P, Thatcher N. 1990. Preliminary experience with quality of life evaluation in patients with lung cancer. Oncology 4:158–162.

71. Hughes JE. 1985. Depressive illness and lung cancer. II. Follow up of inoperable patients. Eur J Surg Oncol 11:21–24.

72. Cella DF, Orofiamma B, Holland JC. 1987. The relationship of psychological distress, extent of disease, and performance status in patients with lung cancer. Cancer 60: 1661–1667.

73. McNair DM, Lorr M, Droppleman LF. 1971. EITS manual for the profile of mood states. Educational and Industrial Testing Service: San Diego.

74. McGeough A, Edwards J, Chamberlain RM, Nogeire C. 1980. Social isolation in lung cancer patients. Social Work Health Care 5:433–436.

75. Cox BG, Carr DT, Lee RE. 1987. Living with lung cancer. Triad: Gainesville.

76. Greenberg ER, Chute CG, Stukel T, et al. 1988. Social and economic factors in the choice of lung cancer treatment: A population-based study in two rural states. N Engl J Med 318:612–617.

77. Mackillop WJ, O'Sullivan B, Ward GK. 1987. Non-small cell lung cancer: How oncologists want to be treated. Int J Radiat Oncol Biol Phys 13:929–934.

78. Blanchard CG, Labrecque MS, Ruckdeschel JC, Blanchard EB. 1988. Information and decision-making preferences of hospitalized adult cancer patients. Soc Sci Med 27: 1139–1145.

79. McNeil BJ, Weichselbaum R, Pauker SG. 1978. Fallacy of the five-year survival in lung cancer. N Engl J Med 299:1397–1401.

80. Simes RJ. 1985. Risk–benefit relationships in cancer clinical trials: The ECOG experience in non-small cell lung cancer. J Clin Oncol 3:462–472.

81. Aaronson NK, Ahmedzai S, Bergman B, et al. 1993. The European Organization for Research and Treatment of Cancer QLQ-C30: a quality-of-life instrument for use in international clinical trials in oncology. J Natl Cancer Inst 85:365–376.

388

82. Fergusson RJ, Cull A. 1991. Quality of life measurement for patients undergoing treatment for lung cancer. Thorax 46:671–675.

83. Slevin ML, Plant H, Lynch D, et al. 1988. Who should measure quality of life, the doctor or the patient? Br J Cancer 57:109–112.

84. Bernhard J. 1992. 'Lebensqualität' in onkologischen Therapiestudien. Konzepte, Methodik und Anwendung am Beispiel des Kleinzelligen Bronchuskarzinoms. Peter Lang: Bern.

85. Hollen PJ, Gralla RJ, Kris MG, Potanovich LM. 1993. Quality of life assessment in individuals with lung cancer: Testing the lung cancer symptom scale (LCSS). Eur J Cancer 29A:S51–S58.

86. Ganz PA, Haskell CM, Figlin RA, et al. 1988. Estimating the quality of life in a clinical trial of patients with metastatic lung cancer using the Karnofsky performance status and the Functional Living Index–Cancer. Cancer 61:849–856.

87. Finkelstein DM, Cassileth BR, Bonomi PD, et al. 1988. A pilot study of the Functional Living Index–Cancer (FLIC) Scale for the assessment of quality of life for metastatic lung cancer patients. Am J Clin Oncol (CCT) 11:630–633.

88. Hürny C, Bernhard J, Joss R, et al. 1992. Feasibility of quality of life assessment in a randomized phase III trial of small cell lung cancer — a lesson from the real world. Ann Oncol 3:825–831.

89. Kornblith A, Anderson J, Cella D, et al. 1990. Quality of life assessment of Hodgkin's disease survivors: A model for cooperative clinical trials. Oncology 4:93–101.

90. Schag CC, Heinrich RL, Aadland R, et al. 1990. Assessing problems of cancer patients: Psychometric properties of the Cancer Inventory of Problem Situations. J Clin Epidemiol 43:75–86.

91. Bergner M, Bobbit RA, Carter WB, Gilson BS. 1981. The Sickness Impact Profile: development and final revision of a health status measure. Med Care 19:787–805.

92. Bergman B, Sullivan M, Sörenson S. 1991. Quality of life during chemotherapy for small cell lung cancer. Acta Oncol 30:947–957.

93. Coates A, Dillenbeck CF, McNeil DR, et al. 1983. On the receiving end-II. Linear analogue self assessment (LASA) in evaluation of aspects of the quality of life of cancer of cancer patients receiving therapy. Eur J Cancer Clin Oncol 19:1633–1637.

94. Schipper H, Clinch J, McMurray A, Levitt M. 1984. Measuring the quality of life of cancer patients: the Functional Living Index–Cancer: development and validation. J Clin Oncol 2:472–483.

95. Kaasa S, Mastekaasa A, Lund E. 1989. Prognostic factors for patients with inoperable non-small cell lung cancer limited disease. The importance of patients' subjective experience of disease and psychosocial well-being. Radiother Oncol 15:235–242.

96. Ganz PA, Lee JJ, Siau J. 1991. Quality of life assessment. An independent prognostic variable for survival in lung cancer. Cancer 67:3131–3135.

97. Ruckdeschel JC, Piantadosi S, and the Lung Cancer Study Group. 1991. Quality of life assessment in lung surgery for bronchogenic carcinoma. Theor Surg 6:201–205.

98. Silberfarb PM, Holland JC, Anbar D, et al. 1983. Psychological response of patients receiving two drug regimens for lung carcinoma. Am J Psychiatry 140:110–111.

99. Fayers PM, Bleehen NM, Girling DJ, Stephens RJ. 1991. Assessment of quality of life in small-cell lung cancer using a Daily Diary Card developed by the Medical Research Council Lung Cancer Working Party. Br J Cancer 64:299–306.

100. Geddes DM, Dones L, Hill E, et al. 1990. Quality of life during chemotherapy for small cell lung cancer: assessment and use of a daily diary card in a randomized trial. Eur J Cancer 26:484–492.

101. Earl HM, Rudd RM, Spiro SG, et al. 1991. A randomised trial of planned versus as required chemotherapy in small cell lung cancer: a Cancer Research Campaign trial. Br J Cancer 64:566–572.

102. Carlens E, Dahlstrom G, Nou E. 1970. Comparative measurements of quality of survival

of lung cancer patients after diagnosis. Scand J Respir Dis 51:268–275.

103. Nou E, Aberg T. 1980. Quality of survival in patients with surgically treated bronchial carcinoma. Thorax 35:255–263.

104. Felletti R, Souhami RL, Spiro SG, et al. 1985. Social consequences of brain or liver relapse in small cell carcinoma of the bronchus. Radiother Oncol 4:335–339.

105. Jaakkimainen L, Goodwin PJ, Pater J, et al. 1990. Counting the costs of chemo-therapy in a National Cancer Institute of Canada randomized trial in nonsmall-cell lung cancer. J Clin Oncol 8:1301–1309.

106. Kaasa S, Mastekaasa A, Naess S. 1988. Quality of life of lung cancer patients in a randomized clinical trial evaluated by a psychosocial well-being questionnaire. Acta Oncol 27:335–342.

107. Kaasa S, Mastekaasa A. 1988. Psychosocial well-being of patients with inoperable non-small cell lung cancer. The importance of treatment- and disease-related factors. Acta Oncol 27:829–835.

108. Coates A, Gebski V, Bishop JE, et al. 1987. Improving the quality of life during chemo-therapy for advanced breast cancer. A comparison of intermittent and continuous treat-ment strategies. N Engl J Med 317:1490–1495.

109. McCorkle R, Benoliel JQ, Donaldson G, et al. 1989. A randomized clinical trial of home nursing care for lung cancer patients. Cancer 64:1375–1382.

110. Goldberg RJ, Wool MS. 1985. Psychotherapy for the spouses of lung cancer patients. Assessment of an intervention. Psychother Psychosom 43:141–150.

111. Pierce JP, Thurmond L, Rosbrook B. 1992. Projecting international lung cancer mortality rates: first approximations with tobacco-consumption data. J Natl Cancer Inst Monogr 12:45–49.

112. Halpern MT, Gillespie BW, Warner KE. 1993. Patterns of absolute risk of lung cancer mortality in former smokers. J Natl Cancer Inst 85:457–464.

113. Wechsler H, Levine S, Idelson RK, et al. 1983. The physician's role in health promotion — a survey of primary care physicians. N Engl J Med 308:97–100.

114. Cummings SR, Coates TJ, Richard RJ, et al. 1989. Training physicians in counseling about smoking cessation. A randomized trial of the 'Quit for Life' program. Ann Intern Med 110:640–647.

115. Cohen SJ, Stookey GK, Katz BP, et al. 1989. Encouraging primary care physicians to help smokers quit. A randomized, controlled trial. Ann Intern Med 10:648–652.

116. Kottke TE, Battista RN, De Friese GH, Brekke ML. 1988. Attributes of successful smoking cessation interventions in medical practice: Metaanalysis of 39 controlled trials. JAMA 259:2883–2889.

Index

Acetaminophen, 47, 50
Acetylaldehyde, 17
N-Acetyl-cysteine (NAC), 46, 47, 49–50, 56–58
Aclarubicin, 175, 185, 186
Acquired immunodeficiency syndrome (AIDS), 275, 383
Actinomycin D, 119, 178, 200
Acute bronchitis, 49
Acute myelocytic leukemia, 166, 180
Acute myeloid leukemia, 207, 215
Adenocarcinoma, 131–140, 193
    atypical adenomatous hyperplasia (AAH) and, 133–136, 137, 140
    bronchial gland cell (BGC), 131–132
    bronchial surface epithelial (BSE) cell, 131
    chemoprevention of, 59
    chemosensitivity of, 147, 148
    Clara cell, 131, 132, 133, 137, 138
    clear cell, 358
    colon, 133, 172
    gastrointestinal, 206
    gemcitabine and, 336
    genetics of, 93, 94, 100, 101, 138–140
    goblet cell, 131, 138, 140
    growth factors and, 120
    growth properties of, 137
    interferon (IFN) and, 296, 303
    in vivo testing of cytostatic agents for, 156–157, 158, 164–165, 166
    mucinous, 136
    multidrug resistance (MDR) and, 196, 205–206
    neuroendocrine characteristics of, 144, 145, 146, 147, 148, 149, 151
    NMU-1, 156–157
    nonmucinous, 136

phenotypic progression of, 136–137
scar cancer concept and, 132
sclerosing bronchioalveolar, 136
smoking and, 9–12, 17, 18, 21, 23, 25–27, 28, 30, 34, 131
staging of, 241
Taxol® (paclitaxel) and, 336
type II pneumocyte, 131, 132, 133, 137
Adenoma, 242
    atypical adenomatous hyperplasia (AAH) and, 133–136, 137, 140
    smoking and, 7–8, 21, 22–23, 28
Adenosquamous cell carcinoma, 47, 136, 149
Adrenal gland metastases, 242
Adrenocorticotropic hormone (ACTH), 145, 373, 374
Adriamycin, see Doxorubicin
Advanced Multiple Beam Equalization Radiography (AMBER) system, 226, 227f.
Aflatoxin B1, 50
Air pollution, 1–3, 365
Alkaline elution assay, 175
Alkylating agents, 184
Alpha-1-antichymotrypsin, 361
Alpha-1-antitrypsin, 361
Alpha-fetoprotein, 356
Alpha-tocopherol, see Vitamin E
4-Aminobiphenyl, 19, 102
p-Aminohippurate (PAH), 102, 103
Amsacrine, see m-AMSA
Aneuploidy, 63, 137–138
Angiosarcoma of the liver, 18
Antagonist A, 121
Antagonist D, 121–122
Antagonist G, 121–122
Anthracyclines, see also specific types

391

neuroendocrine characteristics and, 147, 150
Taxol® (paclitaxel) and, 338–339
Taxoter® (docetaxel) and, 327, 329
vinorelbine and, 341–342
VP-16 (etoposide) and, 333–334
13-*cis*-Retinoic acid, 30, 48–49, 52–53, 58, 103–104
c-*jun* genes, 94–95, 97
CK-BB, 148
c-Ki-*ras* genes, 138, 140
c-*kit* genes, 118
Clara cell adenocarcinoma, 131, 132, 133, 137, 138
Clara cell antigen, 356
Clear cell adenocarcinoma, 358
Cleavable complexes, 177, 185, 209
Clinical staging, 235
Clonal growth, 116–117
Clonogenic assays, 174
CMT64 lung tumor cell line, 157
c-*myb* genes, 95
c-*myc* genes, 138, 296
Cocarcinogens, smoking and, 16, 17, 18t.
CODE regimen, 279
Cognitive changes, 372–373
Coke oven workers, 25, 27
Colchicine, 215
Colon adenocarcinoma, 133, 172
Colon cancer, 46, 47, 50, 61, 101, 104, 155
Colon carcinoma, 156
Colony stimulating factors (CSFs), 273–275, *see also* specific types
Colorectal cancer, 97, 107, 376
Combination chemotherapy, 370, 372
  CPT-11 in, 326–327
  edatrexate in, 330
  etoposide in, 333–334
  fotemustine in, 334
  for pulmonary blastomas, 357, 361
  quality of life and, 379, 382
  Taxol® (paclitaxel) in, 338–339
  vinorelbine in, 341–342
Community Clinical Oncology Program (CCOP), 58
Computerized tomography (CT)
  diagnosis and, 229–231, 233
  staging and, 236–237, 239–241, 242–243, 247
Cotinine, 77, 85, 98
Coumarin, 16
CPT-11, 324–327
c-*raf* genes, 95, 97
CX-1 colon carcinoma, 156
Cycloheximide, 119
Cyclophosphamide, 382

in CAVE, 333
chest irradiation and, 264, 267
edatrexate and, 330
etoposide and, 333
hematopoietic growth factors and, 276, 277, 279, 280, 281, 282, 284, 285, 286
interferon (IFN) and, 297, 307
multidrug resistance (MDR) and, 200
in VAPEC-B, 282
Cyclosporin A, 174, 179, 194, 208, 211, 214
Cystic blastomas, 358–361
Cytarabline, 276
Cytokeratin (CK), 164–165, 356, 361
Cytolysis endpoint assays, 196
Cytostatic agents
  in vitro testing for small cell lung cancer (SCLC), 171–187
  in vivo testing for non-small cell lung cancer (NSCLC), 155–167

Dacarbazine, 276
Dactinomycin, 199
Daunorubicin
  in vitro testing for small cell lung cancer (SCLC), 175, 176, 180, 185, 186
  multidrug resistance (MDR) and, 194, 203, 206, 208
10-Deazaaminopterin, 329
Debrisoquine hydroxylation, 102–103
Denmark, smoking in, 7, 75
Dense-core granules, 144, 147, 356
Depression, 365, 374
Desmin, 357
Detection, 97–103, 104–106, *see also* Diagnosis
Dexamethasone, 338
Diagnosis, 248, *see also* Detection
  adjustment to, 366–368
  screening as applied to early, 224–225
  techniques used in, 223–233, 244–247
  tumor characteristics and, 231
Diet, 9, 34, 44–45, 104
Difluoromethylornithine (DFMO), 50, 293
Digitonin, 206
1,2-Dimethylhydrazine, 47
Diphenhydramine, 338
Diploid DNA, 235
Dithiolethiones, 50
DNA
  antagonists D and G and, 122
  chemoprevention and, 46, 51, 62, 63
  gastrin-releasing peptide (GRP) and, 114

394

interferon (IFN) and, 297
metabolic phenotypes and, 103
nuclear, 134, 137–138
smoking and, 25, 31
topoisomerase I (topo I) and, 324
topoisomerase II (topo II) and, 175–178, 185, 209
DNA adducts, 21, 22, 23, 24, 26, 27, 34, 47, 98, 102
DNA ploidy, 235
Docetaxel (Taxotere®), 327–329
Dopa, 143
L-dopa decarboxylase, 143, 147, 296
Doxorubicin (Adriamycin), 147, 193
  in CAVE, 333
  chest irradiation and, 259, 264
  in CODE, 279
  CPT-11 and, 327
  hematopoietic growth factors and, 276, 278, 279, 280, 282, 284, 285
  interferon (IFN) and, 297
  in vitro testing for small cell lung cancer (SCLC), 172, 176, 184, 185, 186
  in vivo testing for non-small cell lung cancer (NSCLC), 161–162, 164, 166
  multidrug resistance (MDR) and, 194, 195, 199, 200, 201, 202, 203, 206, 207, 209–210, 211, 212, 215, 216–217
  in M-VAC, 282
  in VAPEC-B, 282
  VP-16 (etoposide) and, 333
Drug additivity, 175
Drug antagonism, 175
Drug synergy, 174
Drug transport assays, 178–180
Drug transporter function, 206–208
Dye exclusion assays, 196
Dye workers, 27
Dynorphins, 118–119
Dysplasia, 92, 93
  bronchial, 53, 60
  bronchopulmonary, 151
Dyspnea, 369–370

Early Detection Research Network (EDRN), NCI, 106
Eastern Cooperative Oncology Group (ECOG), 324, 338, 378
Edatrexate, 329–330
egfr genes, 63
Ellagic acid (EA), 50–51
Endorphins, 118–119
Endothelin, 122

Endpoints
  in chemoprevention, 58, 60–63
  development of new, 376–383
  intermediate, 98, 104–106
  quality of life, 381–383
England, smoking in, 44
Enkephalins, 118–119
Environment, genetic interactions with, 96
Epidemiology
  chemoprevention and, 44–45
  of smoking and lung cancer, 7–9
Epidermal growth factor (EGF), 46, 120–121, 122–123
Epidermal growth factor receptors (EGFRs), 60, 94, 95
Epidermoid carcinoma, see Squamous cell carcinoma
Epidoxorubicin, 281–282
Epigallocatechin gallate (EGCG), 31
Epipodophyllotoxins, 209, 210
Epirubicin, 307, 331
Epithelial blastomas, 349–354, 356, 357–358
Epithelial membrane antigen, 356, 361
erbB1 genes, 59
erbB2 genes, 59
Esophageal cancer, 18, 51, 53
Ethylene oxide, 102
Etoposide, see VP-16
Etretinate, 48–49, 54
Euploid tumors, 235
European Organization for Research on the Treatment of Cancer (EORTC), 56, 265–266, 286, 341, 378, 379
Excision, 357
Experimental chemoprevention, 45–47

Fagerstrom Questionnaire, 76–77, 81, 86
Family studies, 96
Fat, dietary, 34, 104
Fatigue, 373
Fiber, 104
Field cancerization, 53
Filter cigarettes, 9, 27, 28–30
Finland, smoking in, 12
Flank tumors, 161–162, 166
Flavone acetic acid (FAA), 161–162
Formaldehyde, 17, 23
Fotemustine, 334
Fractionation schedule, 261–262
France
  increase in lung cancer in, 1, 2f.
  smoking in, 5, 6f., 12
Free radicals, 13, 46, 295
Functional Living Index-Cancer, 379

Functional status, 368–369

Galanin, 115–116, 121, 122
Gallium-67 scintigraphy, 245, 361
Gastinoma, 113
Gastrin, 116
Gastrin-releasing peptide (GRP), 115, 116,
        121, 122, 150–151, 354
    properties of, 111–114
Gastrointestinal adenocarcinoma, 206
Gastrointestinal cancer, 50
Gastrointestinal carcinoids, 146
Gemcitabine, 313, 334–336, 337t.
Gender, see Men; Women
Gene-specific analysis, of multidrug
        resistance (MDR), 196–199, 205–
        206
Genetics, 91–107, see also Oncogenes;
        Tumor suppressor genes
    of adenocarcinoma, 93, 94, 100, 101,
        138–140
    environmental interactions with, 96
    targets for primary prevention and,
        103–104
Genetic suppressor elements, 210
Gene transfer/therapy, 165
Genistein, 206, 207, 208
Germany, smoking in, 5–7
GETCB study, 266
Glutathione-S-transferase, 102
Goblet cell adenocarcinoma, 131, 138, 140
G-proteins, 113–114, 122
Granulocyte-colony-stimulating factor (G-
        CSF), 118, 273, 280–281, 282,
        283–286
    neutropenia and, 275–277, 278–279,
        283–284
Granulocyte/macrophage colony-
        stimulating factor (GM-CSF), 118,
        273, 281–282, 285–286
    clinical applications of, 275–277
    neutropenia and, 278, 279–280, 283–284
Granulocytopenia, 281, 335, see also
        Leukopenia
Growth factors, 111–123, see also
        Hematopoietic growth factors
    neuroendocrine peptides as, 150–151
    non-small cell lung cancer (NSCLC)
        and, 114, 117, 119, 120–121,
        122–123
    small cell lung cancer (NSCLC) and,
        111–123
    therapeutic implications of, 121–123

Halichondrin B, 185

Hand-rolled cigarettes, 7
Head and neck cancer, 54, 58, 61–62, 104,
        107
Hemangioendotheliomas, 158
Hematopoiesis, 275
Hematopoietic growth factors, 118, 273–
        287
    absence of negative impact on
        chemotherapy effects, 280–281
    clinical applications of, 275–277
    dose escalation and intensity of
        chemotherapy, 282–285
    nonrandomized trials of, 278
    optimial dose-on-time delivery of
        chemotherapy and, 281–282
    randomized trials of, 278–279
Hemoglobin adducts, 26, 27, 34, 102
Hemoptysis, 223, 350
Hepatocellular carcinoma, 50
her-2-neu genes, 59, 60, 63, 95, 101
Hilar node metastases, 238–240, 242
Histology/histopathology, 160–161
    neuroendocrine markers in, 144–146
    smoking and changes in, 9–12
HLA antigens, 294, 297, 313
Home nursing care, 382–383
Homohalichondrin B, 185
Hospital Anxiety and Depression Scale
        (HADS), 374
H-ras genes, 94, 100–101
Hydrogen cyanide, 29
4-Hydrox-1-(3-pyridyl)-1-butanone
        (HPB), 23–24
N-(4-Hydroxyphenyl)retinamide (4-HPR),
        47, 49
1-Hydroxypyrene, 22, 34
5-Hydroxytryptamine (5-HT), see
        Serotonin
Hydroxyurea, 276
Hypercalcemia, 370, 373
Hyperfractionated radiotherapy, 261, 310
Hyperplasia, 92
Hypervitaminosis A syndrome, 48

Ifosfamide
    hematopoietic growth factors and, 276,
        278, 284
    interferon (IFN) and, 307
    in vivo testing for non-small cell lung
        cancer (NSCLC), 161–162, 163, 166
    multidrug resistance (MDR) and, 212
Immunohistochemical studies, of
        multidrug resistance (MDR), 198–
        199
Incipient cancer, see Preneoplasia

comparison of small/non-small cell lung
cancer in, 200–201
defined, 194–195
drug transporter function and, 206–208
gene-specific analysis of, 196–199,
205–206
interferon (IFN) and, 297
in vitro chemosensitivity testing and,
195–196
in vitro selection of specific cell lines,
201–208
in vitro testing of cytostatic agents for,
174, 178–187
resistance-modifying agents (RMAs)
and, 211–212, 213–215
topoisomerase II (topo II) and, 195, 201,
203, 209–210, 216
trial design to study relevance of,
212–214
Multidrug resistance associated protein
(MRP), 204–205
Multiple myeloma, 166
Murine lung tumor models, 156–157
Muscle-specific actin, 357
Mutations, 94, 94–95, 100, 101, 105, 225
adenocarcinoma and, 138, 140
chemoprevention and, 61–62
multidrug resistance (MDR) and, 194
smoking and, 25, 26–27
topoisomerase II and, 209
M-VAC regimen, 282
MX-1 mammary ductal carcinoma, 156
myc genes, 59, 63, 97, 138, 140
Myeloid leukemia, 155
actue, 207, 215
Myocardial infarction, 52
Myoglobin, 357

Naloxone, 119
Naltrexone, 119
2-Naphthylamine, 19
Nasal cavity cancer, 21
National Cancer Institute, U.S. (NCI), 11,
30, 44, 50, 51, 75, 104, 106, 107,
171, 172, 264
National Cancer Institute of Canada
(NCIC), 263, 264, 331
National Cancer Institute of Milan, 49, 54
National Council on Radiation Protection
and Measurement, U.S., 19
National Public Health Institute of
Finland, 51
Nausea, 370–371
Needle biopsies, 350
Neo-kyotorphin, 119

Neo® gene, 165
Netherlands, smoking in, 7
neu genes, *see her-2/neu* genes
Neural cell adhesion molecules (NCAMs),
145–146
Neuroblastoma, 119, 215
Neuroendocrine characteristics, 143–152
chemosensitivity and, 146–150, 151–152
multidrug resistance (MDR) and, 196
in pulmonary blastomas, 356, 358
Neuroendocrine markers, 143
in histopathologic diagnosis, 144–146
interferon (IFN) and, 307
pulmonary blastomas and, 356
Neuroendocrine peptides, 114–117, *see
also* specific types
clonal growth stimulated by, 116–117
as growth factors, 150–151
Neuron-specific enolase (NSE), 144, 146,
148, 149, 150, 307, 354
Neurotensin, 111, 115, 116, 121, 145, 148,
151
Neutralizing antibodies, 313
Neutropenia
hematopoietic growth factors and,
275–280, 283–284, 285, 286
Taxol® (paclitaxel) and, 336, 338
Taxotere® (docetaxel) and, 327
vinorelbine and, 340, 342
Nickel vapor, 1
Nicotine, 7, 12–13, 27, 28, 29
addiction to, 75–77
measuring dependence on, 85–86
Nicotine chewing gum, 78–81, 83, 86
Nicotine nasal spray (NNS), 84, 85, 86
Nicotine substitution, 77, 78–81, 85, 86
Nicotine transdermal patch, 78, 79, 81–83,
86
Nicotine vaporizer, 83, 86
Nitrates, 30
Nitroalkanes, 27
Nitrogen oxide, 29
Nitrosamine, 102, 103
N-Nitrosamines, 18
tobacco-specific, 19–21, 22–24, 25–27,
34
N'-Nitrosoanabasine (NAB), 19
N'-Nitrosoanatabine (NAT), 19
N-Nitrosodiethylamine (DEN), 47
N-Nitrosodimethylamine, 24
N'-Nitrosonornicotine (NNN), 19, 26
NMU-1 adenocarcinoma, 156–157
N-myc genes, 296
Nodal metastases, 237–238
Non-filter cigarettes, 9
Nonmucinous adenocarcinoma, 136

402

smoking and, 9-12, 17, 24, 25, 27, 28, 30, 34, 131
staging of, 238
vinorelbine and, 340
Squamous metaplasia, 53
Staging, 223, 233-248
clinical, 235
early diagnosis and, 224
new international system for, 234t.
pathological, 235
techniques used for, 233-247
TNM system of, *see* TNM staging system
Stem cell factor (SCF), 118
Steroids, 211, 373
Stomach cancer, 50, 61
Stomach endocrine cell hyperplasia, 92
Styrene, 102
Substance P analogues, 121-122
Suicide, 373
Surfactant apoprotein, 356-357
Surgery, 235, 236, 237, 357, 368, 377, 381
Surrogate markers, *see* Intermediate endpoints
Survival, chest irradiation and, 256-266
Sweden
increase in lung cancer in, 1, 2f.
smoking in, 5, 6f., 7, 9
Symptoms, 368-369
Synaptophysin (SY 38), 145, 147, 148, 150

Tachykinins, 119
Tamoxifen, 104, 211
Tar (total particulate matter), 7, 8, 17, 27, 28, 29
Taxol® (paclitaxel), 179, 194, 328
current studies of, 336-339
Taxotere® (docetaxel), 327-329
TCNU, 161-162, 163, 166
Tea, green, 31
Teniposide, *see* VM-26
Testicular cancer, 211
Tetraploid DNA, 235
Thoracoscopy, 224, 232-233
Thoracotomy, 224, 233, 237, 239-240, 243, 248
Thrombocytopenia
CPT-11 and, 325
edatrexate and, 329
fotemustine and, 334
gemcitabine and, 335
hematopoietic growth factors and, 283, 284, 286
Taxol® (paclitaxel) and, 336
Taxotere® (docetaxel) and, 327
VP-16 (etoposide) and, 334

Thrombopenia, *see* Thrombocytopenia
TNM staging system, 131, 138, 223, 233, 234t., 235
TNO rat lung tumor model, 157-165
Tobacco carcinogenesis studies, 16-27
Tobacco chewing, 27
Tobacco consumption, *see* Smoking
Tobacco-specific N-nitrosamines (TSNAs), 19-21, 22-24, 25-27, 34
Topoisomerase assays, 175-178
Topoisomerase I (topo I), 175-176
CPT-11 and, 324
in vitro testing of cytostatic agents for, 172, 179, 187
multidrug resistance (MDR) and, 209
Topoisomerase II (topo II), 175-178
in vitro testing of cytostatic agents for, 172, 179, 180, 184, 185-186
multidrug resistance (MDR) and, 195, 201, 203, 209-210, 216
Topotecan, 324
Topothecan, 179
Total body irradiation, 277
Total particulate matter (TPM), in smoke, *see* Tar
Toxicity
of hematopoietic growth factors, 275
of radiochemotherapy, 258-259, 264
*tp*53 genes, 59
Tracheal tumors, 24
Transbronchial biopsies, 224
Transesophageal ultrasonography, 243-244
Transferrin, 117-118
Transforming growth factor-α (TGF-α), 120-121
Transforming growth factor-β (TGF-β), 296
Trans-Thoracic Needle Biopsy (TTNB), 228
Treatment
clinical decision making on, 376-378
MDR1 gene P-glycoprotein expression and, 216
of pulmonary blastomas, 357-358, 361
socioeconomic factors in, 377
Tumor characteristics, 231
Tumor initiators, 16, 17, 18t.
Tumor necrosis factor (TNF), 286, 294, 296
Tumor promotors, 16, 17, 18t.
Tumor suppressor agents, 30
Tumor suppressor genes, 91, 94
as biomarkers, 100-101, 107
chemoprevention and, 59
properties of, 95-96
smoking and, 22

403